Bacterial Virulence

Anthony William Maresso

Bacterial Virulence

A Conceptual Primer

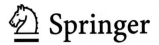 Springer

Anthony William Maresso
Dept. Molecular Virology and Microbiology
Baylor College of Medicine
Houston, TX
USA

ISBN 978-3-030-20463-1   ISBN 978-3-030-20464-8   (eBook)
https://doi.org/10.1007/978-3-030-20464-8

The cover shows an electron micrograph of the attachment of enteroaggregative *E. coli* to the surface of enteroids derived from a biopsy of the author's intestine. Special thanks to Anu Rajan and Jim Barrish at Texas Children's Hospital.

Most of the artwork was done by: Petar Dekic Graphic Designer and Social Anthropologist Senior Curator at the National Museum in Smederevska Palanka Trg heroja 5 11420 Smederevska Palanka, Serbia.

This Springer imprint is published by the registered company Springer Nature Switzerland AG
The registered company address is: Gewerbestrasse 11, 6330 Cham, Switzerland

scientia vinco morbus ("knowledge defeats disease")

To the sick, it is for you.
To today's scientists, your life is for them.
To tomorrow's scientists, may you fear nothing.

Prologue

They Come Unseen

May 2, 2011, Hamburg, Germany. The pain began about 2 AM – wrenching as if someone was ringing the intestines like a soaked sponge. Four AM brought the cold sweat, the linens a swamp. By 6, the urge to defecate was unbearable, which then became inevitable. The explosive release of what seemed actual organs came next, one after another. The toilet became fouled with the most pungent of smell, from the most revolting of form in its base, the form itself unvaried in color. This was bloody, hemorrhagic diarrhea, seemingly relentless in draining the body of precious fluid.

The back pain came next, just above the hip. This was different, not like a pulled muscle or some strain from the back end heaving of waste and water. The constant diarrhea with cramping, although not easy by any stretch, at least became a routine, with some relief every time the bowel emptied. This pain was constant and sharp – a 10-inch needle ever so slowly being inserted down through the kidney. The urine became dark, not the dark yellow one observes if slightly dehydrated. This urine was spent engine oil, a mixture of blood and necrotic tissue that was impenetrable to light. It carried an odor of iron and urea.

The weakness came next and then lethargy. The loss of kidney function coupled to profuse diarrhea turned consciousness upside down, the body conserving energy to support only the most basic of functions and the cells working only half efficiency in a semi-molten state. This was not a transient diarrhea from a spicy meal. This was a life-threatening disease, and its name was hemolytic uremic syndrome (HUS).

HUS manifests via the destruction of kidney cells, and there is no cure. Supportive care via dialysis, which replaces the function of the kidney, is all doctors can rely on, hoping the kidneys retain their normal function with time. It can take weeks of intensive care for full recovery, and even those that survive, any many do not, have chronic damage.

A day passed. Two more cases, nearly identical in clinical symptoms, abdominal cramps, bloody diarrhea, and what looks to be HUS, are reported at the Hamburg Hospital.

Four more cases emerge in German hospitals the next day.

Between May 4 and 8, eight cases are reported. On May 9 alone, there are six cases. For the next 2 weeks, approximately 35 cases per day are reported at German hospitals. On May 20 itself, a single day, greater than 60 cases present.

Sometime during this period, an email goes out to the Robert Koch Institute (RKI), the leading German authority in the investigation of rare diseases. The special minds at the RKI have a knack for a particular type of mysterious ailments – those that are infectious in origin. Like its namesake Koch, they study diseases caused by bacteria. The inference was that this was an outbreak.

In Poland, a father who traveled to Germany notices his son has bloody diarrhea. In Sweden, Denmark, and France, nearly 100 cases are reported; 40 show HUS. Eleven other countries report cases, including the United States and the United Kingdom. Germany announces in mid-May a common element, cucumbers imported from Spain. The Spanish Government denies its foodstuffs are the culprit. Russia responds by banning all produce from the European Union, resulting in 200–400 million dollars per week in lost economy. Germany modifies its statements, linking the disease to bean sprouts produced from a small farm in Bienenbüttel, Lower Saxony. The seeds from some of these sprouts may have been circulating for years.

By the end of July 2011, 4,000 cases had been reported; 50 people had died of kidney failure. Over 3 billion dollars had been lost from the European economy.

This case in particular highlights the sheer power of bacteria. The causative agent of this outbreak was revealed to be a version of a bacterium that is a common inhabitant of the gastrointestinal tract of mammals and birds, termed *Escherichia coli*. "Bacterium coli commune" or *E. coli* as it was later named was first described in an 1886 publication by Theodor Escherich, a German-Austrian pediatrician who was studying the physiology of infant digestion. *E. coli* has since become the face of a microbe revolution that spans human health, industry, and biotechnology. Because it is easy to grow and tolerates DNA from other forms of life inside its cytoplasm, *E. coli* has been the go-to organism for the propagation of DNA, the life-giving molecule of heredity. Thus, nearly every gene ever cloned by scientists has first been amplified in this bacterium. The human genome could not have been sequenced in 2001 without *E. coli* as the replicator of the large plasmids carrying human DNA. *E. coli* also aids in our health. Various strains that live in our intestine make vitamins; and other strains may stimulate our immune system in a positive way. *E. coli* has been engineered to degrade oil from spills (called bioremediation) and to produce beneficial small molecules that aid human health (probiotics).

This outbreak is what microbiologists know in the mind and fear in the heart – that a deadly microbe will emerge from an unknown reservoir, bats, a water well, a dead mammoth after a permafrost thaw, or, in this case, bean sprouts produced near a cattle farm, and ravage an unsuspecting community. In this case, the *E. coli* responsible for these infections is part of a group of closely related bacteria, or pathotype, which is known to be able to cause gastrointestinal illness, principally diarrhea. This pathotype is called entero-aggregative *E. coli*. The "entero" refers to the fact that it was isolated from human stool samples, being Greek for entrails or intestine. The "aggregative" describes what the scientist that first discovered this pathotype, James Natarro, saw when the bacteria were first imaged under a microscope, circa 1987. The *E. coli* aggregated together in a strange, brick-like formation – a pattern not seen before for this, or any, type of bacterial species. Natarro, an infectious disease physician, believed that this pattern of adherence was somehow related to the intestinal diarrhea he was observing in children recruited to a study exploring causes of diarrhea in impoverished communities (we will learn more about how bacteria adhere to cells in ▶ Chap. 7). The aggregative adherence was perhaps a way to better "stick" to human intestinal cells and avoid being washed out of the gut lumen until desired. It seemed that entero-aggregative *E. coli* was a common cause of diarrhea, but, interestingly enough, the disease was self-limiting and could eventually resolve without much medical intervention. It was not as severe as some other diarrheal diseases caused by related pathotypes of *E. coli* that already had been described, such as the more famous entero-hemorrhagic *E. coli* (EHEC). EHEC infection results in bloody diarrhea and made headlines in the 1980s and 1990s for causing outbreaks from the consumption of hamburger meat. Cattle farms, in particular the intestines of cows, are prominent

sources of pathotypes, such as EHEC. Thus, one can see why hamburger meat is sometimes contaminated with EHEC bacteria.

But unlike EAEC (the "aggregative" bacterium), EHEC can cause the deadly hemolytic syndrome associated with kidney destruction and disease. It does so because EHEC makes a toxin, termed Shiga toxin. The toxin is encoded in the DNA of a bacteriophage, a virus that infects bacteria. Somehow, EHEC's survival in the environment was at one point enhanced if it acquired this toxin from the phage, so natural selection favored strains of EHEC that became infected with the phage carrying the DNA from the toxin (we will learn in ▶ Chap. 6 of the incredible adaptive capability of bacteria and how they skillfully acquire new capabilities via mobile genetic elements). Shiga toxin is an amazing protein – after being made by EHEC, it is secreted by the bacterium into the intestinal lumen. There, it can cause cell death of intestinal cells but also enter the circulation and find its way to the kidney. The toxin enters kidney cells and cleaves a key component of the cells ribosome. Since ribosomes are important for the synthesis of proteins, the kidney cell cannot make proteins and dies. We will learn much more about bacterial protein toxins like Shiga toxin in ▶ Chap. 10.

Here we have two pathotypes of *E. coli*, EAEC and EHEC, each being *E. coli* but each having different molecular properties. EAEC can "stick" to intestinal cells very well and likely uses aggregative adherence to avoid being flushed out of the intestinal track. When you ingest it, it stays. EHEC can't stick as well, but it makes a toxin that causes intense diarrhea with kidney damage (HUS) as a by-product of this effect. The diarrhea releases more EHEC into the environment and thus makes it more likely another animal can ingest it, therefore propagating the bacterium to new hosts. Up to 2011, these two features infrequently crossed paths in the same organism. The unique feature about this outbreak was that it was caused by a hybrid *E. coli* that had the ability to adhere to cells *and* produce the toxin. When scientists sequenced the outbreak strain, they were amazed to find that most of the core genome looked exactly like EAEC, with the genetic elements to confer the stickiness present in abundance. But, to their surprise, this strain also had acquired the DNA that encodes Shiga toxin. This generated the perfect storm of a bacterium, one that retained strong pathogenic features of two separate *E. coli* pathotypes, thereby combining the stickiness of the bacteria with the lethality from the toxin. The result was an epidemic of not only significant loss of human life and money but international tension with major world powers assigning blame to the other for the problem. It is quite amazing to realize how our own human evolution and history have been shaped by infectious bacteria. To the evolution of an immune system to combat such invaders to the restructuring of society and culture, bacteria have and will continue to be intimately linked to our past, present, and future. We will learn about the interactions of such amazing, but deadly, bacteria with our immune system in ▶ Chaps. 4 and 5.

The remarkable thing about this event is that it likely was the product of one very rare exchange of genetic information in the intestine of a ruminant on a farm in Germany. It illustrates the power of the genetic evolution of microorganisms, and how even the most simple of creatures such as bacteria, with the right complement of virulence factors, can undo the most complex of beings, such as a human. It took our species a long time to come to this realization. Microbiology, as an organized field, is only about 150 years old. Ninety-nine point nine-nine-nine percent of everything we know about bacteria, the methods to study them and the medicines to heal people from their ravages, have been learned in the past 6 or so human generations out of the something like 10,000–100,000 generations since are species "began." This is rather striking considering 40,000 years ago we painted beautiful art on cave walls and perhaps a million or more years ago, had the capacity to invent tools. Now, with even better tools, we can finally understand the sometimes devious behavior bacteria use to undermine their human hosts (a topic which we approach in ▶ Chaps. 1 and 2).

This brings us to the microbe hunters. Who are they? Maybe who they are is not as important as how they become who they want to be. The microbe hunter is the investigator of all small things – too small, in fact, to see with the unaided eye. They are detectives, but they solve puzzles of a different type. Here, the clues are subtle – a protein on a gel there, a bacterium on an agar plate here, and a whole bunch of graphs in between. Their "evidence" is not a testimony or footprints; it's data. Lots of it actually, the lots needed to convince others, and themselves, they have figured something out. Acquired through long hours,

hunched (and broken) backs, and most often colossal failures in search of the perfect experiment at the perfect time, the microbe hunter lets the world's actions reveal the nature of its true secrets. It comes first out of passion but second to do good for our kind. It is born of a compassion and empathy for the suffering of our kindred and the desire to do something to help ease their sickness. The problem is the right answers can only be found by the most stringent of scientific investigations and the most diligent technical work – and this, for lack of a better description, is just plain exhausting. But it can be exhilarating when the answer is revealed, when the knowledge is shared for all to see, and you were the one that gifted it.

This volume aims to give the microbe hunter – the one wanting to reveal the dirty tactics the pathogen uses to harm us – a guide. Written at a level targeting the most eager and unspoiled of minds (College age) but structured with just enough sophistication so the current microbe hunter can learn about related areas of their craft, and everyone in between including doctorate and medical students, there is one main objective: teach, and inspire, the next generation of talent to consider taking up the fallen pipet and continue the fight. Pathogenic bacteria are not going away, and some would argue they are now undergoing a resurgence. Trapped in the pages herein are descriptions of bacterial trade secrets, from biofilms to toxins, from secretion systems to adhesins, and from microbiomes to the sepsis they can cause to arm the microbe hunter with a knowledge base that can be used against them. The work is not meant to be written like a typical scientific review article – there are enough of those! Instead, a comprehensive and integrated view of what we call bacterial pathogenesis is the task. The creatures we seek to understand that cause these diseases don't do so with all these important elements in a vacuum separated in time and space. They use them all at once! As Science itself trends toward a more integrated approach, so to must the mentality of the microbe hunter. As science moves us to the star and other worlds, we must not forget about the small.

We start first with our world though, one full of giant slayers – the pathogenic bacteria – which come unseen.

Anthony William Maresso

Acknowledgments

Before we begin this 16-chapter adventure, the author must briefly acknowledge some of the people who helped shaped the environment which produced this work, an effort that spanned almost 2.5 years. Squeezed in between grant cycles, student defenses, data meetings, and manuscripts and prodded along under a dim lamp when the world sleeps, the effort would not have been possible without some heroes of the author's past. This includes Dr. Randall Jaffe who taught the author "to verify," Dr. Joseph Barbieri who taught the author "to think," and Dr. Olaf Schneewind who taught the author "to fight." Olaf and family - your own "fight" inspires us to never give up. It also includes current "mentors" of the author, Drs. Janet Butel, who hired him, and Mary Estes, who inspired him. These great scientists are exemplary role models; the author is fortunate. To colleagues at Baylor College of Medicine's Molecular Virology and Microbiology Department (especially the author's current chairperson, Dr. Joe Petrosino), the author is grateful for their collegiality, critical critique, and professionalism. BCM is a special place with special minds that has risen from a fledgling academic experiment in an underdeveloped plot of Houston land to a world-class intellectual powerhouse in medical research. A special thanks should also go to the two outstanding editors at Springer Nature that the author worked with over these years, Drs. Claudia Panuschka and Silvia Herold. Their tireless spirit, enthusiasm, and critical analysis helped shape the work into its current form. The author's past and current students and trainees are owed youthful exuberance and hope for the future. They are the reason for this work. The graphic art skills of one Petar Dekic, who took many of the failed drawings of the author and made them alive, were invaluable. Thank you Petar for your long nights perfecting the artwork throughout this volume. The author's friends, Greg and Matt, remind him there is much more to life than a sense of accomplishment. The author's parents, Sharon and William, and immediate family, Carol, Robert, Michael, James, and Bill, emphasized to follow your interests with passion but humility all the way, letting hard work pave the rocky path. Now, the author has his own family of three, Leo, Christian, and Maxwell; it is for them, and all those as innocent as them, that scientists strive to provide a more enlightened future. Finally, to the author's spouse, Karen, worlds could be moved if everyone had someone like you. Thank you.

Contents

About the Author

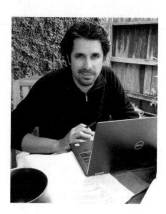

Anthony William Maresso
 is a professor and scientist at Baylor College of Medicine in Houston, Texas. His research aims to understand how bacteria cause disease in their human hosts so as to discover and develop preventative vaccines and therapies for deadly infections. When not in the laboratory or teaching, he enjoys hiking, camping, fishing, woodworking, and gardening with his wife, Karen, and their three sons, Leo, Christian, and Maxwell.

A Short History of Microbiology

© Springer Nature Switzerland AG 2019
A. W. Maresso, *Bacterial Virulence*, https://doi.org/10.1007/978-3-030-20464-8_1

1

Learning Goals

In this chapter, the student is introduced to the evolution in thought, and the thinkers themselves, over the past 500 years that gave rise to the modern theory of the bacterial germ. From Leeuwenhoek's "animalcules" observed under a primitive magnifying lens to Koch and Pasteur's rigorous attention to experimental detail, the foundational principles of the microbe hunter are discussed. The historical trend towards reductionist microbiology is examined in the context of pursuit of the mechanism of action of bacterial molecules made during infection, knowledge which has been used to develop life-saving prophylactics and therapeutics. The chapter closes with the advent of the "omics" revolution and new insights in dynamic modes of host-pathogen interactions that capture many biological states at once.

1.1   Invisible to Visible to Cultured

The discovery of microorganisms has its roots in curiosity and observation. The development of the field of Microbiology, or the study of microbial (tiny) life, begins with sweat, failure, and necessity over a 500 year period. The first formal notation of this curiosity began with Anton van Leeuwenhoek's observation of small single celled life-forms in a drop of pond water – the "animalcules." Leeuwenhoek was not a physician by training – he made cloth. But his desire to observe the quality of his cloth in his shop led him to practice the art of glass shaping to make various lenses that had strong magnifying properties. Amongst his hundreds of letters to the British Royal Society over 40 years, Leeuwenhoek described all types of these microorganisms, including many from the plaque of the human mouth. These were the first observations of bacteria, and they represented a proof of another world unseen to our eyes.

The connection of these animalcules to human disease would be slower to come. For thousands of years dating back to before the great Greek philosopher Aristotle, the dominant belief was that life resulted from spontaneous generation. That is, life came not from other life, but the elements inherent in matter. With perhaps the exception of the first life, this is incorrect; life as we understand it comes from other life, an argument experimentally demonstrated by the great French microbiologist Louis Pasteur (more on him later) in the late 1800s. The belief in spontaneous generation was not insensible. There were examples of what seemed like spontaneous formation everywhere. The production of maggots in rotting meat, the growth of plants from the tiniest of seeds, fungi on moldy bread, all represent examples where one might reasonably conclude that life just happened. Of course, it would take someone to observe flies depositing their eggs in the meat, and the observation of the transformation of the egg to a maggot – events that could not be readily seen during this time – for the theory to be disproven.

Some of the earliest thoughts on there being small things that caused "putrefaction" or infections began with the Italian scholar Girolamo Fracastoro. In 1546, Fracastoro wrote about contagion as "a certain precisely similar corruption which develops in the substance of a combination, passes from one thing to another, and is originally caused by infection of the imperceptible particles." He speculated contagion can occur by direct contact, that the air can divide the particle enhancing its spread, and that not all life was equally suspect to the particle. For example, plants can get diseases animals cannot and vice versa. Here we have some of the earliest writings of an infection being caused by a tangible substance, the transmission of that substance, and that the substance has a tropism, *i.e.* that infectious microorganisms have a defined host or species they are capable of infecting and generally do not cross this barrier unless mutated. Fracastoro's writing are remarkable in the prophetic sense, given the knowledge framework he was working with at the time, and that he could not actually see the "fomes" as he called them. But Microbiology still had a long way to advance in his time. Even Fracastoro believed that certain ocular infections could be caused by making direct eye contact with those afflicted. Investigative science dispels such myths.

Of central importance to society, much of the query into the causes of infectious diseases from this period focused on those that affected agriculture. Although not widely credited with such, the Italian farmer and property owner Agostino Bossi proposed in the 1830s that a disease that afflicted silk worms (which ravaged the silk industry in Italy and France) was caused by an animal that infected the worms. The great German anatomist Jakob Henle would argue in 1840 for support of the germ theory of infection. While considering various theories prominent at that time in European circles, Henle wrote "the second possibility is that the contagion consists of animal elements which can be cultured and isolated from the sickness and which can become free-living entities, from which the infection can spread." In the 1850s, the German physician Ignaz Semmelweis recommended using "chloride of lime" on dirty hands to prevent the spread of deadly infections that afflicted mothers giving birth in a neonatal center in Austria. His efforts dropped the mortality rate by about 4-fold, thereby bringing to consciousness the fact that disease can be cleansed. Infections of these mothers and their neonates were likely caused by Group B Streptococcus, a pathogen we will learn a bit about in this volume. The use of carbolic acid, otherwise known as phenol, by Joseph Lister to sterilize surgical instruments and wounds, a process inspired by the experiments of Pasteur, revolutionized how surgical practice was performed.

Although it would be more than 200 years after Leeuwenhoek's animalcules and 300 years after Fracastoro's fomes for an unknown German country doctor named Robert Koch to deduce that microorganisms were the *cause* of disease, it was his systematic methods and logical deductions that birthed the practice of modern Microbiology. To this day, Microbiologists studying the molecular mechanisms of bacterial diseases use the conceptual framework Koch established to construct their own proofs and ideas. Formed over five papers during the late 1800s, Koch's work would teach us that bacteria can be isolated by growing them in culture, meaning that every cell in the culture was of the same species. He would invent the now commonplace method of growing bacteria on a solid medium, a precursor to deriving his pure cultures. He would attain samples from infected animal tissues, grow them until pure, and demonstrate that their reintroduction into a healthy animal reproduced the disease. This was done with the "tubercule" bacillus, known today as *Mycobacterium tuberculosis*, a lung infection of humans that infects upwards of 30% the world's population. He would pioneer the use of microscopy to observe cell shape and function. In this way, Koch would see the transition of *Bacillus anthracis*, the causative agent of anthrax, from a vegetative cell (metabolically active and growing) to a spore (a dormant version of the cell prepared for long-term hibernation) and the germination of the spore back to a vegetative cell. We learn more of tuberculosis and anthrax later.

1.2 Elucidation of a Molecular Basis of Bacterial Diseases

During this explosion in knowledge in the Microbiological sciences, advances were being made simultaneously in the budding field of Immunology. Leading researchers were starting to become aware of a link between these diseases of contagion and the body's resistance against them. Like the origins of the germ theory of disease, it would be observations in animal husbandry that would prove most revealing. Smallpox was a viral disease that presented with high mortality (upwards of 50% that contracted the disease could succumb to it) and was absurdly contagious. In the 1800s, the disease was prominent in England, and feared, so much that people were willing to be purposely take infected pus and "variolate", or scratch the skin with said pus, in hopes of protecting against the disease. This practice was widely known to somehow guard against catching the disease at a later date. Variolation, however, would often lead to full-blown smallpox, and so the practice was also risky and controversial. Edward Jenner, a country doctor from Gloucestershire England, made the astute observation that milkmaids would develop postules on their hands from cattle infected with cowpox, a virus related to smallpox. It seemed those who first contracted cowpox, which only produced a mild disease in humans, were subsequently protected against smallpox, the more virulent and deadly form. Acting on these observations (and farmer lore), Jenner was the first to systematically prove the idea that vaccinating with cowpox could protect from smallpox, using as his first test subject an eight-year old boy whom he "variolated" from the postules of a milkmaid that acquired cowpox. Upon challenge with smallpox, the boy showed no disease, as did other subjects that Jenner systematically tested. Although Jenner did not understand the molecular basis of these findings, it's clear from the work that cowpox was similar and less "virulent" than smallpox and that people could be primed against the more worrisome smallpox. Eighty years later, Pasteur would convincingly demonstrate the concept of attenuation by showing

that the passaging of a cholera-like bacterium steadily reduced its virulence. The attenuated form could be used to protect against subsequent disease with the more virulent form. We learn of attenuation and the concept of virulence in ▶ Chap. 2.

Around the same time as it was being accepted that there were tiny creatures that were the basis of disease, seeds were sown for many new theories concerning the molecular basis of such afflictions. This is best exemplified by the work of Friedrich Loeffer, an apprentice of Koch who, in 1884, observed the "edema … inflammation … and reddening" of organs of infected animals even though the inoculation with bacteria occurred at a distant site and the organs themselves contained no observable pathogens. To him, a "poison … must have circulated in the blood" and reached these tissues, causing harm. The experimental proof of a diffusible substance that was toxic would come 5 years later when Emil Roux and Alexandre Yersin would demonstrate that animals injected with sterile supernatants from a bacterial culture (in this case, *Corynebacterium Diphtheriae*) produced nearly identical symptoms as infection with diphtheriae itself. With this discovery was born the field of toxin biology, a discipline that would be the foundation of our understanding of the molecular ways in which bacteria cause disease. We learn more about the amazing properties of bacterial protein toxins in ▶ Chap. 10.

The conceptualization of a toxigenic basis of bacterial diseases brought attention to the new field of serology, or the study of blood and its properties. Not a year after proof was presented of a diffusible substance, Emil von Behring and Shibasaboro Kitasato would demonstrate that the serum of rabbits that were previously inoculated with the bacterium that causes tetanus (*Clostridium tetani*), could "render harmless the toxic substance which the tetanus bacillus produces." Yes, indeed, your thoughts are correct! This is a description of the protective effect of antibodies. Here we have the adaptive immune system, knowledge of which would transform medicine wholly and society in part. Thus, if one knew the "poisons" that bacteria made that elicited disease, one could be rendered immune to their action via vaccination with an inactive form of that poison. ▶ Chapters 4 and 5 of this volume cover the immune system.

1.3 Anti-Bacterial Medicines

Not long after the recognition that bacteria could cause disease would researchers begin to exploit this knowledge to kill them. The early days of drug discovery must have been roaring with excitement: so many discoveries, some accidental and some not, came with great ferocity. Paul Ehrlich in 1908 pioneered a concept used today; that a chemical's toxicity could be precisely modified so as to lower its toxic effects towards mammalian cells but still be lethal to the bacterial cells. Thus was born the field of chemical or "Chemo"-therapy, whereby molecules are designed that specifically target the disease in question. From this would come the first marketed anti-bacterial, Salvarsan, generated by Alfred Bertheim, to treat the sexually transmitted bacterial infection syphilis. The momentum of these efforts would later yield the modern field of medicinal chemistry. Chemists could now build unique chemical add-ons around core structures to make them safer or more active or both. Felix de Herelle and Fredrick Twort would, independently in 1915 and 1917, respectively, describe what we know today as bacteriophages, or viruses that infect bacteria. Just as our own cells can be infected with a virus, so too can bacteria. The infection of bacteria by some bacteriophages results in their lysis, a process that leads to new virus progeny. The discovery of bacteriophages was considered a potential medical breakthrough, an effective way to treat bacterial infections, until that now famous day of September 9, 1929. On this date, Alexander Fleming returned from a trip to find a "zone of clearance" around the mold penicillin that had overgrown on his plate full of bacteria. It would take another 16 years, but Howard Florey and Ernest Chain would succeed in finally synthesizing the active chemical, that of penicillin, in 1945, thereby birthing the golden era of antibiotic development, which has carried us to today (Fig. 1.1). From 1950–1970, the major classes of antibiotics used today would be generated and a vibrant drug-making industry would flourish. It would seem that Leeuwenhoek's animalcules and Francatoro's contagions, which for hundreds of millennia were the scourge of our species, had an unbeatable adversary. The miracle of the antibiotic would help the allies win World War II, save countless children, and safeguard all types of people from bacterial peril. But almost as soon as it was discovered, scientists recognized that penicillin was also destroyed by bacteria. Joshua Lederberg in the 1940s would describe how bacteria could engage in a type of primitive sex, exchanging beneficial elements, including those that break wonder drugs like antibiotics. Today's microbe hunter, searching for new ways to cure such deadly infections will no doubt need to address this issue head-on. How vaccines and antibiotics intersect with bacterial virulence is described in ▶ Chaps. 15 and 16.

1.4 Useful Methods and Increasing Sophistication

The tools of microbiology were being developed as well. Christian Gram would in 1884 report a reliable method to stain bacteria, improving upon that of Koch and Ehrlich. The "Gram" stain is taught to first year medical students, nursing students and clinical PhD microbiologists to this day. RJ Petri would improve upon, circa 1887, another of Koch's inventions by "using flat double dishes", one side slightly larger (the lid) than the other, where Koch's gelatin could be poured and solidified. This technique is so practical and inexpensive there has not been any change to it in the last 130 years. There were improvements in microscopy and they fueled the ultrastructural analysis of bacteria. The construction of the electron microscopy by Ernst Ruska and Max Knoll in 1931 opened the door to the visualization of the bacterial form,

and all its wonderful micro-structures. This changed our perspective – now the microbe hunter could see the invaders in all their intimate and deadly detail. We learned that bacteria have defined layers (cell walls and membranes), a dense center (the DNA), and even appendages such as pili and flagella that pathogenic forms use to engage your cells. Black and grey electron microscopic images would soon give way to color and a rainbow of possibilities with the development of fluorescent microscopy. Specific fluorescent probes would tag bacteria and, like a flashlight in the dark, illuminate their sinister activities. In the later part of the twentieth century, the construction of bacterial cells expressing a jellyfish fluorescent protein and live imaging microscopy would help us observe bacterial behavior in real-time. Now, during an infection, we could see where the invaders went, what tissues and cellular components they interfaced, and how they precisely manipulated our own biology to gain an advantage. Thus would be born the field of cellular microbiology, and with it as much knowledge of the inter-workings of our own cells as that of bacteria.

Some bacteria would remain elusive. So much so that the disease they caused were mistakenly, at first, attributed to viruses. There was good reason for this. These bacteria were hiding inside mammalian cells. Bacteria, as it turns out, were not just creatures of blood and tissues; some of them could also invade our cells and even replicate there. The immune system was at its best surveying and destroying foreign entities that were extracellular. Macrophages could pick off lonely bacteria in blood and antibodies could inhibit or disrupt critical bacterial processes. Inside host cells, there were less threats, and more nutrients. The stealth practices of bacteria are discussed in ▶ Chap. 8.

Technology would further enhance our understanding of these fascinating creatures. The revelation that DNA was the unit of heredity, and that its manipulation via the simple changing of any of the bases of a four letter code, would allow researchers to use forward and reverse genetics approaches to deduce the contribution of individual genes to disease and the infection. This would usher in the still-booming discovery of the bacterial virulence factor, a genetically encoded bacterial product (usually a protein), that was important in some way to sustain an infection. Now, strains could be generated that lacked genes suspected of encoding a bacterial toxin, or adhesin, or suppressor of the immune system, or any of the other products used to wage war against its host, and the precise contribution of that factor to the disease or perturbation of host physiology assessed. This molecular version of Koch's postulates would narrow the disease to the sum of these virulence factors, each working at a precise step in the infection, a concept pioneered by the late and great Microbiologist Stanley Falkow. In addition to animal models, now the culturing of human cells, perfected by cell biologists, would provide an avenue to determine how these virulence factors perturbed the normal function of the cell. Simple live or dead, or healthy or sick designations when cells or hosts were exposed to bacteria would be refined. Now, the effect of bacteria might be described as a disruption

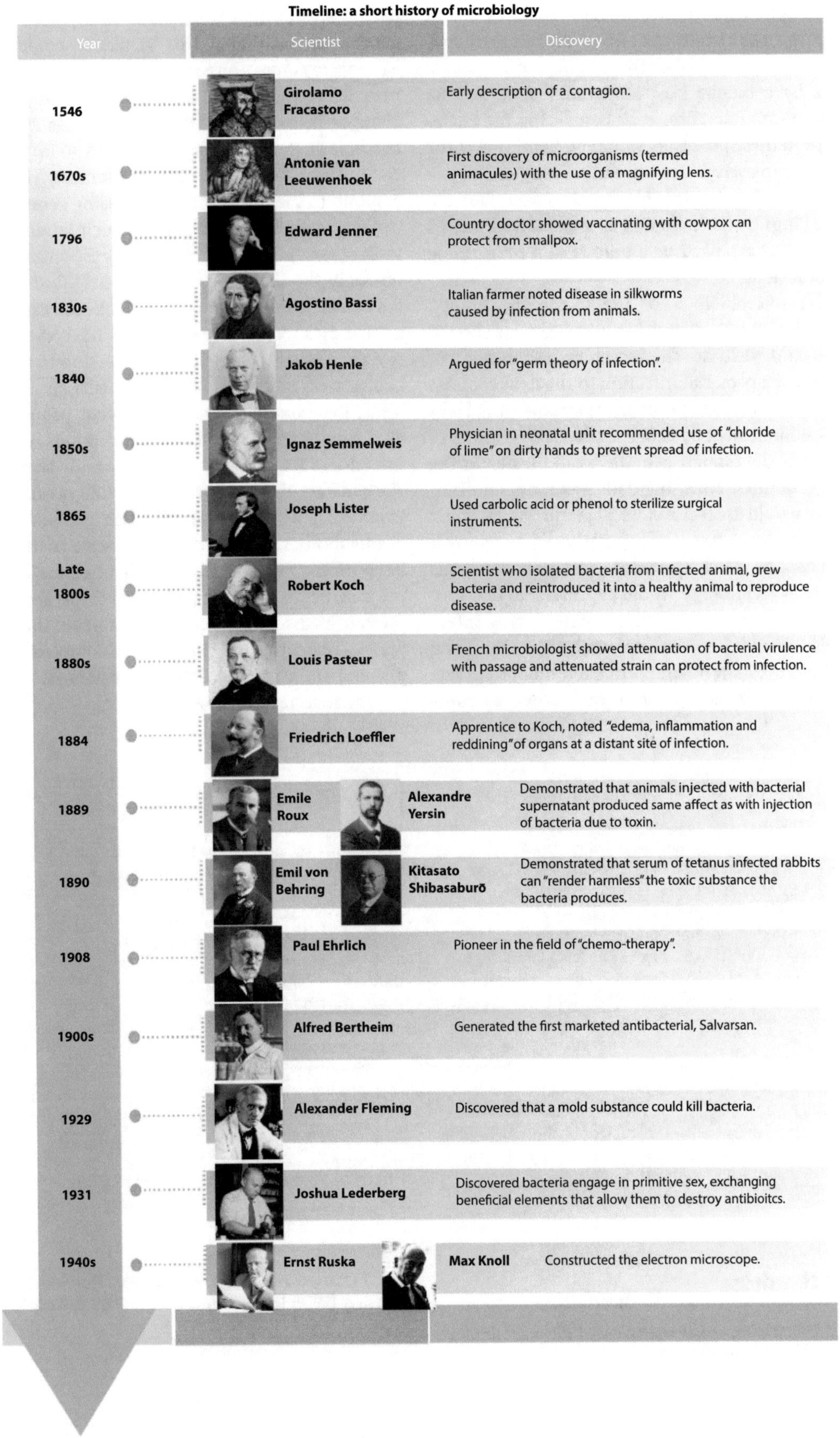

Timeline: a short history of microbiology

Year	Scientist	Discovery
1546	Girolamo Fracastoro	Early description of a contagion.
1670s	Antonie van Leeuwenhoek	First discovery of microorganisms (termed animacules) with the use of a magnifying lens.
1796	Edward Jenner	Country doctor showed vaccinating with cowpox can protect from smallpox.
1830s	Agostino Bassi	Italian farmer noted disease in silkworms caused by infection from animals.
1840	Jakob Henle	Argued for "germ theory of infection".
1850s	Ignaz Semmelweis	Physician in neonatal unit recommended use of "chloride of lime" on dirty hands to prevent spread of infection.
1865	Joseph Lister	Used carbolic acid or phenol to sterilize surgical instruments.
Late 1800s	Robert Koch	Scientist who isolated bacteria from infected animal, grew bacteria and reintroduced it into a healthy animal to reproduce disease.
1880s	Louis Pasteur	French microbiologist showed attenuation of bacterial virulence with passage and attenuated strain can protect from infection.
1884	Friedrich Loeffler	Apprentice to Koch, noted "edema, inflammation and reddining" of organs at a distant site of infection.
1889	Emile Roux, Alexandre Yersin	Demonstrated that animals injected with bacterial supernatant produced same affect as with injection of bacteria due to toxin.
1890	Emil von Behring, Kitasato Shibasaburō	Demonstrated that serum of tetanus infected rabbits can "render harmless" the toxic substance the bacteria produces.
1908	Paul Ehrlich	Pioneer in the field of "chemo-therapy".
1900s	Alfred Bertheim	Generated the first marketed antibacterial, Salvarsan.
1929	Alexander Fleming	Discovered that a mold substance could kill bacteria.
1931	Joshua Lederberg	Discovered bacteria engage in primitive sex, exchanging beneficial elements that allow them to destroy antibioitcs.
1940s	Ernst Ruska, Max Knoll	Constructed the electron microscope.

Fig. 1.1 Some notable figures and events in the history of the field of Microbiology up to the middle of the twentieth century. Credit to Sabrina Green, Baylor College of Medicine

of say the actin cytoskeletal network that maintain the host cell's architecture, or the shutting down of the vesicular trafficking of key cellular proteins, or the modification of one of these proteins by a unique posttranslational modification that altered its normal function – all benefitting the bacterium. The steps in these processes would be examined at the molecular level, with even greater resolution sought. Not just virulence factors being responsible for an effect, but the molecular workings of these factors as a nanomachine, its specific amino acids arranged as a unique fold performing distinct chemical steps.

The cellular microbiology of the twentieth century, dominated by the pursuit of mechanism and reductionist approaches, would yield to the sweeping assessment of global dynamics of a bacterial infection in the next century. This marriage would be fueled even more by emerging technology. The announcement by U.S. President Bill Clinton of the sequencing of the human genome would usher in the revolution in genomics. Now, big data was king, and biomedical science would use technological platforms designed to assess the biological "states" of infected cells, in contrast to the one-gene one-effect approach. The buzzword was "Omics" and each technology would capture a 10,000 foot view of multiple, not just one, cellular state during infection. Genomics would facilitate the analysis of the gene content of bacteria. Different strains of bacteria of the same species could be directly compared to each other. By comparing strains that were virulent to those that were not, genes that facilitated this virulence could be identified. Microarrays, encompassing most or every expressed gene in a bacterium, its host, or both, could be assessed for changes in their level of expression. Genes the bacterium needs to sustain the infection would go up, and these genes were then targets for study. Similarly, the host would respond to the infection by expressing genes needed to protect the cell. We learned from such studies that the host undergoes specific anti-bacterial responses which activate not only the infected cell but its neighbors, and leads to a collective immune response that kills the invader. Genomics approaches would give way to the next level in biology, the presence of the gene and its conversion to a message to the analysis of the product of this message, that of protein. Thus, proteomics would assess what proteins were made, and how their chemical modifications changed during infection, from both bacterial and host perspectives. Proteins are the catalysts of cell biology and their presence would map a state of the cell. Their products, however, that of metabolites, would be the true state of the cell. Thus was born metabolomics, an assessment of the biochemistry of the cell itself. The integration of these approaches would provide an assessment of the dynamics of the host-pathogen fight in real-time and teach Microbiologists how truly complicated and elegant are these associations …

The investigation continues.

Out of the Box

Then, same as now.

Even pre-school children have heard of germs. They may even understand the meaning of the word bacteria and be able to draw an image of one, or explain how they make people sick. Almost certainly prior to circa the 1880s for just about everyone, and even into the twentieth century for most people, the idea that disease can be caused by the presence of another living organism inside of you was unfathomable. It took some towering mind-power, aided by technology, for our species to come to grips with this reality. Now it's household knowledge.

Pondering this topic makes one wonder what kind of barriers to new ideas and knowledge our current generation faces? What kind of boxed thinking traps us and how do we burst from its doldrumic confines? So much of our brain's physical development occurs in the first 10 years of life, and our personality seems to be shaped well into teenage years and young adulthood. If in the first 20 years of life all major neuronal connections are made, representing all our experiences and types of thoughts, opinions, and ideologies, how difficult is it to substantially rewire these connections to gain a different scientific perspective? If past performance is indicative of future behavior, then the script to code over these connections will be built on the elucidation of new knowledge that is fueled by technology that enables us to see the natural world with novel refraction. Staying true to these principles – *i.e.* supporting the tools and endeavors to generate new knowledge – will then allow for our natural reasoning and logic skills to slowly accept new knowledge. Taking perhaps a generation or two to gain acceptance, they eventually do, but then they themselves become the barrier to the next idea. Take a moment this week and discuss with your fellow classmates or learner colleagues how we can break out of the current box and pave the path for new Microbiology ideas for the twenty-second century; and look for the "Out of the Box" segment at the end of each chapter in this volume for an extra push.

Suggested Reading

Beck RW (2000) A Chronology of Microbiology in Historical Context. American Society of Microbiology Press

Brock T (1961) Milestones in Microbiology. Prentice-Hall International

Bulloch W (1938) The History of Bacteriology. Oxford University Press

The Form and Function of a Bacterial Pathogen

© Springer Nature Switzerland AG 2019
A. W. Maresso, *Bacterial Virulence*, https://doi.org/10.1007/978-3-030-20464-8_2

Learning Goals

In this chapter, we discuss the form and function of the bacterial cell. The salient features of bacterial architecture include the cell membrane, peptidoglycan, pili, flagella, and other important structures needed for the organism to survive in its host. This section also includes a discussion of metabolism, energy production and the genome as it relates to pathogenesis. The reader will become familiar with bacteria from an anatomic and metabolic standpoint so as to have a solid foundation to understand basic principles presented in the remaining chapters of the volume.

2.1 Introduction

The Chinese military strategist Sun Tzu, in his ancient book *The Art of War*, is credited as stating, "If you know the enemy and know yourself, you need not fear the result of a hundred battles. If you know yourself but not the enemy, for every victory gained you will also suffer a defeat. If you know neither the enemy nor yourself, you will succumb in every battle."

The wisdom implied in this statement is that only when you are familiar with yourself *and* your enemy will you be successful in battle. Some Microbiologists have used warfare as an analogy to an infection, and for good reason. There are two sides, bacteria and host. One is trying to invade and the other is defensive. Each have armory and tactics and counter-tactics. One side is victorious and the other is defeated. There are casualties. The

site of battle is left a wasteland (inflammation). If this analogy is accepted, Tzu's writings suggest that for Microbiologists to be victorious, we must understand both bacteria and the host. This chapter begins our first foray into a thorough appreciation of the bacterial adversary, starting first with a tutorial on the most basic elements of bacterial cells, how these organisms are structured, and how the components function in the context of their importance to the death-match with the host.

If one had to name the most important macromolecular component of a bacterial cell, DNA would probably top most people's list. There is no arguing the importance of DNA. It begets the cells in its entirety. But all cells contain DNA, and DNA is not what necessarily makes a bacterial pathogen different from all other cells. What does make the pathogen special is the bacterial surface, and all its individual components of that surface. The surface of the bacterial invader is fortified like no other cell. Everything the host throws at the bacterium – toxic peptides and proteins, deadly free radicals, and antibodies - are first encountered at and by the bacterial surface. As a result, the bacterial invader must be specifically adapted to combat the exact tactics the host will use against it. Even more, the surface must also serve as both a sensor and gatekeeper for the exit and entry of nutrients and waste products. To think of how the bacterial surface can achieve these tasks while engaging a host cell combatant a hundred times the size is just one small reason to marvel at what evolution can conjure. To know thy enemy, we must start with their being and with this in hand we look deeply at their form and function (◘ Fig. 2.1).

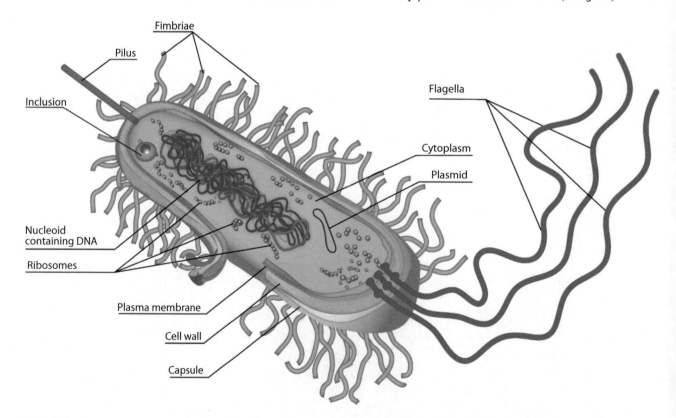

Fimbriae

Pilus

Inclusion

Flagella

Cytoplasm

Plasmid

Nucleoid
containing DNA

Ribosomes

Plasma membrane

Cell wall

Capsule

◘ **Fig. 2.1** Important structures on the bacterial pathogen. The cell body constitutes one or two membranes, a cell wall, ribosomes and DNA. Extra-cellular structures include a flagella (which aids in movement), pili (which may aid in adherence to the host or the exchange of DNA) and fimbriae (which aid in adherence and biofilm formation). Some bacterial pathogens also produce a capsule, often the most external structure that acts as a shield against many host insults. These structures are discussed below

2.2 Bacterial Rebar: The Cell Wall as Scaffold for Virulence

The bacterial surface is also what delineates the two major groups of bacteria; that of Gram-positive and that of Gram-negative. A Gram-positive bacterium, when incubated with the dye crystal violet, binds the dye and retains it. A Gram-negative bacterium does not. The reason a Gram-positive cell retains the violet is because it cannot exit as readily through the thick surface primarily made up of the **cell wall**, or more formally, the **peptidoglycan**. The peptidoglycan is named as such because it is composed of both peptides (peptido) and sugars (glycan). The most common sugars are N-acetylglucosamine (NAG) and N-acetylmuramic acid (NAM). NAG and NAM alternate in a repeat pattern and are covalently linked by a bond between them (◻ Fig. 2.2).

Each NAM is covalently attached to a peptide of amino acids, usually three to five in length depending on the species. In Gram-positive bacteria, each peptide itself is cross-linked to the neighboring peptide by the amino acid, often glycine. The overall array creates a mesh-like pattern of repeating units of NAG-NAM-peptide—peptide-NAM-NAG that surrounds the cell in a crystalline array (◻ Fig. 2.3). In Gram-positive bacteria, the peptidoglycan is in many cases the most distal structure, external to the membrane, is thick (~40 nm) and constitutes most of the weight of the cell. In Gram-negative bacteria, it is a thinner structure (<10 nm) and constitutes less than 10% the dry weight of the cell. In contrast to Gram-positive cells, the Gram-negative peptidoglycan lies between the inner and outer membrane[1] in an area of the cell termed the **periplasm**. The periplasm is an enigmatic bacterial component. Being mostly gel-like in composition, it is heavily saturated with proteins that bridge the structural and functional gap between the inner and outer membranes. Proteins and smaller solutes that are transported in and out of the cell transit the periplasm. A rendering of important surface structures of Gram-negative and

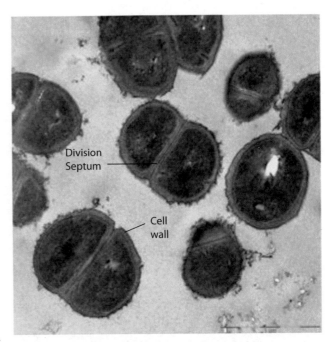

◻ **Fig. 2.3** Electron microscopy of the Gram-positive cell wall. Transmission electron microscopy shows the thick cell wall of *S. aureus* (a cause of many different types of human infections) in dividing cells. Notice a thinner newly synthesized cell wall in the division septum. (Adapted from Frees et al (see *suggested readings*) under a creative commons license (▶ https://creativecommons.org/licenses/by/4.0/))

Gram-positive bacteria is shown in ◻ Fig. 2.4, and an electron micrograph of Gram-negative in ◻ Fig. 2.5.

The peptidoglycan of most Gram-positive bacteria are often the first entity to encounter the host and as such plays an important functional role during infection. Because of its physical location and prominence, not only is it more frequently studied in Gram-positives than Gram-negatives, it also is more likely to be shed from the surface, and thus, is bioactive. In fact, the host has evolved mechanisms to not only detect the cell wall but also degrade it. Intracellular host signaling molecules called NODs can sense peptidoglycan fragments and alert the immune system to the presence of a bacterial invader. In addition, secreted host enzymes such as lysozyme specifically cleave between the NAG and NAM. In response, some bacteria make modified repeating units that resist the actions of this enzyme. In Gram-negatives, the peptidoglycan is sheltered by the **outer membrane**. Thus, its turnover is largely kept internal and there may be little to no external shedding.

The crosslinking peptides and repeating units impart a rigid structure to the cell wall relative to the more fluidic membrane. A main function of the cell wall then is in part to provide structure to the cell, a kind of exoskeleton. It also resists the osmotic forces that may lead to a swelling or collapse of the cell cytoplasm. This role is not necessarily specific to its importance during an infection. These are functions attributable to all bacteria with external cell walls. A more specific role for the cell wall comes in the form as an anchor for bioactive surface proteins. Amongst these,

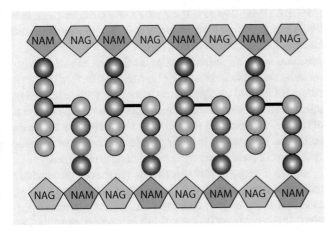

◻ **Fig. 2.2** The structure of the Gram-positive cell wall. The cell wall is composed of repeating subunits of the sugars NAG and NAM (commonly) linked to a string of five amino acids (colored balls) which itself are linked by a crossbridge (black bar) that joins the entire unit to the next one. This generates a lattice like ordered arrangement

2

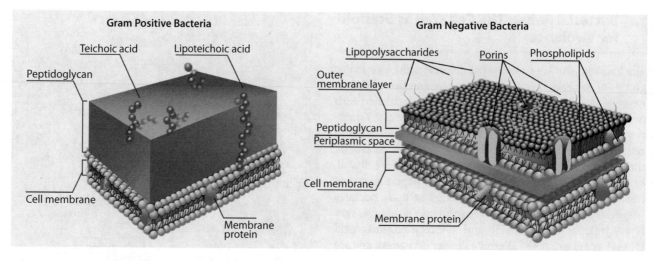

■ **Fig. 2.4**   The surface organization of the Gram-positive and Gram-negative bacterial cell

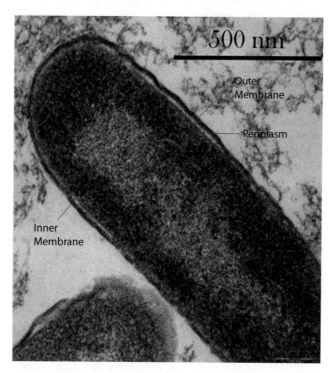

■ **Fig. 2.5**   Electron microscopy of a Gram-negative cell. Thin section transmission electron microscopy of *E. coli* (a cause of systemic and intestinal infections) shows the surface arrangement of a typical Gram-negative bacterial cell. Visible are the outer membrane, a clear periplasmic space, and a dark inner membrane. (Adapted from Klaus et al (see *suggested readings*) under a creative commons license (► https://creativecommons.org/licenses/by/4.0/))

pertaining to pathogenesis, it serves as a scaffold for surface proteins that intersect with the host. We discuss a few themes here because the cell wall is an underrated target for new antimicrobials.

There is great diversity in the function of the proteins linked to the cell wall. Some of them include **nutrient transporters**. Nutrient transporters are any bacterial surface protein that partakes in the uptake of key molecules necessary for the growth and physiology of the cell. Unlike the lipid bilayer that constitutes the membrane, the cell wall is thought to be permeable to most small solutes. But some nutrients can be large, bulky and relatively insoluble. Amino acids, sugars, and metals are examples of compounds or atoms bacterial cells acquire during infection. Some are essential, like metals. Cell wall attached nutrient transporters effectively steal these metals from the host and use them to serve the needs of the pathogen. We learn more about all the ways bacteria raid your nutrients in ► Chap. 11.

The cell wall and outer membrane is also a site of attachment of **adhesins**. Adhesins are extracellular bacterial proteins that directly, and often very strongly, bind to receptors on host cells, tissues, and/or extracellular matrix components. Adhesins are so important for disease and infection that they are a common target for the development of new vaccines and small molecule drugs. We discuss the general classes of adhesins and their function in ► Chap. 7 but for the purposes of this discussion, one should consider the cell wall as an important base platform for the anchoring of adhesins, including the family of surface adhesins termed the **microbial surface components recognizing adhesive matrix molecules** (MSCRAMMs). Tissue extracellular matrix, the material that binds our cells together, includes collagen, fibronectin, and laminin, and are common host receptors for MSCRAMMS. In addition, some adhesins function as the first site of engagement between bacteria and the host thereby facilitating close combat. Fighting in tight spaces may help the bacterium to inject deadly toxins into the host cell or promote the invasion of the cell. By invading the host cell, the bacterium may gain additional advantages, including protection from the immune system and access to higher levels of diverse nutrients.

Another group of proteins attached to the cell wall include those that confuse or divert the immune response. Here, we can label them as **immune modulators**. As the name suggests, these proteins do something to prevent the immune system from engaging or otherwise killing the pathogen. Some cell wall linked immune modulators gobble up host antibody and arrange it in a way that renders it useless. Others inhibit phagocytosis by host macrophages, the major pathogen-killing special operations soldier of the human body[2]. By avoiding phagocytosis, the bacterium eliminates one of the most important of all immune functions your body uses to rid itself of invaders. Other cell wall immune modulators fool the body into degrading complement. Complement is a protein complex present in our blood that binds to the surface of bacteria. Complement deposition involves a cascade of blood proteins that form a complex on the surface of the invader which attacks the bacterial membrane. By avoiding the deposition of this landmine, bacteria resist one of the more efficient and widespread toxic activities blood has on bacteria.

The cell wall is also a nucleator of bacterial communities termed **biofilms**. Specialized surface proteins attached to the cell wall promote not only the association with the host, but also other bacteria of the same species. Millions of bacterial cells may eventually group together in a carbohydrate-rich structure that not only protects them from the immune system but is also impervious to the penetration of some antibiotics. Biofilms are common occurrences on implanted medical devices such as catheters, artificial joints, stents and the like. The formation of biofilms on these devices can lead to a deadly infection and is one of the more feared types of infections clinicians encounter. We explore biofilms in ▶ Chap. 12.

Before moving on to the cellular membranes of bacterial cells, we should consider one additional important surface structure, the **capsule** (◻ Fig. 2.6). Its name implies its function – it literally encapsulates the bacterial cell being the outermost structure to the outer membrane in Gram-negatives and the cell wall in Gram-positives. The capsule varies in structure and composition quite widely, even between strains of the same species. However, it is primarily made of repeating units of carbohydrates or in some species certain amino acids. The glycan variety makes sense. As the outermost structure of many pathogenic bacteria, it will often be the structure that comes into contact with the host. This includes antibodies, macrophages, complement, antimicrobial peptides and more. We learn in more detail about these host immunological factors in later chapters but suffice it to say at this point that all of them are detrimental to the bacterium. The capsule, though, can resist them. Its main function in the context of pathogenesis is that it can prevent phagocytosis by immune cells and act as a type of force field against killer host molecules like complement and antimicrobial peptides. When it comes to antibodies, the myriad of different structures various assortments of glycans can arrange into acts as a kind of decoy to immunological detection. This is one of the main complicating issues behind the making of universal vaccines against some bacterial pathogens. With not every capsule being the same between different strains, a one-antigen one-vaccine model does not fit all. We learn more about this in ▶ Chap. 16 on vaccines.

Out of the Box
The Mysterious Cell Wall
The peptidoglycan of Gram-positive bacteria lies external to their single membrane, yet, it is meant to provide structural support and rigidity (shape) to the cell. Proteins tens of thousands of daltons in size are somehow secreted through this structure and smaller molecules that fuel metabolism head in the opposite direction. How does a supposed repeating unit of sugar and crosslinked peptide with little malleability accommodate such dynamic biology? Or is the cell wall not homogeneous throughout? Perhaps there are local microdomains of functionality, somewhat deconstructed in rigidity, to allow for two-way traffic through the membrane. Or maybe during cell division there is a narrow window of opportunity, or region, where the membrane is continuous with the environment? Some of the most substantial human pathogens, your staphylococci, streptococci, and enterococci that live on you, have a thick external cell wall. A world of knowledge has yet to be uncovered into the mysterious biology of the bacterial cell wall. Answers to these questions will aid efforts to improve infectious disease medicine.

2.3 Organized Fluid: The Membrane

As mentioned, Gram-negative bacteria house an inner and outer membrane, whereas Gram-positive bacteria contain only a single membrane inside the outer cell wall. ◻ Figure 2.3 shows the difference in the Gram-positive and Gram-negative surface. Similar to the cell wall, the membrane participates in several general functions common to all bacteria, including serving as a permeability barrier, the selective transport of important solutes, and is the source of an electrochemical gradient of ions that generates energy for the cell (the proton motive force). Unlike what was true for Gram-positive bacteria

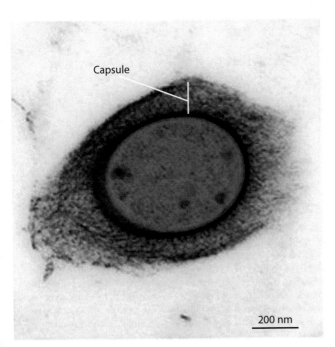

Capsule

200 nm

◻ **Fig. 2.6** The bacterial capsule. Electron microscopy of *K. pneumoniae* (a cause of human blood and lung infections) showing its thick capsular structure. In some areas, the width of the capsule is nearly a quarter of the diameter of the cell. (Adapted from Short et al (see *suggested readings*) under a creative commons license. (▶ https://creativecommons.org/licenses/by/4.0/))

2

and the peptidoglycan, most of what we understand about the bacterial membrane comes from the study of Gram-negatives and their two membrane system. Like the cell wall, the membrane is also critical for pathogenesis.

The outer membrane serves several important roles in pathogenic bacteria. First, and foremost, the outer membrane is the anchor site for one of the more important molecules studied in the context of diseases caused by bacteria, that of "endotoxin." Endotoxin is the name given by the German physician Richard Pfeiffer in the early twentieth century to describe a substance produced as a result of the lysis of bacteria that causes harm to injected animals. We now know the substance as **lipopolysaccharide**, shorted to LPS. LPS is composed of three main components: the outer polysaccharide (sometimes called the O antigen because of its immunogenic properties), the core oligosaccharide, and membrane anchored lipid A (☐ Fig. 2.7). The outer polysaccharide is highly variable and its carbohydrate structure changes between species and even within strains of the same species. This region interacts directly with the host. It is believed that the variability in the sugar structures is one way bacteria escape cross-species recognition by the immune system. The core structure is unchanged much from bacteria to bacteria. The anchored portion (lipid A) is highly hydrophobic and as such embeds itself in the membrane. Lipid A is also very toxic to mammalian cells and when released, either through lysis or normal turnover of LPS, acts as a potent **pyrogen** (induces fever) and stimulator of the host immune system. Specific immune cells, especially macrophages and monocytes, have receptors on their surface termed **toll like receptors** or **TLRs** that bind lipid A, thereby activating cell signals that promote the release of small inflammatory mediators such as cytokines and chemokines[3]. One of the hallmarks of bacterial infections is fever; in many cases, lipid A is the reason for this response. Too much lipid A has dire consequences for the mammalian host and can result in an immune system that transforms into one that is protective to one that is overstimulated, and therefore dangerous. The most serious consequence of too much bacteria and its products is a condition termed **sepsis**. Sepsis results when a serious infection combines with a massive immune response to this infection. The body is overwhelmed; substantial damage to major organs and tissues occurs. It is widely believed that released lipid A, due to its immunostimulatory properties, is a prominent component of the onset of systemic sepsis, but other bacterial molecules including DNA and secreted toxins and effectors also contribute. Sepsis occupies our thoughts in ▶ Chap. 14.

The second major component of the outer membrane are **porins**, first described in *E. coli* in the mid-1970s. Porins are classified into two types based on function. Generalized porins allow the transport of a wide-range of small solutes, mostly sugars, amino acids, and vitamins. Specialized porins have certain structural features that make them more selective. The porin structure consists of anti-parallel β sheets arranged in a cylinder embedded in the membrane. Two porins may pair together in a structure termed a dimer, or three may pair in a trimer. The center of the cylinder is the "molecular sieve", a

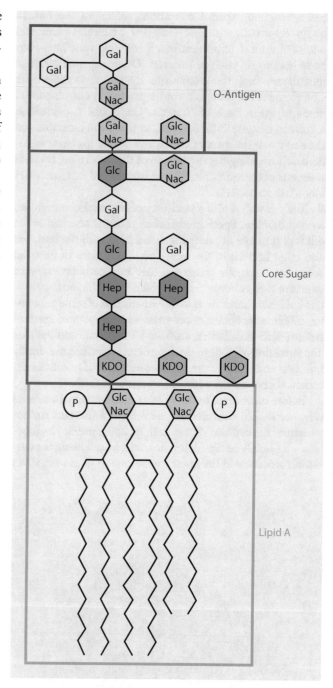

☐ **Fig. 2.7** Bacterial lipopolysaccharide. The Gram-negative LPS is often recognized as a three part structure. The most distal component is oligosaccharide antigen, or O-antigen. As its name implies, the structure of this component can vary widely between species and even strains, largely to confuse the immune system. The O-antigen can have a repeating nature of this component, upwards of 40 units at times. The central component, or core oligosaccharide, is often consistent between species, and single in its unit structure. The most proximal portion is lipid A, its aliphatic chains of carbon units embedded in the outer membrane

channel that small solutes can pass through to either enter or leave the cell. This center is **hydrophilic** (water loving), lined with the side chains of polar amino acids so that water-loving solutes will be attracted to its channel. Intermixed among these are amino acids whose **hydrophobic** (water afraid) side chains are oriented away from the central channel towards the lipids of the outer membrane. They serve to promote attraction to the membrane lipids with similar properties and keep the porin in the membrane. Specialized porins often contain an eyelet, an extracellular flap that functions as a gate to regulate entry into the centralized channel.

A remarkable feature of many porins is their high level of expression in each cell, sometimes as high as one million total molecules. The expression of each type of porin is usually regulated by the concentration of the solute it helps move into the cell. Environmental conditions such as changes in the pH, temperature, and molecular status of proteins that control transcription also regulate porin production. Given their abundance and surface localization, it should not be surprising that the host has developed ways to exploit their presence. Lactoferrin, a secreted protein present in bodily fluids such as breast milk, and which chelates iron away from growing pathogens, binds to surface porins on *E. coli*. Complement, the innate immune complex that attacks bacterial membranes leading to their lysis, also uses porins as an anchor site. In *Neisseria gonorrhoeae*, the cause of the sexually transmitted disease gonorrhea, outer membrane porins cause host cell apoptosis and also serve as important nutrient importers[4]. In invasive enteric bacteria that cause diarrhea, outer membrane porins are adhesive molecules. They also promote entry into the host cell. The nutrient uptake and adhesion roles are similar to proteins that are anchored to the cell wall (above) and thus highlight a common feature for surface structures.

Unlike the outer membrane where porins allow small solutes to enter the periplasm, the bacterial inner membrane is much more selective. Acting as a true diffusion barrier, the transport of solutes is active and thereby must couple to a process that liberates energy to overcome this barrier. This energy then drives the import of solutes against a concentration gradient into the cell. The process is mediated by a larger family of proteins conserved in all domains of life termed **ABC (ATP-binding cassette) transporters**. These transporters are composed of an extracellular domain that binds the ligand for import, a transmembrane domain that spans the inner membrane bilayer, and an intracellular domain that binds ATP. Upon the ligation of a solute, the intracellular domain cleaves the high energy terminal phosphate from ATP, converting it to ADP and free phosphate. This energy is transduced by a series of conformational changes along the length of the transporter such that the extracellular domain squeezes the bound solute down a protected channel to the cytoplasmic side. Using this energy coupled mechanism, solutes can be concentrated against a gradient into the bacterial cell.

Transporters are not often considered in the discussion of true virulence factors but some of them are essential for the sustenance of a bacterial infection. They are the main mechanism by which bacteria eat, and their uptake of all types of nutrients fuels the growth of the cell, its physiology, and ultimately is binary division to make daughter cells. Transporters are directly responsible for securing scarce nutrients in the hostile and sometimes nutrient limiting environment of the host. From metals to peptides providing amino acids, there are numerous reports of the importance of such transporters during infection. Transporters are also strictly regulated, both in terms of their expression as well as function. Their versatility in responding to various environmental stimuli depends on the nutrient composition of the host niche they occupy and drives **patho-adaptive** (metabolic adjustments in response to the host environment) changes as the infection progresses. The direct link between transporters and transcriptional and metabolic regulators provides the pathogen the ability to quickly pivot to meet its nutritional needs. In the host, where each niche may be a world apart in terms of key building blocks, these patho-adaptive traits are the difference between survival and death.

2.4 The Bacterial Heart: The Cytoplasm

The bacterial cytoplasm is the engine of the cell and the place for much of the cell's metabolic output. In pathogenic bacteria, the efficiency of the engine is of the utmost importance. As such, conserved intracellular functions have often been co-opted or modified to fit the pathogen's ultimate narrative: survival in the host. The three main components of the bacterial cytoplasm that have special prominence include the DNA, the ribosomes, and its protein enzymes and regulators.

Deoxyribonucleic acid, or **DNA**, is the chemical name for the structure that begets life. Inherent in its four nucleoside bases of adenine (A), guanine (G), cytosine (C), and thymine (T), covalently bound like beads on a very long string, are the instructions to create a protein, all its components via those proteins, the cell itself, and ultimately, an organism. Each bacterium contains a slightly different code and thus yields a slightly different cell; the diversity of all the different bacterial genera, species, and strains is a reflection of the diversity of the DNA code. In fact, the diversity of all life is reflected in the linear arrangement of these four letters. The code is read by an enzyme termed RNA polymerase. Along with specialized proteins termed transcription factors, the RNA polymerase converts the DNA code into an RNA message in a process termed **transcription**. The ribonucleic acid (RNA) message is complimentary to the DNA code, which ensures the fidel conversion of the message contained within that code. Once the RNA message is complete, it is recognized by a 30-protein complex – the **ribosome**. During **translation**, the ribosome machinery reads each RNA message and recruits one of the twenty amino acids, one for each three **codon** combination of RNA bases, to the complex and links them end on end until a protein is formed. Conserved from the simplest cell to the most complex organism, all life uses this basic script to build cells. There are entire volumes written about the properties and function of DNA and RNA – we won't attempt to cover it all here. What is of importance to the microbe hunter is that what distinguishes a non-pathogenic

2

and thus harmless bacterium from one that can lead to your demise is what is encoded in its DNA. Therefore, the content of the DNA of bacterial pathogens, the arrangement of all those "A"s, "T"s, "G"s, and "C"s linearly along the code, is different than for bacteria that do not cause disease. Knowing these differences is one strategy the microbe hunter can use to classify, and understand, dangerous bacteria.

2.5 Movement

A number of pathogenic bacteria have the ability to move, that is, travel to a new location within their host. There are many benefits to being able to re-locate. First and foremost, bacteria that can move can go to an area where nutrients are more plentiful. In fact, bacteria have the ability to sense the concentrations of nutrients in their immediate environment and chemotax to locations of high nutrient levels. Second, movement also allows bacteria to flee. More accurately, tumble and roll away from approaching immune cells. Phagocytic cells like macrophages and neutrophils chase bacteria down and grab them with outstretched tentacles, the purpose ultimately to engulf and kill them. Bacteria use movement to avoid this fate. Finally, a number of pathogenic bacteria will actually invade their host cells, propelling themselves into the host cell (to live) or back out the cell to infect neighbors. All of these actions are mediated by what is called the bacterial **flagellar system**. Looking like a whip on one pole of the bacterium, the flagellum can rotate, either clockwise or counter-clockwise, to move and change its direction. The main component of the whip filament is a protein termed flagellum. The whip is anchored to a hook, which has a slight kink, and is localized in the outer membrane of the cell. The kink gives the organism the ability to rotate the whip in a manner that will propel it forward. These structures are anchored in the periplasm and inner membrane through a series of rings which encase the motor complex. As its name implies, the motor complex harnesses the energy from the bacterial proton motive force to transmit physical changes to the whip structure, which results in its rotation. The importance of the flagellar apparatus in bacterial virulence is illustrated by the fact that loss of these genes renders the pathogen less harmful in animal models of infection.

2.6 The Pathogenome

Most pathogenic bacteria have a single, large circular molecule of DNA, the bacterial **chromosome**, that encodes, depending on the species, between 2500 and 6000 total genes. These genes are usually tightly packed along the chromosome. There is not much non-coding DNA (does not give rise to a protein) between these genes, unlike eukaryotes (like us) where the majority of DNA is non-coding. Genes of similar function are often a part of an **operon**, or genetic unit. An operon is under the control of a single promoter; thus, all the genes in the unit are transcribed at approximately the same time and at the same level. For example, if the genes encode proteins that constitute a secretion system whose parts depend on each other for overall function, having them made at the same time and at similar levels makes the assembly of the system more efficient. Thus, the bacterial chromosome can be considered highly efficient in its use of space and coded genes. Most of the DNA of the chromosome encodes proteins that function as "housekeeping" genes; that is, they perform duties that are routine for most cells. DNA replication, membrane biogenesis, and energy production are a few examples. These functions are necessary for the bacterial pathogen but they are not unique to it. All bacteria carry out these functions. In addition to these essential genes, the chromosome of bacteria that engages a living host has additional genes. These genes somehow confer the ability to infect the host and survive its defenses. Very rough estimates put the percentage of genes from a bacterial pathogen that are bonafide virulence factors at about 25% of the total genes in the genome. When the genes of an operon or genes that are otherwise near to each other along the length of the genome encode for virulence factors, this is sometimes referred to as a **pathogenicity island**. These islands are of the utmost importance in the causation of bacterial diseases. Unlike some stand-alone virulence factors that may not require any other component for its function, proteins transcribed and translated from pathogenicity islands often work together. Their collective action may even cause a particular type of disease or symptom of the disease. Secretion and adhesive systems are good examples (◻ Fig. 2.8).

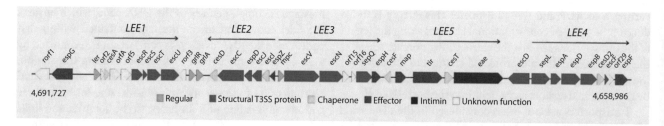

◻ **Fig. 2.8**   A classic pathogenicity island. Clusters of genes that encode factors important for virulence are often referred to as pathogenicity islands. A classic example is the locus of enterocyte effacement (LEE) that is observed in pathogenic and diarrhea-causing strains of *E. coli* such as enterohemorrhagic *E. coli* (EHEC). This locus encodes the components to make an injection system (secretion system) that delivers toxins to host cells, the toxins (or effectors) themselves, and adhesins. We learn about secretion systems, toxins, effectors, and adhesins and their role in pathogenesis in the coming chapters. (Adapted from Hansen et al (see *suggested readings*) under a creative commons license. (▶ https://creativecommons.org/licenses/by/4.0/))

The chromosome is not the only DNA element that codes for the production of bacterial virulence factors. One common feature of pathogenic bacteria is that they often contain in their cytoplasm accessory pieces of DNA in the form of a **plasmid**. A plasmid is a small circular piece of DNA that typically encodes less than 100 genes. Plasmids are thought to confer an advantage to their carrier in a certain environment. In the context of this discussion, a plasmid that allows a bacterium to colonize our gastrointestinal tract, or kill immune cells, or break down an antibiotic, would be selected for in a human host and likely be maintained by the patho-

gen. Here we find one of the more important reasons bacterial pathogens are as successful a form of life on Earth as any - the mobile and mutable **pathogenome**.

Unlike many other parts of the genome, the pathogenome is any set of genes that confers virulence to its bacterial host and is more readily transferred across species or genera. Humans (or any other eukaryotes for that matter), cannot readily take in or lose foreign DNA. Not true for bacteria. Arguably, the ability to acquire and discard useful or non-useful DNA is what makes bacteria so special (◘ Fig. 2.9). They are artful in this skill, and do it better than

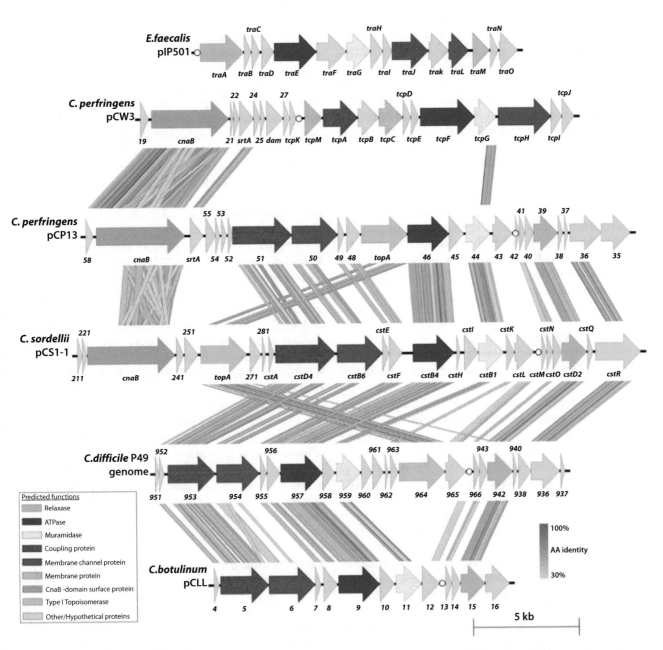

◘ **Fig. 2.9** Mobile genetic elements such as plasmids carry virulence factors. Plasmids are extrachromosomal elements of DNA that are often transferred between pathogenic strains of the same, and even different, species. Shown above is a plasmid identified in the bacterial pathogen *C. sordellii* (causes infections of the lung and heart) that has spread amongst other members of the clostridial genus, including *C. difficile* (a common cause of colitis which has adopted this gene set onto its chromosome) and *C. perfringens* (which causes gangrene), and other enterococci, including *E. faecalis*, a cause of drug-resistant bloodstream infections. Gene functions are color coded (legend). (Adapted from Lyras et al (see *suggested readings*) under a creative commons license. (► https://creativecommons.org/licenses/by/4.0/))

any other form of life. From the wellspring of diversity inherent in the DNA code comes change, and if that change benefits the pathogen, it will be retained and passed to its progenitors. The ability to change one's biological state simply by changing the content of its DNA, either plasmid or otherwise, is as powerful a driver of virulence as any. This is an area of biology where many bacterial pathogens, especially those adapted to humans, thrive. For some of these deadly microbes, the genes of the plasmid are the primary determinant of virulence and loss of that plasmid or gene renders the infecting bacterium avirulent. The causative agent of anthrax, *B. anthracis*, which houses two large plasmids, is an example of this point. One plasmid encodes a deadly toxin, the other a protective capsule. Loss of these plasmids substantially attenuates the virulence of this organism. That is not to say all virulence is contained with the plasmids of bacillus, but many of the genes on these plasmids seem to have no other function except to fight the host. For other pathogens, notably the spirochetes that cause Lyme disease, there may be half a dozen plasmids or more, each contributing some important function but heterogeneous enough as to be unique to certain strains. Like a tank that can instantly change the caliber of its gun, the mobile pathogenome, combined with a core set of housekeeping genes located on the more stable chromosome, provides the bacterium with an adaptable arsenal to confront its host. The virulence factors themselves are certainly the effectors of disease; they are the action molecules. But it all starts with the elusive pathogenome. In ▶ Chap. 6, we discuss these points in more detail.

2.7 Metabolism

The bacterial cytoplasm is also the site of most of the biosynthetic and regulatory functions of the cell, powered by the proteins produced from translation. Most pathogenic bacteria fuel their metabolism through the use of carbon-containing molecules that yield energy when broken down. For pathogenic bacteria, this consists of acquiring molecules the host makes or eats, including host proteins as a source of amino acids and host proteoglycans such as mucins as a source of sugars. We will discuss soon enough how an armory of secreted proteases is one way pathogenic bacteria liberate these important host molecules for bacterial consumption. When more complex molecules are degraded so that their products can be used as metabolites or for energy it is termed **catabolism**. This contrasts with the construction of larger molecules from smaller precursors, which is **anabolism**. Both catabolism and anabolism are necessary metabolic processes for deadly bacteria. By far, the most commonly used catabolite for energy is the sugar glucose. Just as a high-sugar drink can ramp up your activity level during sport, so too does glucose for bacteria. When bacteria acquire organic

(carbon-containing) molecules from their environment, they are **heterotrophic**. "Hetero" is Greek meaning "different" while "trophic" means "to feed." Thus, heterotrophic bacteria feed on a wide array of different compounds. All pathogenic bacteria are heterotrophic, and for good reason. They must be versatile in using the nutrition that is available to them in a host to be successful pathogens.

As mentioned, the most sought after small molecule of energy for many pathogenic bacteria is glucose, which is directed into a pathway for its degradation, **glycolysis**. During glycolysis, glucose is converted by eight steps into pyruvate and two high energy molecules of adenosine triphosphate (ATP). Very little goes to waste with bacteria. The pyruvate can be utilized in many ways but some of it is diverted into the **tricarboxylic acid cycle** (TCA).[5] This results in more ATP for energy, as well as reducing agents that neutralize free radicals the cells make as a result of their respiration. In addition, the products of the TCA cycle are used to make some amino acids, the building blocks of proteins, and hence, virulence factors. An auxiliary pathway to glycolysis is the **pentose-phosphate pathway** (PPP), with also uses glucose metabolites but mostly for the purpose of building the precursors to make nucleotides, the building blocks of DNA, as well as "closed" or aromatic amino acids. Thus, PPP uses glucose to anabolize critical molecules for pathogenic bacteria to make more of themselves.

Some pathogenic bacteria use an alternative to glycolysis, termed the **Entner-Doudoroff** (ED) pathway. ED also uses glucose to generate ATP and reducing equivalents, but less so then traditional glycolysis. The prominent lung pathogen *Pseudomonas aeruginosa* uses the ED pathway instead of glycolysis, for example, thereby highlighting how different pathogenic bacteria enable the metabolism best suited for their environmental niche they find themselves. Finally, when bacteria cannot attain glucose from the host, they need to synthesize it. This process is called **gluconeogenesis**. Here, glucose is synthesized from non-sugar sources of carbon, derived from the breakdown of host proteins or lipids, which can be shunted into glycolysis to generate energy. Gluconeogenesis is a commonly utilized process for bacteria that prefer to live inside host cells since the substrates for this pathway are found in higher concentration that glucose. ◻ Figure 2.10 summarizes the energetic output and important molecules of these various pathways.

2.8 Regulation

The final cytoplasmic component important in the life-style of a bacterial pathogen is its **regulatory system**. This group of proteins are linked by their function, namely, to mediate the balance between events that generate a virulent cellular state and those that control central metabolism. When pathogenic bacteria are faced with starvation, or a change in

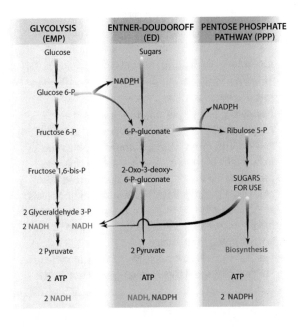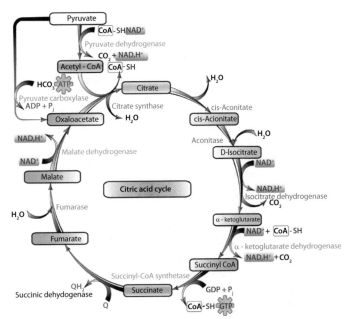

Fig. 2.10 Summary of bacterial metabolic pathways. Pathogenic bacterial employ numerous metabolic pathways to utilize various sources of carbon. Sugars like glucose are the primary and preferred source of energy and are processed through glycolysis, ED or PPP pathways, each generating the high energy molecule ATP and a source of reducing power (NADPH). They also generate pyruvate, GTP, and other complex molecules that are building blocks for biosynthesis or energy sources. Only the enzymes of the citric acid cycle (with each input substrate and reaction products produced) are shown so as to give the reader an appreciation of the complexity of these processes. ATP adenosine triphosphate, GTP guanine triphosphate, NAD nicotinamide adenine dinucleotide, CoA coenzyme A, Q coenzyme Q

host conditions, or one of any other seemingly limitless host changes that can affect their survival, the microbe must be able to quickly adjust its metabolism to respond to these host changes. Regulators are the proteins that mediate this conversion. As such, these regulators link an environmental or host signal to DNA transcription, thereby providing a conduit by which the signal is converted into changes in the expression of gene products involving metabolism or virulence. Regulators control every major arm of virulence, from adherence to the production of toxins and secretion systems. We discuss this topic at length in ▶ Chap. 6.

2.9 Dangerous Accessories

It is not sufficient to discuss how bacteria cause disease without knowing what constitutes the enemy in the first place. A discussion around a surface protein that inactivates your protective antibody is meaningless unless one understands how that surface protein is attached to the cell wall, when the bacterium decides it should make that surface protein, and whether that protein is present in all or just one type of bacterial species. The basic cell components that are the scaffold for the action of virulence factors are as much a target for new drugs as the factors are themselves. All cellular life has form. If one can know the details of the form, one can interpret the generalities of the function.

Summary of Key Concepts

1. The bacterial cell is a highly-organized organism equipped to rapidly adjust to the many challenges of the mammalian host. This is most evident in the unique surface structures that insulate the cell from harmful host insults and the diverse metabolic pathways that drive bacterial physiology.

2. The surface of Gram-negative bacteria encompasses a two membrane system that sandwiches a thin cell wall and periplasm. Gram-positive bacteria harbor a thick well wall external to a single membrane. Both types of bacteria may also contain flagella (for locomotion), pili (for adherence and the transfer of genes), and capsular polysaccharide that protects from attack by the host's immune system.

3. Mutation and the exchange of genetic information is a hallmark of many pathogenic bacteria which can acquire virulence factors and genes that make them resistant to antibiotics.

4. Pathogenic bacteria power their cell by both the uptake of host nutrients and the synthesis of key metabolites. The breakdown of sugars is a major generator of energy and reducing equivalents, both of which feed into biosynthetic pathways.

❓ Expand Your Knowledge

1. You are a college student assigned to present to your class peers on the bacterial surface. Compare and contrast the bacterial surfaces of Gram-negative and Gram-positive bacteria. Consider in your answer the structural and chemical differences between the two. Armed with this knowledge, search the scientific literature for published papers that describe their isolation, ultrastructural details, and differing functions in bacterial physiology and disease. Read one of these papers and include a short presentation of this paper to your class or colleagues.

2. As a new post-doctoral fellow at the National Institutes of Health in Bethesda, Maryland, you are tasked to understand the patho-adaptive changes that occur as Salmonella transitions from the lumen of the human intestine to the blood. Read about the nutrients present in these two environments and prepare a short report on how this organism will need to shift its nutrient sources and metabolism as it transitions between the two niches.

3. The Center for Disease Control hires you, a computational biologist, to analyze the genome of a strange strain of klebsiella species isolated from a contained outbreak in a hospital in New York. This strain is associated with deadly infections of the peritoneal cavity in those undergoing abdominal surgery. A comparative analysis indicates that unlike all other sequenced strains of klebsiella in Genbank, a public genome repository, this strain harbors a large 10 kilobase DNA element with at least 6 encoded genes not present in other klebsiella strains. Interestingly, passage of this strain in LB media in the laboratory facilitates the loss of this DNA. Provide an explanation as to how this strain arose and became deadly.

Notes

1 = A Gram-positive bacterium only contains a single membrane, and it resembles in form and function the inner membrane of Gram-negative bacteria.

2 = Phagocytosis literally means "cell-eating." It is the process by which certain immune cells of your body wrap themselves around a pathogen, leading to its engulfment and internalization. The internalized bacterium, in most cases, is then dissolved by the actions of a specialized organelle termed the lysosome, which bombards the bacterium with membrane-destroying free radicals.

3 = These molecules, including TLRs, are discussed in more detail in ▶ Chap. 4.

4 = Apoptosis, or "programmed cell death" is a purposeful attempt by eukaryotic cells to commit suicide. This often happens when they become infected by pathogens and is a way to clear the pathogen via the sacrificing of the infected host cell. Other pathogens purposely trigger apoptosis by hijacking the signaling pathways that activate the process. This is a way for the pathogen to further invade a host niche.

5 = The TCA cycle is also called the citric acid cycle or Kreb's cycle, after its discoverer Hans Adolf Krebs.

Suggested Reading

Achouak W, Heulin T, Pagès JM (2001) Multiple facets of bacterial porins. FEMS Microbiol Lett 199:1–7. https://doi.org/10.1111/j.1574-6968.2001.tb10642.x

Aunins TR et al (2018) Spaceflight modifies. Front Microbiol 9:310. https://doi.org/10.3389/fmicb.2018.00310

Bæk KT et al (2016) The cell wall polymer lipoteichoic acid becomes nonessential in Staphylococcus aureus cells lacking the ClpX chaperone. MBio 7. https://doi.org/10.1128/mBio.01228-16

Boneca IG (2005) The role of peptidoglycan in pathogenesis. Curr Opin Microbiol 8:46–53. https://doi.org/10.1016/j.mib.2004.12.008

Dorman MJ, Feltwell T, Goulding DA, Parkhill J, Short FL (2018) The capsule regulatory network of. MBio 9. https://doi.org/10.1128/mBio.01863-18

Foster TJ, Geoghegan JA, Ganesh VK, Höök M (2014) Adhesion, invasion and evasion: the many functions of the surface proteins of Staphylococcus aureus. Nat Rev Microbiol 12:49–62. https://doi.org/10.1038/nrmicro3161

Gottschalk G (1979) Bacterial metabolism. New York, Springer

Neidhardt F, Ingraham J, Schaechter M (1990) The physiology of the bacterial cell. Sunderland, Massachussets, Sinauer Associates

Raetz CR, Whitfield C (2002) Lipopolysaccharide endotoxins. Annu Rev Biochem 71:635–700. https://doi.org/10.1146/annurev.biochem.71.110601.135414

Robertson CD, Hazen TH, Kaper JB, Rasko DA, Hansen AM (2018) Phosphotyrosine-mediated regulation of enterohemorrhagic. MBio 9. https://doi.org/10.1128/mBio.00097-18

Vidor CJ et al (2018) Pathogenicity locus plasmid pCS1-1 encodes a novel clostridial conjugation locus. MBio 9. https://doi.org/10.1128/mBio.01761-17

Ziebuhr W, Ohlsen K, Karch H, Korhonen T, Hacker J (1999) Evolution of bacterial pathogenesis. Cell Mol Life Sci 56:719–728

The Practice of the Microbe Hunter

Learning Goals

In this chapter, the basic methodological tenets of the study of pathogenic bacteria are discussed. This includes the analysis of the growth, properties, and behavior of bacteria, as well as the tools and methods used to assess pathogenesis *in vitro* (host cells) and *in vivo* (animal models). The basic definition of virulence is introduced, and model systems that faithfully recapitulate infection, both present and those likely to be a part of the future, are highlighted. The reader will be armed with the tools of microbiology so as to frame the origins of the knowledge presented in forthcoming chapters.

3.1   Introduction

To fully understand how pathogenic bacteria can unravel as complex an organism as a human being, we must start with what is practical. We learned with Koch that the development of strict procedures and the use of reliable implements help shape the discipline of Microbiology into the quantifiable, the reproducible, and ultimately the believable. Like any tradesman with hammer or wrench in hands, good Microbiologists use the tools of their trade to their advantage, while generally being bound by well-established practices and unwritten codes. These practices are understood amongst all members of the field even though their native tongues may not be, and they may not change from scientist to scientist. It builds trust and confidence in the work of the field as a whole. The tools too are similarly shared in design and function. This chapter is intended to introduce you to the brick and mortar of these practices, including why and how they are used, with the hope of equipping the next generation of microbe hunters with the skills to continue the consistency of the trade.

3.2   Growing Bacteria

All bacteria share as a fundamental unit of their existence the purpose of reproduction of their being. They must grow and divide. Depending on the conditions of their environment, some faster than others. The way one bacterium makes two is a process termed **asexual division**. It is asexual because a partner is not needed – a single cell gives rise to two daughter cells, which are said to be **clonal**. In theory, in the absence of any mistakes in replicating the DNA, the daughter cells are exact copies of the parent. They are true clones, genetically identical. In reality, the DNA-making machine of bacteria is imperfect. Mistakes are made. Microbiologists will often loosely state that clonality has been established after a few passages of a single bacterial colony on solid medium[1].

Asexual division is a powerful evolutionary process that allows pathogenic microbes to clone without having to wait for a mate. Two daughter cells beget four more cells, those four yield to eight, and so on. With a doubling time of 20 min for some bacterial pathogens, in as little as 8 h millions of daughter cells are made. This fact is the first attribute the

microbe hunter should never overlook. Unless their growth is purposely stopped, or their nutrient supplies limited, most bacterial pathogens will grow, and fast. As they grow, the levels of their toxic byproducts, and virulence factors, will increase to. If the bacterium can continue to grow, and the host's immune system cannot clear it at the rate equal to that of asexual division or greater, a diseased state may ensue. Of course, this is a simple model that assumes all bacteria divide at their fastest possible rate inside their human hosts. This is not usually the case for reasons we will see later. Imagine fighting an army that multiples every 20 min. You encounter four enemies but those four make eight more before you even engage. This is one challenge the host faces during infection, and it is substantial.

The measurement of bacterial growth is fundamental to the field of Microbiology. The more growth, the more damage, the more inflammation, the more disease and so on. The effect of any stimulus or modification of the bacteria, be it chemical or genetic, can alter the growth of bacteria. Growth measurements are to Microbiology what reaction products are to Chemistry or dividends are to Finance. To understand bacteria is to understand their need for growth.

Most of what we know about bacterial growth comes from studies using homogenous populations of bacteria in some type of growth medium. Microbiologists have made many of these types of mediums. In general, they are osmotically balanced in salts, contain a source of energy, have near neutral pH, and have the building blocks needed to catalyze and build more cells. In a **defined medium**, the exact components and concentration of those components are known. That is, they are defined. Defined mediums are sometimes classified as **minimal**. They contain only the minimal amount of nutrients to support growth. In a **complex medium**, some components may be known, but others may not. Complex mediums often contain an additive; a magical factor that provides a specialized enrichment the bacterium needs. The addition of blood to a minimal medium is an example of an enrichment that enhances the growth of some pathogenic bacteria. Because the exact components of blood are not all known and can vary, this new medium is a complex medium. With such mediums, the Microbiologist has a powerful tool to make as much as the pathogen as one needs, a useful element in their study.

But not all bacteria are easily grown. In fact, most cannot even be cultured. Others need specialized upgrades. For example, **strict anaerobes** need the culture conditions to be void of oxygen. This is true for some pathogens of the gastrointestinal tract where the lumen is relatively anoxic. *Clostridium difficile*, a spore-forming bacterium that can colonize our colon and is a leading cause of nosocomial infections, is an example of a pathogenic anaerobe. A **facultative anaerobe**, however, can grow in the presence of oxygen or its absence, although one condition may be preferred. Other bacteria won't grow freely in liquid culture but instead need a cellular host. They are **obligate** to their cellular host and will only grow inside this host, usually the cells of the host. The cause of the deadly spotted fever, *Rickettsia rickettsii*, is an example. *R. rickettsia* can only grow in the cytoplasm of mammalian cells. Finally, some bacteria that may be pathogens or are associated with a human disease have yet to be successfully cultured. This is especially true for some residents of the human gastrointestinal tract. There may be an indirect association with a particular disease, but the specialized niche in which they live (the intestine) has not been modeled well enough in culture to support their growth.

3.3 Stages of Growth

When bacteria have plentiful nutrients (a complex medium) and one takes measurements of their cell numbers and plots that value against time, a characteristic pattern of growth is observed (◘ Fig. 3.1). The first phase, termed the **lag phase**, is defined by the bacteria adjusting to the environment in which they find themselves. This may include a complete rearrangement of their central metabolism to maximize the resources available to these new conditions. It takes time for the cell to change in this manner; growth is thus delayed or very slow. If the medium is a rich complex medium and the environment a controlled culture flask, this period of adjustment may be short since nutrients are plenty. After the adjustment is made, especially in a closed and controlled system such as a culture flask, the population enters a second phase, termed **logarithmic or exponential phase**. Here, division is accelerated and may be at the bacterium's maximal capacity such that the expansion kinetics are characterized by an exponential increase in bacterial numbers. Under these conditions, nutrients are rapidly utilized and potentially toxic byproducts accumulate unless replenished or released, respectively. The population then begins to reduce its growth rate until the number of replicating bacteria either stops altogether or is in equilibrium with the number of dying cells. Here, the population exists in a kind of suspended existence, termed the **stationary phase**. When the nutrients have all been exhausted or byproducts become toxic or both, there is

a net loss of cells, and the population enters the **decay phase**. Left without replenishment or wash out, all the cells will either die off or enter a state of hibernation.

3.4 Measurement of Growth

The above description applies to bacteria grown under controlled conditions in an enclosed flask, a scenario most Microbiologists would prefer because of the ease of experimentation the practice affords. But in nature, the truth is that every infection is a clash between two very divergent worlds, two very different evolutionary lineages. Understanding this clash requires different approaches that move beyond the culture flask. In an infected host, the situation is much more complex. Let's take the example of human blood. Depending on the species of bacteria and particular strain, as well as the species of the host and even the individual, other factors, not present in a culture flask or defined medium, dramatically affect the growth of the pathogen. The bacterium may need to upregulate a transporter to sequester very scarce host nutrients, or it may need more redox enzymes to deal with the oxidative stress of this environment, or anti-immunity factors to fend off complement in serum or macrophages primed for murder. Under these conditions, growth may never start, may occur slowly and linearly, or undergo wavelike transitions that fluctuate between high and low states. In this limited example, the boundaries between the four phases are blurred, and thus, the microbe hunter's ability to extract meaningful data, more difficult. For bacteria that replicate inside host cells (intracellular replication), the standard growth curve has almost no bearing on the reality of the kinetics of growth. In the case of *Mycobacterium tuberculosis*, the cause of the lung infection tuberculosis, the bacterium may lay dormant inside one's alveolar macrophages for decades. Upon a stimulus, the mycobacteria may suddenly initiate growth, albeit at a slow pace with perhaps just a few divisions. One must understand that the assessment of the replication of bacteria under laboratory conditions is useful for meeting the routine needs of the scientists that study them. The challenge for the next generation of Microbiologists, however, is to develop growth mediums that better approximate the conditions bacterial pathogens often encounter when infecting their mammalian hosts. These systems will more accurately describe the bacterial state during its direct engagement of the host as disease develops, and likely also lead to a greater understanding of how they cause said diseases.

The composition of the medium will also determine the instrumentation and method best suited for measuring bacterial levels. Laboratory cultures in most standard bacterial mediums can be quickly assessed using optical approaches. Here, a spectrophotometer is used to measure the amount of light passed through a diluted sample of culture. The more light that fails to reach the detector, the greater the number of particles (bacteria) in the sample, the light having been absorbed by the particle. Since this method provides a quick

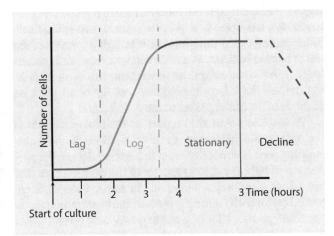

◘ Fig. 3.1 The commonly observed growth phases of a bacterium in a medium with plentiful nutrients under controlled conditions

3

approximation of bacterial levels, it sometimes is necessary to correlate the level of absorbed light (the absorbance) to either the number of **colony forming units** (**CFUs**) in the same sample or the total dry weight of the cellular fraction. CFUs are determined by simply applying a sample of the culture, often diluted, onto a solid medium of agar, a method termed **bacteriologic plating**. By plotting the number of colony forming units or dry weight of cells verses the absorbance over a dilution range, the cell number at any recorded absorbance can be determined, as long as the relationship is linear.

For blood and fluids, mammalian tissues, and infected mammalian cells, optical measurements are not possible. There simply is too much turbidity for any light measurements to have accuracy. In these latter cases, the sample is usually diluted and then plated. By simply counting the number of colonies that grow the next day, one can report the number of colony forming units per volume or mass of the original sample. This is currently the most common way of determining the levels of bacteria during the infection of a host.

Whereas optical readings and colony counting are tried and trusted methods to measure bacteria in culture or tissue samples, the complexity that comes with each infection sometimes requires surveys just as dynamic. When more than a snapshot in time is required, it's also possible to follow bacteria that have been labeled with **fluorescent tracers** or **probes**. These probes allow the investigator to use specialized imaging equipment with sensitive detectors that capture the emitted light from the probes. Such investigation is made possible by the remarkable advances in the engineering of proteins produced by deep see creatures, such as the Green Fluorescent Protein from the jellyfish *Aequorea victoria*. By expressing these genes in pathogenic bacteria and introducing these now fluorescent microbes to the cells or host organisms they infect, one can measure the bacterial levels by measuring the total output of light and dividing this number by the light emitted per cell (presumably already known). A correction may be needed to account for visible light absorbed by the tissues of the host (if working with animals). In practice, most microbiologists omit this sometimes difficult step. Overall, however, the advantage to this method is that one does not have to sacrifice the infected host. In this sense, the method is not invasive and can be used repeatedly throughout the entirety of the infection. Such a technique offers a comprehensive assessment of the state of infection with less labor and less experimental subjects and, importantly, with time as a component.

Quantification of the numbers of bacteria in real-time in as complex an environment as a living host is not the only useful feature of this approach. One can also record the movement and behavior of bacterial cells. Some pathogens are equipped with specialized structures termed flagella[2] that facilitate a swimming action. The prominent food-born pathogen *Listeria monocytogenes*, which sometimes contaminates milk and is dangerous to pregnant mothers, uses flagella to penetrate and spread from host cell to host cell. The

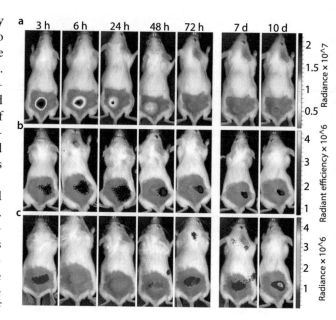

□ **Fig. 3.2**   In vivo imaging a bacterial infection and immune response. In this study, the authors imaged the growth of a bacterial pathogen (*P. aeruginosa*) engineered to express a bioluminescent probe. The top panel shows the growth of bacteria at the infection site. The middle panel represents the same animals imaged with another probe (near infrared) that detects neutrophils. The bottom panel shows data from injection of a third probe (chemiluminescent) that detects the killing activity of neutrophils. (Adapted from Hancock et al (see *suggested readings*) under a creative commons license. (▶ https://creativecommons.org/licenses/by/4.0/))

movement between cells can be tracked if the listeria are fluorescent. Some bacterial pathogens do not have flagella and their movement inside a host is dictated by the movement of the host cells themselves. A macrophage is a common host cell targeted by bacterial pathogens. Some species of salmonella, a food/water-born pathogen, specifically infects intestinal macrophages and are often spread in this organ by the movement of these infected macrophages throughout the tissue, and further. If bacteria are non-motile and do not infect host cells, they may also spread throughout the body by blood and/or lymph fluid. If the bacterium is fluorescently tagged, the investigator can follow where in the host body the bacterium has spread, a process termed **dissemination**[3]. More recently, **real-time infection imaging** combines the use of labeled bacteria, a suitable animal model, and specialized cameras to monitor these movements in a living, breathing host as the infection progresses. □ Figure 3.2 gives an example of the use of probes to image infection.

Probes also are used to report on the biological state of the pathogenic bacterium during infection. If the light-emitting gene is physically fused to a bacterial gene, the production of light is a direct reporter of the expression of that gene. Such a technique allows one to assess what genes are turned on (and off) during growth in the host (or under any condition really). Knowing the expression of certain genes under a set of conditions gives the investigator an idea of how the bacterium is trying to adapt to its host. Other genes report on the metabolic activity of the pathogen by coupling the production or depletion of a metabolite to the emission of light. Metabolites, which include sugars, lipids, amino acids, phosphates, peptides, and other small molecules typically less than 1000 daltons in molecular mass, are the products of a cell's activity or normal working function. As such, they report on the physiological state of the bacterial cell, information that can be used to determine how bacteria expend energy when combating host defenses.

Out of the Box

Domesticated Bacteria

The main emphasis of this book is to discuss the ways in which bacteria make us ill. But not all bacteria are bad. In fact, the vast majority of them cannot harm us at all and some of them are really important in our daily lives. We discuss in ► Chap. 13 how the bacteria of our intestinal microbiome keep pathogenic bacteria out, help our immune system, and even make vitamins we need. Bacteria are also important in industry, food production, molecular biology, and the construction of medicines. For example, bacteria are sometimes added to an important industrial step to help make a product, including ethanol. Some bacterial enzymes are used in household products. Lactobacillus is used to make everyday foods, including cheeses and yogurt. It is tempting to speculate that our ancestors were probably trying to avoid contamination of milk and accidentally discovered that sometimes the fermentation of milk by bacteria can make substances that are still edible and safe. Bacteria have been proposed as a natural garbage disposal to clean up spills of toxic chemicals and oil (termed bioremediation), whereas others can be added to soil to improve plant growth in agriculture. A type of bacillus is an insect pathogen and its spores are used to kill crop-eating caterpillars. This is a natural type of pesticide that avoids harmful chemicals. The biomedical revolution that occurred in science over the past 70 years has been fueled by the use of *Escherichia coli* to shuttle and amplify DNA. This species is also used by scientists to make certain proteins, including insulin. It is exciting to think about other potential uses of bacteria to aid human quality of life. Will artificially constructed bacteria one day be used as little medicine factories engineered in a way to make any kind of small molecule in high amounts? Can we use modified bacteria to eat the Martian soil with oxygen being a byproduct? Will bacteria one day be controllable by computers, little cellular androids that swim to a part of the body and repair a lesion or dysfunctional human cell or tissue? The only thing for certain is such work will be exciting.

3.5 Bacterial Virulence

The ways in which Microbiologists measure the pathogenicity of any given bacterium is by studying its **virulence**. The more virulent the pathogen, the more likely it will cause a particular disease, infect a particular host, or otherwise be harmful to other organisms. The basic unit of virulence is referred to as a **virulence factor**. A virulence factor is any bacterial product, usually a protein, whose presence enhances the disrease-causing ability of the pathogen during infection of a suitable host. Although the term is broadly applied and anything that is important for the fitness of the pathogen *during the infection* may also be considered a virulence factor, the term is more practically applied to a gene or set of genes whose products are made only during the infection (or whose synthesis is induced by host signals or environmental conditions), directly engages the host or functions specifically within it, and whose elimination is expected to attenuate the organism and thus reduce disease severity. Many housekeeping genes (like DNA polymerase) may technically fit this definition but they are generally not considered specific virulence factors if found across all genera of bacteria including in those that are harmless. In this sense, virulence factors can be viewed as an additional genomic toolkit that enhances survival of the pathogen in the host environment. The bulk of virulence factors described to date are most often secreted protein toxins, injected protein effectors, the injection systems themselves, surface proteins that engage the host in some manner, factors that protect against the immune system, and factors that promote nutrient uptake or metabolic adjustment to the host.

Virulence factors often directly counter the host's attempt to clear or otherwise kill the bacterium. Microbiologists, for the most part, are interested in identifying virulence factors whose contribution to the diseases they cause are significant. The reason is simple: these factors are high priority targets for the development of countermeasures against the pathogen, including vaccines. A significant level of virulence of several historically important bacterial pathogens can be attributed to just one or a few virulence factors. Tetanus, for example, is a disease whereby intense muscle spasms can lead to dysregulation of the diaphragm's ability to regulate ones' breathing, sometimes resulting in death. The causative agent of tetanus is the bacterium *Clostridium tetani*, which inhabits the soil and can enter the body via a wound. The disease is entirely caused by the production of a single toxin, tetanus toxin. The toxin works by enzymatically modifying neuronal proteins that regulate how the muscles of the body contract. Vaccination with an inactivated form of the toxin is very effective in preventing the disease. In this regard, tetanus toxin is a clear example of a virulence factor. In the absence of the toxin, *C. tetani* does not cause disease, and measures taken against the toxin eliminate the disease. Young children are often protected against tetanus through the administration of what is called the DTaP vaccine. DTaP is also composed of inactivated toxins from the bacteria that cause pertussis ("whooping cough") and diphtheria ("true croup"). Thus, vaccination with these three virulence factors, which themselves are the primary causes of the disease, protects against three different yet quite serious ailments. The microbe hunter's primary task is the search for the virulence factors that constitute the disease.

3

3.6 The Search for Virulence Factors

How does the microbe hunter determine if a particular bacterial gene encodes a bonafide virulence factor? The answer lies in our use of **infection model systems**, sometimes just described as *a model* or *a system* (◘ Fig. 3.3). Infection model systems do what their name implies; they model in part or in whole the infection so humans do not have to be used in the experimentation[4]. Human samples may be used, however, and during the final stages of the evaluation of a treatment for the disease, humans must be used. Generally, there are as many model systems used to study bacterial pathogenesis as there are pathogens themselves, and each one has its virtues as well as its limitations. We can consider this line of experimentation at two levels. The simpler level takes advantage of cells of the host's tissue that are primarily targeted by the pathogen. These are **in vitro cellular systems**. For example, if studying the lung pathogen *M. tuberculosis*, one may use cultured lung epithelial cells or lung macrophages as the infection "host." The advantages of using in vitro cellular systems are plenty. They include; (i) *reproducibility* – more experiments can be performed and thus the rigor of the conclusions drawn from many replicates is higher; (ii) *cost* – generally speaking, cells are not as costly as animal subjects and this too improves the rigor of the studies by eliminating barriers to reproduce the experiments; (iii) *complexity* – by having a simpler system with less variables effecting the outcome, the ability to draw accurate and clear conclusions is also higher; (iv) *manipulability* – one may be able to fine-tune the host cell to help meet the objectives of the study, including chemical or genetic treatments; and (v) *specificity* – one can examine the effects of the infection on a single cell type, preferably the host cell type also effected during the infection. Each of these concepts are important in aligning with the modern day version of the scientific method. This is the reason why cell cultures, as "models", are useful in understanding the pathogenesis of bacterial diseases.

Performing an infection in an in vitro system is technically straightforward. One simply delivers the desired dose of bacteria to the cultured cells and the infection begins. The dose of bacteria is important in this context; too much and the host cells may die quickly, too little and the infection may not take. The dose of bacteria used is referred to as the **multiplicity of infection** or **MOI**. The MOI is the ratio of the bacteria to the cultured cells. A typical MOI ranges

◘ **Fig. 3.3** The many modalities that model microbial maladies. The rendering is displayed as a circle by which increasing complexity in the model is illustrated clockwise. The ultimate objective is to understand bacterial disease in *H. sapiens*, and develop preventions or treatments that demonstrate efficacy against these diseases. Except for humans, no one model is "better" than another; each model has its advantages and should be chosen to best address the question at hand

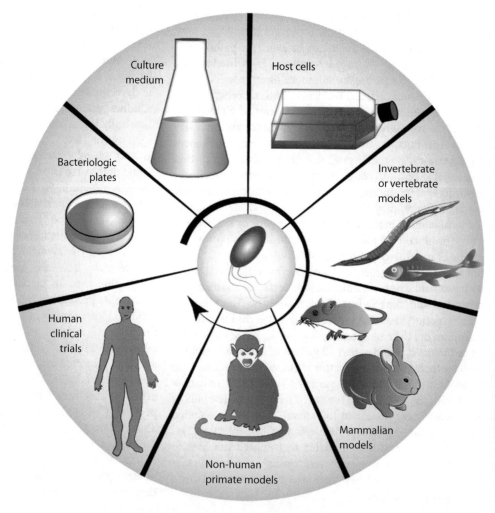

from 1 to 100 depending on the needs of the investigator. Virulence is often measured by determining the effect of the infection on the cultured mammalian cells. The effect may vary on the one extreme to complete death of the cultured cells to on the other extreme some type of perturbation of cell function or physiology (*e.g.* actin rearrangements, ion flux, protein trafficking, etc). Both cell death and cell disruption are an example of an **infection output**, that is, a precisely measured parameter whose intensity is generally indicative of the effect the infection is having on the host cells. There are many common ways to measure cell death but measurement of the disturbance of cell physiology can be quite specific and also numerous. For example, if a particular bacterium disrupts the cytoskeleton of the host cell, this can be assessed by visualizing the actin network by fluorescence microscopy. If one makes mutants in the bacterium in question, the effect of these mutations on the status of the actin is a proxy for the importance of these genes in disrupting actin. These effects are often proportional to the MOI so in culture infection experiments, dosing of the bacterium, is of high value.

Not all in vitro culture experimentation requires bacteria. Indeed, with the advent of technologies to introduce DNA into mammalian cells, it became possible to express bacterial genes in the very host cells they may infect during the natural course of disease. Since bacterial virulence factors comprise a secreted or injected toxin that enters host cells, Microbiologists learned that they could simplify the analysis by simply expressing the bacterial gene inside the host cell using **transfection**, or the use of lipid micelles to promote the uptake of foreign DNA into a cell. An approach like this allows the intracellular actions of a single bacterial protein to be examined without the many other effects that occur when bacteria interact with host cells; and, should this protein be linked to an observable effect, one can make further mutations in the gene to determine the precise structural factors comprising that protein (amino acid residues) that mediate the effect. This **reductionist approach** distils the complexity to its most basic of terms so that the variables are less confounding. In turn, the data becomes a bit interpretable. Like most biomedical investigation, scientists seek to understand the **molecular mechanism** (how a cellular process works on the most basic of levels) of disease causation in hopes they can fine tune this mechanism to achieve beneficial clinical outcomes.

There are disadvantages of in vitro systems too. Whereas on one hand their simplicity is advantageous in one context, on another it may be a liability. In the above example, if one wanted to know how the blood in the lungs altered the infection of *M. tuberculosis* while inside the host cells, the answer could not be found using a culture system. If one wanted to know how the infection of lung cells was recognized by the immune system or how the infection effected other tissues or organs of the body, again, a simple cell culture system would be insufficient. To best answer these questions, an **in vivo system** or approach is required. This takes us to the next section.

3.7 Modeling Bacterial Diseases

In vivo host infections entail the use of a living, breathing organism. Like in vitro systems, the advantages of using a living organism are also numerous, but for different reasons. Unlike cultured cells, the infection does not occur in a vacuum, separated from the real world. A living organism contains all the complexity a bacterium would normally encounter during an infection of its native host in the environment. If the experimental model system is say a rodent, a common choice to model mammalian infections, then the experimenter has a system that integrates all the dynamics of multi-tissue higher level organisms at once, with host responses of several organ systems working in unity. In our earlier case of the lung infection, the circulatory system delivers the immune system to the respiratory system, each bathed not in a synthetic medium but an environment where temperature, dissolved gases, nutrients, and thousands of other metabolites fluctuate with time. Architecturally, the simplicity of the local village yields to a city, towering upwards now in three dimensions, each compartmentalized and with their own unique environment. This complexity, as mentioned above for cultured cells, can work against the experimenter because it is difficult to precisely change one variable without other unseen variables effecting the outcome. In most cases, this is an acceptable risk; plus, the gratification and excitement that comes from revealing even the slightest bit of insight into how bacteria navigate these challenges provides immense central intelligence for the microbe hunter.

An in vivo system also has another advantage – clinical outcomes can be measured. After all, most microbe hunters wish to understand disease to one day prevent it. Clinical outcomes are what allows the investigator to make clear conclusions about the type and strength of a disease a particular bacterium may cause. These outcomes are often directly proportional to the amount and virulence of the bacterium. The amount of bacteria that yields a certain clinical outcome is a number and can be compared to other amounts when a variable is changed. The most simple of assessments is that of life or death. A **survival study** is one in which a fixed number of bacteria are delivered to a suitable host and the proportion of the host that survives is plotted with time (◻ Fig. 3.4). All things being equal (an assumption made to simplify things), the shorter the time period needed to have most or all of the test subjects succumb to the disease, the more virulent the bacterium can be considered. In such a study, it is important to have a suitable number of replicates in each experimental group so that meaningful conclusions can be reached.

Another way to measure virulence is to determine the bacterial dose (ideally the number of cells) at which 50% of the test subjects fail to survive. The term for this is the **lethal dose 50**, often abbreviated to **LD$_{50}$**, and its number can be compared between bacterial species, strains, or mutants of a strain for a gross level assessment of the virulence of a pathogen in question. The lower the dose at which half the subjects succumb, the more virulent the bacterium (◻ Fig. 3.5). The LD$_{50}$ has been and is still as useful a measurement as any in the bacterial pathogenesis field, and it is the staple of knowing what does or does not constitute a virulence factor. For example, if a Microbiologist has data to support the claim that a mycobacterium gene prevents an infected lung cell from telling the immune system that the lung cell is infected, it is expected that the deletion of this gene from the mycobacterial genome would compromise the ability of this bacterium to survive long-term in the host. By deleting only this gene and comparing its LD_{50} to that of the unaltered, wild-type strain, one can numerically assign a level of importance of the gene to the mycobacterial infection. Should the LD_{50} be higher than wild-type, it is reasonable to conclude the gene is a virulence factor. A similar but less used value is the **infectious dose 50**, or **ID_{50}**. This term describes the number of bacteria that are required to cause an infection in half the test subjects. When using the ID_{50}, one must precisely specify what constitutes an infection. Generally speaking, the ID_{50} does not necessarily have to result in death of the subjects, unlike the LD_{50}.

An infection is also a process that changes with time. Thus, time becomes a variable one can use to measure virulence. The most common quantifiable parameter of time to gauge the importance of a virulence factor is **mean-time-to-death**, or **MTD**. The MTD is the mean length of time, usually in hours or days, required for all the test subjects at a fixed dose of bacteria to succumb to the infection. In our example from above, if the putative mycobacterial gene is an important virulence factor, than a strain that lacks this gene will demonstrate an increased MTD when compared to the wild-type strain. Both the MTD and LD_{50} are hallmark measurements of virulence but sometimes the effect of a virulence factor on these measurements may be subtle. When more sensitize approaches are needed, the Microbiologist may mix the wild-type and mutant strain in equal proportions and inoculate *both* into the animal host. The total bacterial cell number of each is then recorded with time using the methods described above. This is called a **competition** or **fitness assay**. Should the mutant strain be less fit in the host than the wild-type strain because it lacks the gene in question, there will be less of the mutant than the wild-type because the wild-type will have outcompeted the mutant. The quantitative unit of this assay is the competitive index, usually the fraction of mutant to wild-type cells. The approach does require that each strain be delineated from the other (usually by selective growth, PCR, or expression of different light-emitting probes), and this difference cannot effect the fitness of the strain while in the host. ◻ Figure 3.6 lists some common techniques to assess the virulence of bacteria.

3.8   The Omics of Infection

Other approaches, popularized during the beginning of the new millennium as the sequencing of bacterial genomes ramped up, is to use "Omics" type technologies to understand the basis of bacterial disease. The omics approach had its foundation in **genomics**, the use of large data sets of gene contents (really, DNA sequences of entire bacterial chromosomes and their plasmids) to help shine light on the gene content that may define a bacterial pathogen. Comparison of

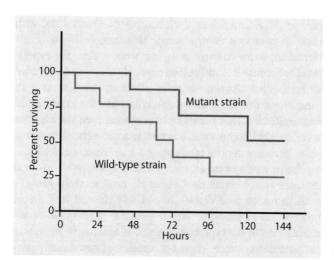

◻ **Fig. 3.4**   Survival curve for a hypothetical virulent wild-type and mutant strain of the same species of bacteria. The mutant strain, otherwise identical to the wild-type strain except for a single change in its DNA code (e.g. single deleted gene proposed to be a virulence factor), is attenuated in the infection because of the absence of this gene

◻ **Fig. 3.5**   Assessment of the lethal dose 50 of a bacterial strain or mutant. A reduction in the number of bacteria required to kill half the experimental test subjects suggests the strain has become more virulent. An increase in this number suggests the strain has become attenuated or less virulent

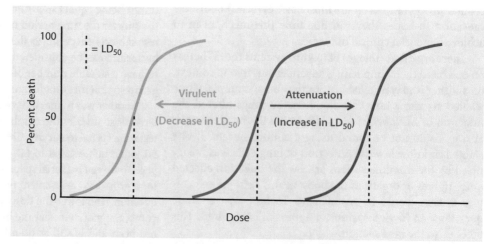

Method or technology	Description	Purpose
Common methods to identify/characterize		
Culturing	Growing bacteria under controlled conditions.	• Increase bacterial numbers • Identify
Optical density	Spectrophotometric measurement.	• Quantify particles in a liquid.
Plating	Culturing bacteria on solid media.	• Isolate pure colonies • Identify
Common methods to visualize		
Light microscopy	Using visible light to detect.	• Quantify bacterial numbers • Identify • Determine morphology
Electron microscopy or EM	Using electrons to detect.	• Determine ulrastructural details and subcellular structures.
Fluorescent microscopy	Using fluorescence of luminous molecules to detect.	• Determine cell localization, movement, metabolism and gene expression.
Cryoelectron microscopy	EM under cryogenic temperatures.	• Determine oligomeric structures.
Common methods to test pathogenicity		
In vitro host culture	Growing bacteria outside host e.g. cells	• Investigate host-pathogen interactions.
MOI[1.]	Bacterial cells to host cells.	• Determine bacteria to cell dose in vitro.
Animal models	Infection model using live animals e.g. mice	• Investigate host-pathogen interactions.
LD 50[2.]	Dose when 50% infected succumb to disease.	• Determine lethality of pathogen.
ID 50[3.]	Dose when 50% become infected.	• Determine pathogenicity of bacteria.
Mean time to death	Time when 50% infected succumb to disease.	• Determine lethality of pathogen.
Common methods to characterize, genetically		
Reverse genetics	Remove genes and test phenotype.	• Identify gene responsible for phenotype.
Forward genetics	Mutagenize genome and perform a selection.	• Analyze phenotype of mutant.
Complementation	Reintroduce deleted gene back into mutant strain.	• Restore wildtype phenotype.

[1.] Multiplicity of infection
[2.] Lethal Dose 50
[3.] Infectious Dose 50

◻ **Fig. 3.6** Some common technologies or methods used in the study of bacterial virulence

say virulent strains to non-virulent strains will reveal genes present in one or absent in the other that may be direct contributors to virulence. This period was fueled by an intensive level of sequencing of as many pathogens as one could get their hands on. Entire databases where generated, publically available and mineable by scientists, to aid the search for these virulence genes. The genomics revolution gave way to the **proteomics** period, which had in concept the same basic idea but took it one step further. Now, infected tissues (or cells) could be analyzed by mass spectrometry and all the proteins present in these tissues (compared to uninfected controls) identified as ether belonging to the pathogen or the host. In this way, genes that were expressed as protein products during an actual infection could be identified. If we go back to our concept of a virulence factor as being something that aids the bacterium in its survival in the host and is thus also made in that host, this was a way to identify novel bacterial factors (and host ones as well) that are likely to be made only in the context of the infectious process.

The natural progression from genomes to proteomes almost mandated that scientists would also consider the **metabolome**, that is, the study of all the cell's metabolites. The metabolites are the product of protein activity, and, as such, represent the sum of all biochemistry occurring at any time in the cell. Perturbations in the metabolites are indicative of changes in overall metabolism. Changes in metabolism have profound effects on cell physiology. Bacteria, especially intracellular bacteria, can and will divert host cell metabolism to meet the bacterium's basic needs. Thus, changes in metabolites are indicative of the activity of virulent bacteria. There are other omes that are important for virulence. The epigenome may affect the expression of genes; **epigenetics** is the study of how modifications of DNA or its structure effect gene expression. We address in ▶ Chap. 6 how methylation (an example of an epigenetic effect) of bacterial DNA can substantially alter its virulence potential. Finally, more recent studies have focused on the **transcriptome** of bacterial infections. The transcriptome encompasses the conversion of genes to message (mRNA), the precursor to the conversion to proteins. It is assumed in many cases that synthesized message will eventually be translated into proteins; thus, a transcriptome is an indirect snapshot of the

3

V1 (acute Lyme disease diagnosis, pre-treatment)

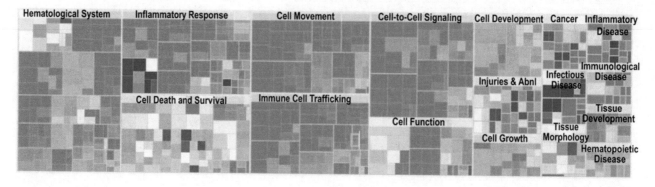

V5 (6 months after completion of treatement)

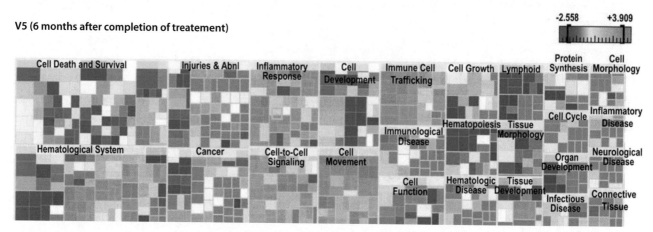

■ **Fig. 3.7** Transcriptomics of human samples before and after treatment of Lyme-disease. Lyme disease is caused by the spirochete bacterium *Borrelia burgdorfori* and is characterized by fever, extreme fatigue, and inflammation. In some patients, the infection and symptoms can last for months or years. The top panel shows the changes in RNA expression in patient's blood prior to treatment of Lyme-disease in genes grouped together by biological pathway or function. The bottom panel is the same analysis 6 months after treatment. Notice the changes in color, which represent changes in gene expression, between the two groups (color indicator range located on the top right of each panel). (Adapted from Chiu et al (see *suggested readings*) under a creative commons license. (► https:// creativecommons.org/licenses/by/4.0/))

"eventual" protein expression of that cell. Because RNA is nucleic acid, which generally is more amenable to large-scale high-throughput analysis, a transcriptome analysis is often used in place of proteomics to compare infected and uninfected samples. An example of a type of omics experiment is presented in ■ Fig. 3.7.

3.9 Next-Gen Organotypic Cultures and the Right Model for the Right Infection

The dichotomies of in vitro and in vivo systems seems to leave nothing in between. You either have cells or you have whole organisms. There is growing concern that rodent models, or any living animal model for that matter, does not accurately reflect human biology. The divide between these models and the successful use of a treatment in humans is full of the corpses of failed medicines that did not translate to the level that matters. Human experimentation is often a last resort option set aside for the direst of cases, or simply not performed at all due to safety, regulatory, societal, monetary, and other ethical concerns. Scientists have still sought to build this bridge. As such, organotypic culture systems are becoming more and more used as an experimental option to study the etiology of disease. An **organotypic system** is exactly what its name implies. It is comprised of a cellular system that resembles the complexity of an organ. Organotypic systems have a few features that separate them from cultured cells, including a (i) *higher level architecture* – cells grown on a plate are, for the most part, two dimensional. Organotypic cultures often are grown in three dimensions, multiple cell layers thick and in some cases layered into a tissue; (ii) *heterocellularity* – organotypic cultures are not, like most cell cultures, comprised of only one cell type. They may contain many cell types and these cell types work together to more fully constitute the tissue; (iii) *integration of systems* – they often also contain multiple

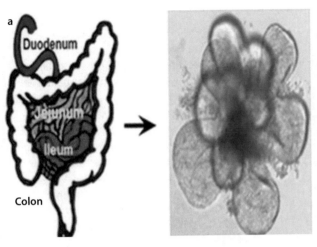
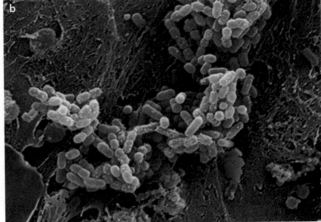

Fig. 3.8 Human intestinal enteroids and bacterial adherence. In addition to cultured host cells and animal models, organotypic culture systems such as human intestinal enteroids offer the promise of increasing the physiologic relevance and thus a greater understanding of human infectious diseases. **a** A sample of human intestine (isolated via either endoscopy or colonoscopy) is grown in culture in the presence of certain growth factors that promote the differentiation of crypt stem cells into an absorptive intestinal epithelium with 3-dimen-sional features and a defined lumen (3D enteroid). **b** 3D enteroids can be used directly for infection studies or made into 2D monolayers. Shown is a 2D enteroid monolayer from the colon of the author with a cluster of adhering enteroaggregative *E. coli* (a common cause of pediatric diarrhea). (Adapted from Maresso et al (see *suggested readings*) under a creative commons license. (▶ https://creativecommons.org/licenses/by/4.0/))

systems integrated, including vasculature, immunity, and extracellular matrix which allows one to assess how such systems influence infection dynamics. In the past 30 years, these systems have been extracted from the animal model (or even human) in question and kept "alive" for just enough time to do an experiment. A good example is a small section of biopsy from the intestine that is placed in culture media and kept functional for about 8 h. But as of late, advances in technology have revolutionized this practice. It is now possible to develop organotypic cultures from stem cells of a given tissue and culture them indefinitely. These are termed organoids, the "oid" often affixed to the tissue being studied. Organoids of the intestine ("miniguts"), the lung, bladder, and even brain have been developed. The great promise and hope is that these advanced systems will add more physiology and complexity to the experimenter's toolbox and, as such, yield novel insights into the underlying causes of disease. One example of the use of organotypic cultures is shown in ☐ Fig. 3.8.

Ultimately, there is no perfect model for all bacterial diseases. The decision of which model system to use depends on the question being asked. What may aid in one particular area of inquiry may not be suitable for another, and vice versa. For example, if one is interested in examining only the adherence to the host for a bacterium that causes diarrhea, the use of intestinal cells in culture might be the best approach. If, however, one wishes to understand how adherence may induce diarrhea itself, a complicated pathophysiology with multiple systems integrated, an animal host will be necessary. The number and scope of models used for such studies varies greatly, from zebrafish, to worms, to pigs and even primates. Zebrafish and worms tend to be very useful in performing screens whereby a large number of subjects are needed. Primates, on the other hand, are often used to model the immune response to the bacterium, but because of their cost only a limited number can be used. Here, the number of animals is traded for the resemblance of the primate system to us. The microbe hunter may also choose one model to answer one question and another model for a different question, both with the same pathogen.

Microbiologists are also becoming increasingly good at applying the tools of geneticists to arrive at mechanisms of disease, the desired goal. Using CRISPR-based technology[5], cultured cells, organotypic systems, most animal hosts can be rendered deficient (knock-out) or competent (knock-in) for many host genes. This allows the investigator to determine the contribution of that gene to the infection, using the very methods described above. These methods also allow the investigator to "humanize" the model system, thereby making it more human-like in the response to the pathogen. Making a mouse express a human immune system, a strategy becoming more accepted and technically feasible, will help Microbiologists make better vaccines, rely less on primates, and increase the scientific rigor while lowering costs. Organotypic cultures may use human tissues connected in parallel (say an intestinal system to a liver) to model disease and also test experimental drugs without having to use people in clinical trials. Just as the tools of Leeuwenhoek and Koch and Ruska revealed a world unseen and advanced medicine while doing it, these next-generation model systems, fused with advances in technology, automation, and computational power, will answer the questions not yet written for the microbe hunters that come to age with them.

3

Summary of Key Points

1. A foundational technique in the study of bacterial pathogens is the ability to cultivate them as clonal cultures to high density. The growth characteristics of bacteria under defined conditions allows one to understand their behavior when these conditions are varied.
2. The basic unit of bacterial disease is a virulence factor. The use of appropriate cell culture or animal model systems for example, often coupled to reverse genetic approaches applied to the pathogen, allows the investigator to quantitatively assess virulence.
3. Other models, techniques, and tools facilitate a molecular understanding of host-pathogen dynamics, including the use of real-time imaging and omics approaches.

❓ Expand Your Knowledge

1. You are fresh off a trip from the Amazonian delta with soil samples you have screened for new antibiotics for your pharmaceutical company. You now wish to know if one of the samples with a unique compound can inhibit the growth of bacteria in culture and in an animal model of infection. How can you test this?
2. As a new Assistant Professor, you have just generated a *Staphylococcus aureus* strain deficient in the ability to make a novel secreted lipase. You wish to know if this gene is important for Staphylococcal virulence in a murine abscess model. How can you determine if the strain is attenuated compared to wild-type *S. aureus*? How can you measure its growth in the host?
3. A mysterious disease arises in lumberjacks clearing forest in central Congo. Your investigative team determines it to be infectious in origin, likely bacterial. What type of tests can you perform to isolate the organism, determine its identity, and determine if it is virulent/causes disease?

Notes

1 = Later in this work, we will learn that these mistakes, or mutations, are one way to give rise to new pathogenic variants, or strains resistant to antibiotics or vaccines.

2 = Flagella are a truly fascinating structure of evolution. On microscopy, they look like a nanomachine. They are also important for some bacterial pathogens.

3 = Dissemination is the term used to describe the spread of bacteria from one localized area of the body to a secondary site and beyond. Often, if dissemination occurs, the host may be in dire trouble.

4 = Gone are the days of Jenner inoculating farm children in a barn with a pathogen in hopes of testing an experimental vaccine. The evaluation of a disease caused by a bacterium (or any pathogen for that matter) and a possible therapeutic solution to the disease are nowadays performed almost entirely in cells or animal model systems. Only after rigorous testing and proof of safety and efficacy of the experimental approach in these systems can controlled, and tightly regulated, clinical trials on humans commence. This is for good reason. Safety is paramount and having experiments do more harm than good has lasting negative effects in the public mindset.

5 = CRISPR stands for Clustered Regularly Interspaced Short Palindromic Repeats. The system was discovered in bacteria as a mechanism to recognize and destroy foreign DNA, particularly phage DNA, that enters into the bacterial cell. It is based on short segments of the foreign DNA being recognized by complimentary sequences processed by the bacterium during current or past phage infections. It has been called a type of bacterial innate immunity. Foreign DNA is recognized by a key protein, termed CAS9, which cleaves the foreign DNA after recognition. The system is highly amenable to control and specificity and has been used to "edit" the genomes of many higher forms of life, including plants and animals, and now humans.

Suggested Reading

Bouquet J et al (2016) Longitudinal transcriptome analysis reveals a sustained differential gene expression signature in patients treated for acute lyme disease. MBio 7:e00100–e00116. https://doi.org/10.1128/mBio.00100-16

DeLeo F, Otto M (eds) (2008) Bacterial pathogenesis: methods and protocols. Springer Science, Totowa

Kaplan E, Meier P (1958) Nonparametric estimation from incomplete observations. J Am Stat Assoc 53:457–481

Monod J (1949) The growth of bacterial cultures. Annu Rev Microbiol 3:371–394

Pletzer, D, Mansour, S et al (2017) New mouse model for chronic infections by gram-negative bacteria enabling the study of anti-infective efficacy and hostMicrobe interactions. mBio 8:e00140-17. https://doi.org/10.1128/mBio.00140-17

Rajan A et al (2018) Novel segment- and host-specific patterns of enteroaggregative. MBio 9. https://doi.org/10.1128/mBio.02419-17

Reed H, Muench L (1938) A simple method for estimating fifty percent endpoints. Am J Epidemiol 27:493–497

Stavrakis AI et al (2014) Combination prophylactic therapy with rifampin increases efficacy against an experimental Staphylococcus epidermidis subcutaneous implant-related infection. Antimicrob Agents Chemother 58:2377–2386. https://doi.org/10.1128/AAC.01943-14

Zwietering MH, Jongenburger I, Rombouts FM, van't Riet K (1990) Modeling of the bacterial growth curve. Appl Environ Microbiol 56:1875–1881

Innate Immunological Defenses Against Bacterial Attack

© Springer Nature Switzerland AG 2019
A. W. Maresso, *Bacterial Virulence*, https://doi.org/10.1007/978-3-030-20464-8_4

4

Learning Goals

In this chapter, the microbe hunter will learn about the first-line of host defense against invading pathogenic bacteria – the innate immune system. These host counter-measures include physical barriers present in important locations of the human body exposed to the outside world. They also include chemical defenses that slow or kill the bacterial invader as well as an assortment of different innate immune cells that directly engage bacteria in mortal combat. The structure and organization of the innate immune response to the invading microbe is discussed so as to inform the reader of the molecular processes that shape the outcome of these encounters.

4.1 Introduction

In medieval Europe, a castle was a place where its residents felt safe, most if not all their needs met from within its sturdy stone walls. A castle was also a fortress, meant to deter even the fiercest of attacks by plunderous outsiders. To siege a fortress, one must breach each layer of defense, and when speaking of a castle, they are numerous. Castles have an outer mote, a physical obstacle that slows the attacker's movements. They have archers shooting razor sharp arrows from great distances. The wall is tall so as to not be scalable and thick so that one can't simply break through it. There are turrets, localized areas of concentrated artillery which serve not only as a source of more defenders and weapons, but also as local areas of coordinated planning. Once inside the castle grounds, there are additional defenses. Here, hand-to-hand combat might occur, and the invaders will still need to get through the many locked doors and hallways leading to the castle center.

To bacteria, the human body is such a fortress, only much more complex. Take the skin for instance. The keratinized skin is hard and thick, like castle walls. There are small molecules on the skin that directly poke holes in the bacterial membrane, like an archer's arrow. Sebum (oils) slow bacteria like motes and in some cases the content of this material is toxic. Localized areas of immune cell congregation represent castle turrets in form and function, a source of reinforcements and distress calls. Even if the skin is breached, there are layers upon layers of additional measures that stop bacteria dead in their tracks. Yet still, as insurmountable as the odds may seem, bacteria sometimes breach these defenses. To appreciate this bacterial version of David overcoming Goliath, we must first learn the basics of our own immune system. We start with what is inherent to us, commonly referred to as the **Innate Immune System**. The innate immune system represents the physical barriers to invasion as well as the first line of guard, an elite special force armed with various generalized weapons systems, that responds to invaders quickly and with ferocity. The methods of this response are not specific, but they are no less effective.

The innate immune system is composed of physical, chemical, and cellular defenses that form a collective anti-bacterial response. They are constantly at work, every second of your day, protecting you from being consumed by billions of bacterial cells. What the microbe hunter must appreciate is that a human being is essentially a bag of nutrients. It has taken much energy to assemble these nutrients, store them, and put them in forms that can be utilized. Every meal you consume is a source of energy and essential molecules. You expended work and energy to locate your meal. The nutrients are then consumed which both immediately powers your cells as well as traps these nutrients inside of you for when you later need them. Bacteria cannot hunt like you can, cannot move great distances to find diverse chemical compounds or atoms. Instead, they must rely on local, more creative ways. To overtake a human and gain access to the biomass of precious compounds would be equivalent to winning a country-wide lottery. Not all do it; some bacteria, like the many that are a part of the native microbiome that lives in and on you, have formed an agreement with your immune system to live either as symbionts or at the very least not cause disease[1]. But the ones that can, they are the concern. One need to only observe how fast a body decomposes (whereby the body is essentially eaten by bacteria) in the summer heat to find evidence of this process. Here we find the reason why bacteria have evolved to be pathogens in the first place. From their perspective, it might just be a worthwhile gamble to attempt to breach the human fortress, even at the cost of its life. Since the bounty is so plentiful, if it wins, maybe yielding millions upon billions of progeny, evolution may have selected for this to be a strategy under the right context. On the flip side of the equation, we also see why your body invests so much energy in keeping these invaders out.

4.2 The First Line: A Barrier

To appreciate the challenge the bacterial invader faces in its quest to overcome us, we first consider the most obvious of defenses, the skin. The skin is effectively an amorphous wall that surrounds your body. Taking a bacterial-eye view as we peel back the numerous defenses designed to keep them out, we learn our skin is home to many different species of bacteria (termed the skin microbiome), and no two areas of the skin are exactly alike in ecology. The skin is colonized by both commensal and pathogenic bacteria, but the host does not care. None are welcome on the inside of the barrier. Some dangerous bacteria live on the skin, including one of the more concerning bacterial pathogens of humans: *Staphylococcus aureus*. *S. aureus*, sometimes referred to as MRSA (methicillin-resistant *S. aureus*) is responsible for a significant number of human mortalities each year and often harbors extensive resistance to antibiotics. Killers like "staph" colonize certain areas of the skin, and probably prefer to exist in such a state, but can also be invasive, *i.e.* enter the body where the bounty of nutrients lie. *S. aureus*, and its related cousins such as *S. epidermidis*, are a wonderful example of a bacterium knowing that a close association with a human host is dangerous but worth it. *S. aureus'* numerous mechanisms to survive on human skin, and its ability to quickly become invasive when conditions favor it, is a testament to the concept that there is an evolutionary advantage to overtaking the host, feeding on it, and producing many progeny to hopefully repeat the cycle.

The first barrier our bacterial invader encounters is the outermost layer of the skin, termed the **epidermis**. The epidermis consists of a thick layer of dead cells and an inner **stratified squamous epithelium**. It is stratified because there are multiple layers of cells built on each other like a stack of bricks. It is squamous because of the shape of these cells – flat, like scales on a fish. In addition to vertical depth, the cells themselves arranged in a stratified manner excludes intercellular crevices. This is good for two reasons. First, it prevents the formation of **microniches**, localized areas of bacterial congregation that are suitable for their habitation. Second, it prevents bacteria from squeezing between the cells all in one location, which could cause a deeper infection[2]. The cells of the skin also turnover a bit faster than the average cell of the body, and these dead cells get sloughed from the surface (the dead layer), taking would-be bacterial intruders with them. This is a constant theme at the epithelial surface; the cells of the gastrointestinal tract, for instance, also slough off quickly, taking adhered bacterium with them. On average, the epidermis is about 100 times the length of a typical bacterial cell, a formidable obstacle to penetrate. Thus, the wall is too thick to simply migrate through without some help. Wounds, cuts, and punctures that lie deeper than the epidermis are a way for bacteria to breach the wall, and this is the reason such injuries should always be handled with aseptic care. But a physical opening that bypasses the epidermis is not the only way bacteria can access deeper areas. Evolution has also produced other clever ways bacteria can breach the skin, including their delivery past the epidermis via the bite of an arthropod such as a tick or flea. By adapting to live in these vectors, bacteria can be transferred from one host to another, getting past some of the host barriers in the process. Lyme disease (caused by a spirochete bacterium living in a wood tick) and the bubonic plague (caused by a rod-shaped bacterium that is carried by a flea) are good examples of bacteria recruiting another organism, a kind of living weapon, to get past the Great Wall formed by your skin (◘ Fig. 4.1).

4.3 The Second Line: Molecular Artillery

As if a thick layer of tightly-sealed cells was not enough of a physical barrier, a plethora of harmful chemicals also awaits the bacterial invader. We can refer to this defense as a chemical barrier. Not quite burning oil thrown over the castle wall on helpless assailants, but the skin does contain an oily substance termed **sebum** whose fatty acids can disrupt the bacterial membrane, which prevents bacterial division; and, its oily nature can trap bacteria thereby neutralizing their movement. The cells of the epidermis also secrete **lysozyme**, the protein glycan hydrolase that cleaves between the NAG and NAM of the bacterial cells wall. We learned in ▶ Chap. 2 of the importance of these linkages. The invader must also contend with more poignant assaults, including one of the more prominent of all innate weapons, the **antimicrobial peptides** (or AMPs). Amps form a large collection of structurally unique polypeptides ranging from 10–50 amino acids that are often composed of positively charged and hydrophobic amino acids. The positively charged amino acids bind to the negatively charged molecules on the bacterial surface, including lipopolysaccharide, teichoic acid, and the phosphatidyl head groups located in the membrane (also discussed in ▶ Chap. 2). Once anchored via surface charge, the hydrophobic residues promote the insertion of the AMP deep into the fatty core of the bacterial membrane. This action likely disrupts critical membrane functions, including depolarizing the membrane, and also creates holes that may lead to lysis of the cells (◘ Fig. 4.2). The production of AMPs, as well as other chemical attacks, by cells of the skin occurs after skin cells have sensed molecules on the bacterial surface. Bacterial molecules that are recognized by the host and in turn help direct an immunological response against them are termed **Pathogen Associated Molecular Patterns** (PAMPs). We will return to PAMPs shortly; for now, suffice it to say that PAMPs are a clever way to tell self from intruder, and quickly. The host recognition of PAMPs sounds the alarm so that localized defenses and coordinated assaults contain the bacterial intruder.

The AMP host missile is certainly an effective measure to kill bacteria, but it is not infallible. Counter evolution to

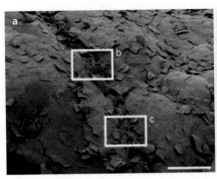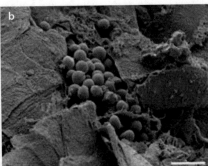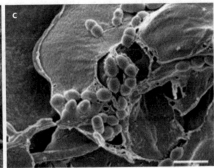

◘ **Fig. 4.1** The skin and its inhabitants. Electron microscopy of the epidermis (and its outermost layer termed the stratum corneum) showing embedded microcolonies of *Staphylococcus aureus*. Panel A demonstrates two regions of staphylococci in a ridge in the skin. Panel B = a higher magnification of box b and Panel C = a higher magnification of box c. (Adapted from Schmidtchen et al (see suggested readings) under a creative commons license. (▶ https://creativecommons.org/licenses/by/4.0/))

4

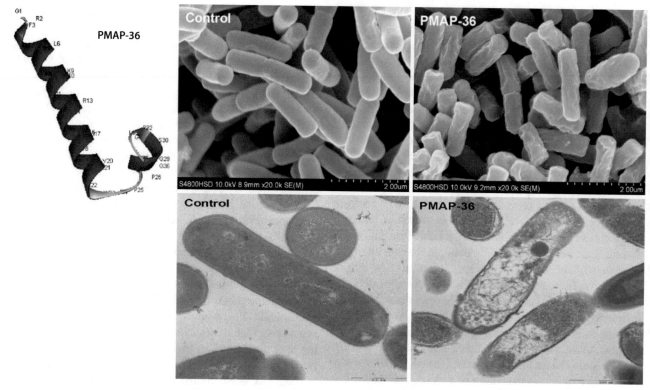

Fig. 4.2 The power of the antimicrobial peptide. Shown in the left panel is a structural rendition of the cathelicidin antimicrobial peptide termed porcine myeloid antimicrobial peptide-36, or PMAP-36. Cathelicidins are a large class of AMPs commonly found in macrophage and polymorphonuclear leukocytes that phagocytose and kill bacterial pathogens. The top and bottom panels demonstrate scanning and transmission electron micrographs images of *E. coli* either treated or left untreated (control) with PMAP-36. Notice the ruffling of the cells treated with PMAP-36 (top), suggestive of membrane damage, and membrane disintegration and loss of cell cytoplasmic contents (bottom) compared to controls. (Adapted from Shan et al (see suggested readings) under a creative commons license. (► https://creativecommons.org/licenses/by/4.0/))

AMPs has been occurring since they first appeared. As such, bacteria use a highly effective missile defense system. The most commonly employed counter defense is to change the bacterial surface, in this case, by modifying LPS, LTA, or the membrane itself, with charged molecules that will repel the AMPs. This effective measure is employed in one way or another by several important bacterial species that look to breach the skin or other mucosal surfaces. Other bacteria take more dramatic measures like something out of a science fiction movie. For inclusion here is the construction of a force field, made almost entirely of commonly available or easily synthesized sugars. The **capsular polysaccharide** as it is called, is one such structure, creating a nearly impenetrable shield that encapsulates the entire bacterial cell (see ► Chap. 2). The AMP missile may hit the capsule, but with no consequence. The bacterial membrane is thus saved. Still yet, other bacteria go on the offensive and even go so far as intercepting the incoming AMP in route. This is accomplished via the secretion of proteases which bind the AMP and cleave it. Destruction of the AMP is a castrating effect; the critical properties of the AMP that allow it to either associate with the bacterial surface, insert in the membrane, or both, are lost. Other proteases are localized on the cell membrane and perform this action at the bacterial surface. Some bacteria downregulate the production of AMPs by altering the host cells that make them.

As our bacterial intruder uses cell surface modifications to become impervious to AMPs, it is not out of the shark-infested water yet. It seems that the invader is not the only one recognizing that the host has plentiful nutrients, for there are at least a dozen or so additional species that routinely colonize and or cause an infection of the skin. For the most part, it's every bacterium for itself and as such, they wage war against each other to better position themselves to be the sole recipient of the bounty. For example, *S. aureus*, perhaps the most deadly of all skin bacteria, is a common cause of atopic dermatitis (AD), an infection that results in painful, red boils on the surface of the skin. Another staphylococcus species, *S. epidermidis*, is less invasive and pathogenic than *S. aureus*, but competes with *S. aureus* for housing on the skin. To do this, *S. epidermidis* secretes an antimicrobial peptide which inhibits the growth of *S. aureus*. **Bacteriocins** are the term given to secreted chemicals, usually proteins, peptides, or other compounds, that have antibacterial properties against other bacterial species. In the case of the competition described above, this compound is so effective that those colonized with high levels of *S. epidermidis* are not as frequently colonized with *S. aureus*; it has even been proposed as a treatment for staph skin infections. *S. epidermidis* also stimulates skin cells to make more AMPs which also negatively affect more pathogenic species such as *S. aureus*.

Our bacterial intruder, scaling giant walls of dead cells, fighting off waring bacterial fractions, and using surface modifications to shield from remote assault, may feel as though it has triumphed.

4.4 The Third Line: Orchestrated Turrets

The first layer of the skin is only the beginning.

Below the epidermis lies the **dermis**. This is where the real battle will be waged for in the dermis lies the pathway to the blood. The systemic circulation of the blood is a subway system to nutrient heaven. For that matter, it is a passageway to any other part of the body. If bacteria can ride these trains to other body locales, they might just gain access to a favorable niche and gain a stronghold, making it harder for the host to clear. The underlying dermis also houses the base of glands and hair follicles, as well as having local areas of immunological strength. These areas are called the **Skin Associated Lymphoid Tissue** or **SALT**. The SALT is a command center, a place where wartime activities are coordinated and critical intelligence and counter-intelligence are attained without being too physically distant from the main battle. One key resident cell of the SALT and other lymphoid centers localized at mucosal barriers throughout the body is a specialized cell termed the **dendritic cell** (in the skin, its specific name is a Langerhan's cell). The dendritic cell is an immune cell whose primary job is to learn about the tactics of the invader, taking in clues about its weaponry and defenses, and relaying this information to larger command centers that ultimately coordinate and stimulate a much greater wartime response (◻ Fig. 4.3). The clues in this case are **antigens**, a bacterial molecule that serves not only as proof an invasion is occurring but also as a source of information to exploit any vulnerabilities the invader may have. In this context, antigens are any molecule that can be turned into an immune response. The antigens are taken up by the dendritic cell in a process termed **phagocytosis** (literally means "cell eating"). During phagocytosis, the dendritic cell either engulfs the entire invading bacterium, or engulfs molecules the bacterium has secreted, and then breaks the bacterial cell or molecules into smaller pieces which can be presented to other specialized cells of the immune system.

These specialized cells that present the antigen comprise part of the **adaptive immune system**, the focus of the next chapter, and their charge is to mount an all-out attack on invader vulnerabilities using the knowledge acquired during the sampling process. As such, the dendritic cell is like a mobile scout, sent out from the SALT command center (in the case of skin), to sample portions of the dermis that might be under attack. Long extensions of the cell, which resemble the dendrites on neurons, finger their way between dermal and epidermal cells looking for any sign of PAMPs. Should the dendritic cell find and phagocytose an invader, the processed pieces are brought back to the SALT for testing. There, the decision will be made to further inform other immune cells that a breach has occurred and reinforcements are needed, as well as stimulate cells of the adaptive system that will form a greater more specific attack. This theme – sound the alarm, take up antigens, process them for the development of more specific anti-bacterial weapons – will repeat itself in many other tissues of the body that come into contact with bacteria, including the airways of the lung, the lining of the nasopharynx, the gastrointestinal tract, and the lining of the urogenital tract. This is an important paradigm of innate mucosal immunity.

4.5 The Fourth Line: Alarms

Despite the bacterium's best attempts to move undetected in and about the layers of the skin, most of the host cells that come into contact with the invader will have sounded the alarm to its presence. The host alarm system comes in many forms but the one that is the loudest of all are the secretion of molecules termed **chemokines**. Chemokines are small ~ 10 kDa proteins that form a Greek key structure that is internally stabilized by disulfide bonds. At least a dozen human chemokines have been described. They are functionally classified as a **chemoattractant**; that is, they are a chemical that attracts other cells, like phagocytes, to the area, a process known as **homing**. After epithelial cells recognize PAMPs on the invading bacterium, host cellular pathways are activated. This results in the production and secretion of chemokines into the area where the bacterium has been detected. A concentration gradient of the chemokine radiating outward from the point of secretion is established, and this serves as a type of chemical beacon or distress call. It is what happens next that is one of the most splendid higher-order cellular responses that characterize complex eukaryotic systems. Specialized phagocytic cells recognize the chemokine via a receptor on their surface and follow the path of increasing concentration to locate the invader. Well past the walls, missiles, and competition with other microbes, the attraction of phagocytic cells to the bacterial invader initiates another phase of the battle. This phase consists of direct hand-to-hand combat between the invader and the host's specialized elite killers. The task: kill the invader at the point of contact, fast and efficiently. The result of this confrontation is what we call **inflammation**, an all-out battle where the virulence factors of the bacterium engage the weaponry of the phagocyte, leaving behind a graveyard of dead cells on both sides. The outcome of this direct interaction will often determine the fate of the infection, and, just maybe, the fate of the host.

4.6 The Fifth Line: Elite Soldiers

The elite guard of a human host that respond to chemokines is made up of several different immune cells with distinct functions. Collectively, these cells are grouped under the name of leukocyte, otherwise known as "white blood cell." White blood cells are a common component of blood. They can be viewed as the first responders to trouble. There are five main types of leukocytes, and each of them has an important role in

4

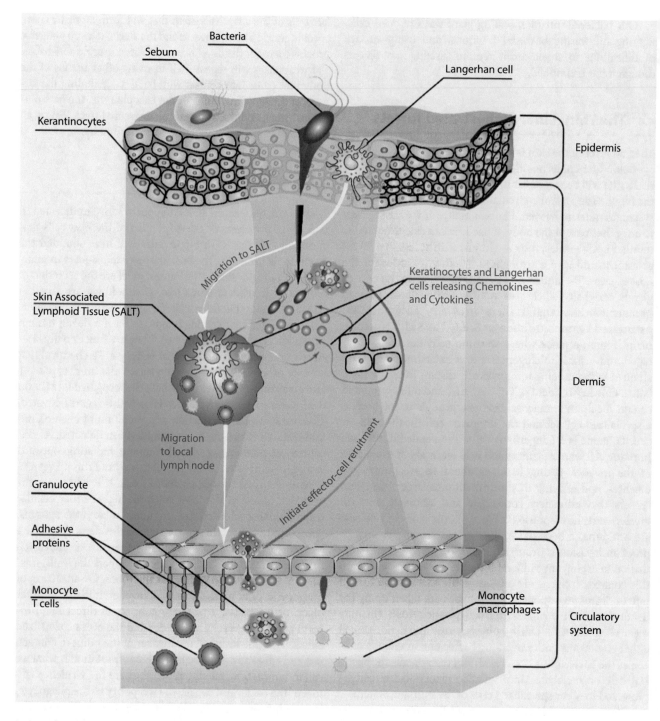

□ **Fig. 4.3**   Bacterial invasion and the innate immune response (example of skin). The host epithelial cells of the skin are termed kerantinocytes. A cut in this layer allows bacteria to enter the breach. The surrounding epithelial cells release chemokines which attract many immune cells to the area, including dendritic cells. Dendritic cells will migrate to local lymphoid centers like a SALT and present phagocy- tosed bacterial antigen to cells of the adaptive immune system. During this process, more chemokines are released, which may attract leukocytes from the blood. These leukocytes, such as neutrophils and monocytes will directly engage the bacterial invader in hand-to-hand combat

responding to pathogens. The most abundant of them are **neutrophils**. Neutrophils can be considered the standing army of the host. They are produced frequently, there are many of them, and they are often the first cell to answer the call to arms. Neutrophils are phagocytic cells; their main mechanism of killing bacteria is through **phagocytosis**.

Phagocytosis, or the process of cell eating, is of central impor- tance in protection of the body from bacterial invaders. Many immune cells are phagocytic, with neutrophils being quite proficient. Upon recognition of the bacterium, likely through a PAMP, the neutrophil extends a cellular arm, an extension of their cytoplasm really, known as a filopod or **filopodia**. This

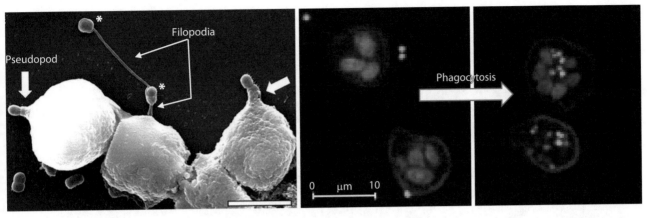

Fig. 4.4 The phagocytosis of bacteria. In the left panel, a neutrophil is shown extending a filopod to capture the bacterial pathogen *Acinetobacter baumannii* (a dangerous cause of drug-resistant pneumonia and bloodstream infections). *A. baumannii* is also engulfed by a leading-edge pseudopod. In the right panel, neutrophils are shown binding to and phagocytosing *S. aureus*. Green = green fluorescent protein expressing *S. aureus*. Red = wheat germ agglutinin staining the neutrophil membrane, and blue = Syto82 binding to DNA. (Adapted from Ramos-Vivas (left) and Strijp (right) et al (see suggested readings) under a creative commons license. (▶ https://creativecommons.org/licenses/by/4.0/))

tentacle latches onto the invader and begins to wrap the cellular body of the neutrophil around the entire bacterium until it is completely engulfed. Neutrophils closer to the bacterium extend a part of their plasma membrane termed a pseudopod which also engulfs the pathogen (◻ Fig. 4.4). The compartment trapping the bacterium in the neutrophil is the **phagosome**. Once inside the neutrophil cytoplasm, the phagosome fuses with another cellular compartment, the **lysosome**. This brings the death blow to the bacterium (◻ Fig. 4.5). The lysosome contains the enzyme NADPH oxidase which adds electrons from NADPH to O_2 to generate H_2O_2 (peroxide). The peroxide itself is deadly to the bacterial cell but can also be converted by another enzyme (myeloperoxidase) to hypochlorite, otherwise known as bleach. Hypochlorite is an extremely reactive free radical having an unpaired and thus unhappy oxygen electron. The bacterium is bombarded by these reactive free radicals. The bacterial membrane likely takes the brunt of the damage via a process termed lipid peroxidation. Proteins and DNA also react with the free radicals. These reactions destroy these structures and the bacterium dies. The infantry of your immune system, neutrophils and other types of phagocytic cells such as macrophages, essentially dissolve bacteria in a cellular bag of bleach. Although one might think of our use of bleach as a disinfectant in our everyday lives as a human invention, nature did it first.

The second leukocyte one must consider as a first responder to a bacterial attack is the **monocyte**. Monocytes have two primary roles in combating bacterial infections. First, like neutrophils, they are also phagocytic and will kill bacteria using the mechanism described above. But unlike neutrophils, monocytes seems to be much more promiscuous in what they will phagocytose, which leads to their second important function. In addition to whole bacteria, monocytes will also engulf bacterial parts spewed on the battleground at the site of inflammation. This activity is akin to learning a bit about the enemy's tactics, behavior, and technology. Monocytes collect this information, store it, and display these bacterial parts as antigens to the adaptive immune system (next chapter). The intelligence learned from examining the structure and weapons (virulence factors) of bacteria is used by the adaptive immune system to develop counter weapons that precisely neutralize these bacterial virulence factors. Monocytes that perform this activity also can become permanent guardians of the land by differentiating into **resident macrophages**. These soldiers are charged with securing the area on a long-term basis so that should another invasion or attack occur, the response can be quicker. Alveolar macrophages of the lung or intestinal macrophages of the GI tract are examples of this.

4.7 Support Staff

Every army also has its support staff. These individuals are technically a part of the army but are not considered infantry and thus do not directly engage the enemy in combat. For example, damage to the battlefield by mortar or other bombings might result in the loss of key infrastructure, perhaps a bridge, and this damage may prevent the occupying army from advancing forward. Engineers and workers may, under the guard of the infantry, repair the bridge so it becomes an asset in the overall war effort, thereby allowing more soldiers to move to the front line. This leads us to the **basophil**, a third leukocyte type. Unlike the neutrophil and the monocyte, the basophil does not phagocytose the bacterial intruder. Instead, it assess the need for geographic or structural changes in the host to occur to facilitate the access of phagocytic and other immune cells to the front line. To do this, basophils secrete the chemicals histamine and heparin. **Histamine** increases the flow of blood to sites of infection. Molecularly, histamine acts to make the endothelial cells that line the walls of blood vessels more permissive to **extravasation**, *i.e.* the passing of immune cells through the vessel wall so they may access the fight. **Heparin**, on the other hand, prevents the clotting of blood so as to not slow the recruitment of said immune cells.

4

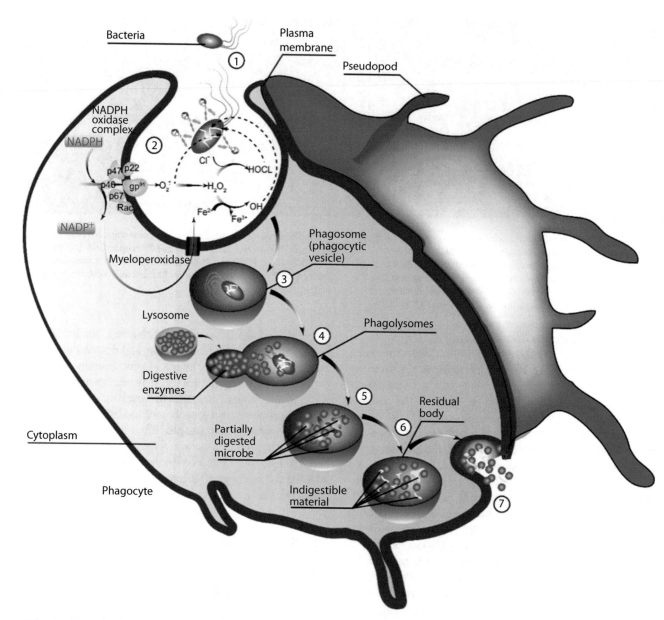

■ **Fig. 4.5** Bacterial phagocytosis and digestion by phagocytic cells. Phagocytic cells such as macrophages or neutrophils recognize bacteria via PAMPs or antibody complexed to the bacterial surface. The bacterium is ingested into a phagosome which matures to a phagolysosome after fusion with a lysosome. During this process, the NADPH oxidase system will have been bombarding the ingested bacterium with highly damaging free radicals, which may occur concomitantly with digestion with host enzymes such as lysozyme (which targets the cell wall). The sequences are ordered for clarity but in reality many of these steps may be occurring at the same time

Both processes act in support of the overall war effort by triggering changes in the host microenvironment so reinforcements have better access to the battle.

A fourth leukocyte is the **eosinophil**. The interaction of bacteria with eosinophils is an area of study that lacks much knowledge, but in general, eosinophils are thought to primarily function to amplify an immune distress call. In addition to the chemokines secreted by localized cells at the site of infection, the eosinophil can amplify these signals by secreting even more chemokines. In addition, eosinophils harbor granules packed of enzymes harmful to bacteria and may release them like giant napalm bombs designed to destroy everything in their path. These enzymes include proteins that attack the bacterial cell wall, as well as enzymes that generate membrane-damaging radicals. The proteins bind to extracellular nets synthesized by neutrophils that capture bacteria like a fly in a web, thereby immobilizing the bacterium for optimal damage. The eosinophil is also associated with the allergy response, an immune action consistent with the sensing of viruses. But in the context of a bacterial infection, the allergy response can be considered a general amplifier of inflammation with the select purpose of decimating breached areas. It should be noted that another cell, termed the **mast cell**, also performs a similar function. In the case of the mast cell, it can be decorated with a specific antibody once the antigen is encountered upon reinfection. As we will

◘ Fig. 4.6 The specialized soldiers of the innate immune system. Each of the leukocytes that respond to bacterial invaders bring a distinct functional element to the battle. See text for details

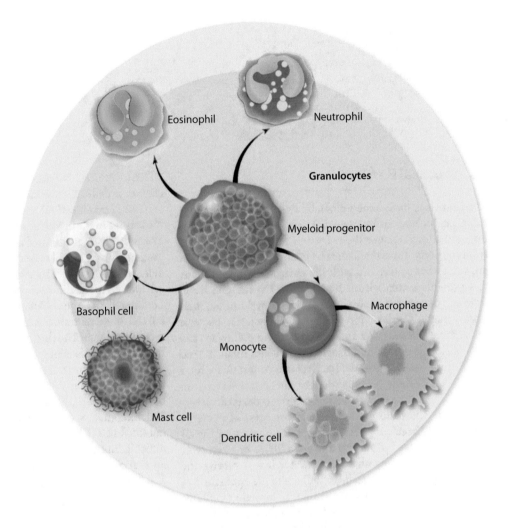

see with the adaptive immune system, antibodies represent a multi-faceted weapon that not only recognize specific pathogens, they also can neutralize their virulence factors. Decoration of the mast cell surface allows for the recognition of a bacterial pathogen to be quickly conveyed to the interior of the cell where pathways can be activated that sound the alarm. ◘ Figure 4.6 illustrates the various leukocytes of the innate immune response.

The final leukocytes to consider include the **lymphocytes**. It can be argued that there is no more extraordinary a cell than the various lymphocytes that constitute the adaptive immune response. So ingenious a creation they are, and the adaptive response they make, the entire next chapter is dedicated to them. Suffice it to say that should the wall, the burning oil, missiles, the competition, the alarms and the hand-to-hand combat fail, it is the adaptive immune system, led by these cells, that will command the next level of attack. The host's ability to analyze its bacterial opponent's weaknesses, and develop a strategy to expose and attack those weaknesses, constitutes the second major component of all of immunity.

Out of the Box
Troublesome Tubes
Tube – *noun*,
    .. a hollow, usually cylindrical body of metal, glass, rubber, or other material, used especially for conveying or containing liquids or gases,
    It is accurate to say that almost every bacterial infection of humans begins via their passage through a tube. Bacterial pneumonias: these are infections that begin after bacteria are inhaled through a tube, the trachea. GI Infections: well, they begin after you ingest bacteria that travel down the tube to your stomach and intestines (alimentary canal). Urinary tract: same thing, these bacteria moved through your urethra, which, you guessed it, is a tube. Ear

canal, nose, etc – all tubes in one way or another. Even in-dwelling devices, often a source of biofilm growth and deadly infections, are for the most part tubes. A puncture wound is also a tube so to speak, albeit it is not designed that way, unless of course a physician places a tube in it to drain excess, infected fluids.
    We need tubes. There is no getting around them. Oxygen exchange and nutrient and energy adsorption are favored with a tube model of anatomy. A tube is required to access the outside world, and bring key molecules inside. Of course, tubes are wormholes for pathogen access as well. We have probably been evolving with bacteria that have become so uniquely adapted to our tubes they may not exist anywhere else. Some intestinal microbes come to mind in this context. What do we have to

4

consider moving forward? The first is we need to know much more about tube biology. All major infections begin via tubes but we have only scratched the surface in our understanding of topics like colonization and immune tolerance or clearance at these surfaces. We also need technology to make better tubes. A cyborg is a human with mechanical or robotic parts. We are not close to full cyborgs walking amongst us, but we are trending that way.

Pacemakers, prosthetics, catheters, etc allow us to live longer, better. As we age, we can envision many parts hanging from us, all at once. If they are tubes, bacteria will find a way to get in them. We should probably think about materials that disincentive colonization of the tubes of the future, or ones that can be made sterile in real-time. But before all this, we need a better molecular understanding of our *natural* tubes.

4.8 Mucosal Barriers

The host does have some vulnerabilities, however. The host must eat, breathe, and excrete. Each of these critical physiologic functions requires the entry and elimination of matter from the body. Thus, there must be openings in the body that are somewhat continuous with the environment. Of course, this presents a conundrum for the host. On the one hand, food and oxygen are an absolute necessity. On the other, their intake may also allow for the entry of bacteria. Bacteria understand this very fact and exploit it. Lung pathogens can hitch a ride on aerosolized droplets that, when inhaled, seed the bacteria inside the body. Bacteria can contaminate food and water. The simple ingestion of these provisions can deliver a large dose of pathogenic bacteria to the gastrointestinal tract. These are not accidental properties of bacteria. Some enteric bacterial pathogens (bacteria that infect the GI tract) have evolved to survive and even thrive in a reservoir that will likely be ingested (say a water hole), survive the harsh low pH of the stomach, and adhere to the epithelium of the intestine. A cough or sneeze response may eject millions of water droplets containing bacteria that flow about a room (sometimes taking hours to settle) until they are inhaled by another host. All is not lost. The host understands that bacteria use these tactics to gain easy access to inside the body and has thus evolved counter measures to protect itself.

What are these measures? The most significant is the **mucosal barrier**. Unlike the somewhat rigid barrier we observed in our discussion of the skin, the mucosal barrier is full of life and activity. Because the intestine and lungs are absorptive organs, the host can't afford to have them so impassable that important nutrients are kept out. As such, the barrier must be selective – one where absorption can occur but not so indiscriminately that bacteria do as well. Instead of a rough keratinized epidermis many cells in thickness, mucosal barriers are typically comprised of a single columnar epithelial cell. The one-cell thick approach allows for nutrients to pass through that cell so as to easily enter into the blood. Instead of a dry and rigid environment, the mucosal barrier is wet, inhabited often by many microorganisms, and in constant motion. Instead of only the deeper layers allowing for the recruitment of immune cells, in a mucosal surface the immune cells can advance as far forward as the columnar epithelium itself, even sampling the **apical** (side facing the lumen) of the mucosal surface. The cells of the mucosal barrier also are quite dynamic and can self-fortify in a way that does not disrupt absorption but does provide an effective barrier to pathogen entry. The remainder of this chapter is dedicated to understanding this dynamic surface.

The gastrointestinal tract is a representative example of the actions of the innate immune system at a mucosal surface. The most distal portion of this barrier is **mucus**. Gooey and gross as it may be, like dead skin, mucus is the first line of defense against bacteria. Mucus is produced by a specialized cell located in the mucosal epithelium named the **Goblet cell**. Looking like a large goblet amongst the much smaller epithelial cell, these cells are fewer in number but pack a big mucus-secreting punch. The thickness of the mucus layer varies with the mucosal surface in question. In the small intestine, where there is less bacteria, it spans a width of about 200 micrometers. In the large intestine, where the density of bacteria can be as high as 10^{12} per gram of feces, the thickness spans up to 700 micrometers. Just like the keratinized epidermis, the spatial thickness of this barrier makes invasion that much more difficult. The mucus also differs in density. The outer layer, the layer in contact with the most bacteria, is loosely constructed. The inner layer is tighter, allowing far less movement or penetration, and has very few bacteria as a result. Perhaps the most associated and well known feature of mucus, however, is its sticky nature. This property serves mainly to slow the movement of the bacterial invader. Some bacteria are highly motile, and this motility is a prominent feature of their pathogenesis. Bacterial movement is largely the result of the actions of the flagellum, the motorized tail we addressed in ► Chap. 2 whose high speed rotations are like the propeller on a boat. The texture of mucus inhibits the propeller. The sticky property of mucus also serves as a net to anchor host molecules secreted by the underlying cells, including AMPs and antibodies. These anti-bacterial agents embed in the mucus, thereby bringing them in direct contact with the already-slowed bacteria. ◘ Figure 4.7 illustrates the architecture of a typical mucosal surface.

4.9 Mucosal Architecture

Mechanophysical properties also work to dispel the bacterial invader. In the nasal passages and trachea, pathogens killed by chemical missiles embedded in mucus, as well as live bacteria trapped by the stickiness, are swept away by the beating of tiny, hair-like projections termed **cilia**. The pathogens are propelled down to the lower GI tract where rhythmic muscle contractions, **peristalsis,** usher food, waste, mucus, and trapped bacteria towards the rectum for excretion. In the

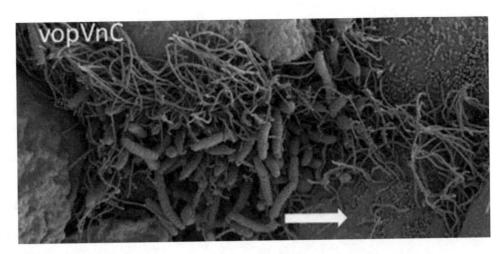

Fig. 4.7 The mucosal surface. Electron microscopy showing *Vibrio parahaemolyticus* (a cause of gastrointestinal illness) cuddled in an invagination of the intestinal mucosa. The arrow shows a microvillus that has become effaced. (Adapted from Waldor et al (see *suggested readings*) under a creative commons license. (▶ https://creativecommons.org/licenses/by-nc-sa/3.0))

respiratory tract, the cough reflex expels mucus that has accumulated in the lungs. The movement of mucus is like tiny conveyer belts propelling a tidal wave of sticky goo away from privileged areas. The **three-dimensional architecture** of the mucosal surface provides pathogen-limiting terrain. For example, to maximize the absorptive function of the intestine, mainly by increasing the surface area of contact points, an undulating morphology has evolved. Here, the most distal cells reside in a villus tip while the most proximal cells lie at the bottom of a crypt. This pattern repeats, peak and trough, along the length of the tissue. At the bottom of the crypt lie **stem cells**, so-named because they give rise to all other cells types in the intestinal epithelium. As stem cells differentiate into the absorptive epithelium that lines the intestinal tract, these cells slowly migrate up the villus shaft until they reach the tip. There they **exfoliate**, or slough off, taking any attached mucus, and bacteria, with them. All of it is expelled down the tract by peristalsis. Because of the rapid turnover of intestinal cells, the shedding is continuous, non-stop kamikazes taking entire bacterial communities with them as they bud from the central tissue. Very few bacteria gain access to the crypts. If they do, the stem cells are guarded by another cell type termed the **Paneth cell** (described below). The continuous process of exfoliation combined with the undulating architecture that makes access to the crypts difficult is just another example of the many lines of defense mucosal surfaces have evolved to contend with microbial communities.

4.10 Sticky Traps

An understanding of mucus biology is important for the microbe hunter. Mucus is at the forefront of the interaction with pathogenic and commensal bacteria, and this interaction has profound implications for human health and disease. This giant tar field is composed of a secreted class of sugar-conjugated proteins termed **mucins**. The protein domain of a mucin is first made in the endoplasmic reticulum of the Goblet cell. In the Golgi apparatus, its sugar moiety is then attached to an oxygen atom from one of the amino acids in the protein (this is called O-linked glycosylation),

and then packaged into granules that are secreted to the apical side of the epithelium. The process is **constitutive**, that is, it is always occurring. However, it is well known that the contact of bacteria with the epithelium also stimulates the production and secretion of mucins, no doubt a way for the host to double-down on the strengthening of the barrier.

The stickiness, thickness, and entrapment of the mucus minefield is the most prominent way this defense repels would be invaders. The host also dwells in the art of illusion and deception. There are over 20 different types of mucin proteins that are encoded in the human genome, and many mucosal barriers express more than one of these different types of mucins. This means that bacteria encounter all types of mucin structures with various properties, some of which are not redundant. To make matters worse from the bacterial perspective, it is the glycosylation of the mucins that introduces the real confusion. Hundreds of different O-linked sugar structures can be added to the protein mainframe of mucins, each with a subtle but important difference in structure. Bacterial adhesins, the surface proteins that mediate most of the adherence of bacteria to the host, have an affinity for sugars. The decoration of mucins with many different sugars ensures that bacteria, regardless of the strain or species in question, will be bound and trapped by the mucus layer. Some mucins also have their proteinaceous component adopt a structure similar to AMPs. Mucin number 7, for example, has a domain that resembles a prominent antimicrobial peptide found in human saliva. Mucin number 6, which is associated with the gastric epithelium in the stomach, is linked to N-acetylglucosamine (NAG), the very same sugar that comprises the cell wall of bacteria. It is thought this mucin inhibits the synthesis of the cell wall of the prominent stomach pathogen *Heliobacter pylori*, thereby limiting its growth.

4.11 Team Defense

The Goblet cell is one player dedicated to microbial defenses, but not the only one. Mucosal barriers are fortified with local arms factories to ensure the mucus is well stocked with deadly molecules. In the intestine, at the base of the crypt,

4

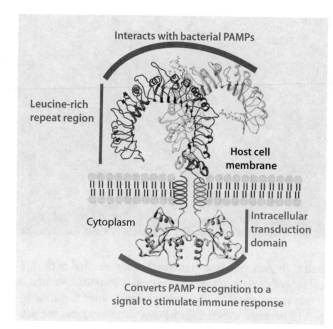

Interacts with bacterial PAMPs

Leucine-rich
repeat region

Host cell
membrane

Cytoplasm

Intracellular
transduction
domain

Converts PAMP recognition to a
signal to stimulate immune response

Fig. 4.8 A pattern recognition receptor (PRR). Shown is a representative structure of a toll-like receptor (TLR) and its extracellular leucine-rich repeat (LRR) and intracellular signal transduction domain. The TLR recognizes bacterial pathogen associated molecular patterns (PAMPs), which induces a conformational change that is transmitted to the transduction domain and eventually converted into a downstream signal that alters gene expression. (Adapted from Yang et al (see *suggested readings*) under a creative commons license with TLR components labeled for clarity. (▶ https://creativecommons.org/licenses/by/4.0/))

lies a specialized cell termed the **Paneth cell**. Upon stimulation with bacterial surface components such as LPS or cell wall, this cell produces granules full of antimicrobial molecules, including the AMP alpha-defensin (inserts into the bacterial membrane), lysozyme (cleaves the bacterial cell wall), and phospholipase (cleaves the bacterial membrane). Although these molecules are found in the mucus layer, the close proximity of Paneth cells to the intestinal stem cells (remember they replenish the cell barrier and in doing so slough off bound bacteria) suggests they may act as personal garrisons for this critical cell niche. The epithelial cells themselves also secrete AMPs, but their main contribution to defense is likely structural and as alarmists. The gaps between cells, termed **gap junctions**, are impenetrable to the passage of bacteria. The apical surface of the mucosal epithelium also contains many different **toll-like receptors** (TLRs), each responsive to a different microbial PAMP (▣ Fig. 4.8). TLRs will bind PAMPs such as LPS, and this triggers the downstream action of activating host gene expression. For bacteria that try to invade these cells, **nod-like receptors (NLRs)** detect the entry of bacteria in the host cytoplasm. Like TLRs, they then activate gene expression, often times innate immune factors that lead to inflammation. Both receptor classes, when bound to their bacterial ligand, activate downstream signaling pathways that culminate in the release of chemokines and cytokines, the signals of infection. And, just as we observed for the skin, the release of these pro-inflammatory molecules promotes the recruitment of

additional immune cells, including phagocytic cells, to the mucosal surface. They also stimulate the strengthening of local defenses; for example, Goblet cell production of more mucin and Paneth cell production of more AMPs. **B-cells**, the antibody-producing cell of the body, will secrete a specialized type of antibody, termed **immunoglobulin A**, into the luminal side of the surface. IgA, also known as secretory IgA, will bind to the mucus layer through its long tail while capturing bacterial surface antigens via its high-affinity head. This further acts to trap bacteria and in some cases neutralizes key virulence factors. We concentrate more on the production of antibody in the next chapter about the adaptive immune system.

The mucosal surface also has an important function in suppressing mutiny. Because of the preponderance of bacteria of all different forms and function that these surfaces encounter, there is the chance that an overblown immune response may damage the epithelium. Such damage may only exacerbate the problem by destroying barriers that keep pathogens out, thereby further stimulating the immune system which may snowball into an avalanche of harmful inflammation. In the colon of the intestine, as high as 10^{12} CFUs of bacteria are present at the mucosal surface. With such a robust number of PAMPs present, of all varieties and kinds, it would seem that the intestine should exist under a state of constant inflammation. Generally, the converse is true. The reason homeostasis is maintained in the face of such seemingly heightened tension is because the immune response is compartmentalized. Specific command centers are localized to mucosal surfaces whose function is to maintain the right amount of attack for the job, a sort of immunological surveillance system. These command centers, known as **lymphoid follicles**, are localized throughout the mucosal surface into distinct structures. Perhaps the most understood lymphoid follicle associated with a mucosal surface is that of the **Peyer's patch** (PP) in the small intestine. The PP serves as a good example of how the many components of the host's military coordinate their action to maintain the mucosal barrier. The immune cells in these regions also become educated on how to direct a response proportional to the level of invasion. We also learn about this concept, termed tolerance, in the next chapter[3]. ▣ Figure 4.9 represents an integrated schematic of the interaction of the host intestinal mucosa and bacterial pathogens.

4.12 Detection

When commensal or pathogenic bacteria are able to pass through the physical and chemical defenses at the most distal part of the mucosal surface, they then access the cells of that surface that formed those barriers. In our example of the intestinal tract, the process begins with the recognition of a bacterial PAMP by the intestinal epithelium via either toll-like receptors (on the host cell surface) or nod-like receptors (inside the host epithelial cell). In this context, the epithelium acts as a group of scouts charged with sounding the alarm

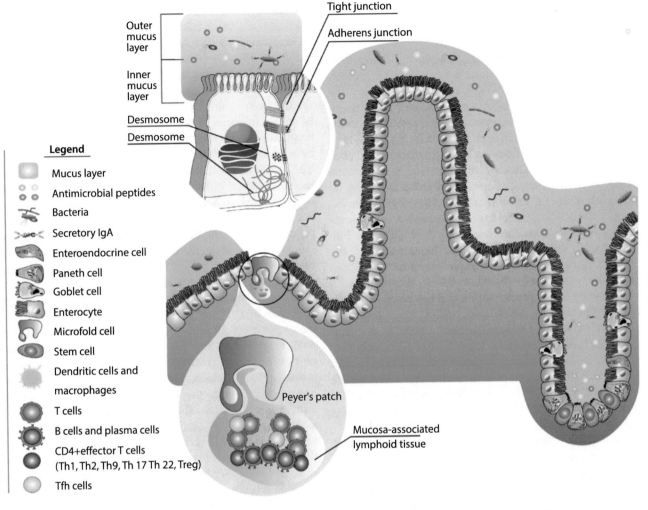

Legend

- Mucus layer
- Antimicrobial peptides
- Bacteria
- Secretory IgA
- Enteroendocrine cell
- Paneth cell
- Goblet cell
- Enterocyte
- Microfold cell
- Stem cell
- Dendritic cells and macrophages
- T cells
- B cells and plasma cells
- CD4+effector T cells (Th1, Th2, Th9, Th 17 Th 22, Treg)
- Tfh cells

Outer mucus layer
Inner mucus layer
Tight junction
Adherens junction
Desmosome
Desmosome
Peyer's patch
Mucosa-associated lymphoid tissue

☐ **Fig. 4.9** The mucosal surface (intestine as example). A coordinated combination of secreted molecules, structural architecture, and immune cell function keep pathogenic bacteria at mucosal surfaces at bay. Mucus, made by Goblet cells, serves as a thick, sticky substance that traps bacteria. Antimicrobial peptides, made by Paneth cells, kill bacteria. Various innate and adaptive immune cells phagocytose or make antibodies against bacteria. Bacterial antigens are brought to lymphoid follicles in Peyer's patches, which further stimulates the adaptive immune response of B and T cells

that danger is approaching. Too ramped an alarm leads to unnecessary inflammation, especially since these cells may be in very frequent contact with **commensal** bacteria, *i.e.* the bacteria that normally live on the host that are not usually considered pathogenic. Only the most egregious of bacterial offenders need an alarm signal, and this is why the TLRs are localized to the **basolateral** surface, that is, the surface that faces away from the lumen and interfaces the underlying **lamina propria**, where lymphoid follicles are present and interfaces the vasculature. This way, the production and secretion of chemokines by these scouts occurs right next to the command center. Not only does this mechanism directly stimulate the specialized immune cells in the command center, it also does so only for those bacteria that have accessed the basolateral surface. Such a property keeps the cells lining the mucosal surface from sending out false alarms at the apical surface for every commensal organism that happens to make its way there, either by accident or directly.

The underlying lymphoid command centers include dendritic cells who, upon being stimulated by the chemokines secreted by the epithelium, embark on a migratory path from the lymphoid follicle to the invading bacterium. In addition, mucosal surfaces also have specialized cells embedded in the intestinal epithelium that perform a similar function as the dendritic cell. In our example of the small intestine, these cells are termed **microfold cells**. Reaching with their cellular arms to the surface, like dendritic cells, they extract antigens from the invaders. The primary purpose of this activity is to generate an appropriate response for the threat at hand. As we will see in the next chapter, it is the presentation of these antigens to cells of the adaptive immune system that allows for the effort to be scaled up on a more systemic level. If there is an immediate threat that requires quick action, specialized resident macrophages localized in the mucosal surface will move in for the phagocytic kill.

4

4.13   The Final Line: Breach, Blood, and Beyond

But what happens when chemical and physical defenses are breached and the first responders are defeated? In this case, the surrounding host cells will continue to amplify the response via the secretion of more cytokines and chemokines. This serves to recruit even more first responders to the battlefield. It also functions to bring in the lymphocytes, neutrophils and company, from the blood. Circulating lymphocytes will detect some of the chemokines that leach into the blood. They will upregulate specific adhesion molecules on their surface and roll across the endothelial cells that line the vessel wall until they detect the wall is passable. In a process termed **extravasation**, they leave the vessel and move into the tissue in the direction of the higher concentration of chemokine. Lymphocytes like neutrophils are first rate killers; when they enter the battlefield, as before, they strike with their ferocity of super radicals, nets, and proteases. Mast cells amplify the response, and more circulating lymphocytes are recruited to the area. Despite all of this, bacteria press on and can resist these mechanisms. Some, after phagocytosis, prevent the formation of the phagolysosome and thus are not degraded. Others secrete soluble toxins that intercept the neutrophil in route, lysing its membrane and leaving it a slow death via loss of water. Others still destroy the chemical signals. We will address all of these throughout this work.

It is at this point that the body may be in trouble. Once the bacteria enter the blood, they have a one-way ticket to just about anywhere. Equivalent to actually entering the castle main hall and being able to run freely to any room whatsoever, bacteria now have access to the very organs and systems that give life to you; the liver, heart, kidneys, even brain. We now enter the final phase of the battle, the fight for the transit system – the roads, waterways, and railways that lead all over the country, or the halls, corridors, and rooms that are the main stay of the castle interior. The blood is an amazing organ. It gives life to you, delivering critical nutrients to all the cells of the body. Despite having a rich bounty of said nutrients, most of them are generally inaccessible to bacteria. As such, we can consider nutrient limitation as another arm of the innate immune system. We take here the example of the metals. All bacterial pathogens, all life for that matter, need metals to fuel basic cellular chemistry. Metals are catalysts for enzymatic reactions. Iron, zinc, magnesium, calcium, etc are co-factors bound to proteins that carry out very important cellular functions, including those leading to replication of DNA, redox balance, and energy metabolism. Metals are the stuff of stars; they cannot be synthesized. Thus, when entering into the host, bacteria must steal these metals from you or, more specifically and in the case of blood, proteins that bind them in circulation.

The host keeps the free levels of most of these metals very low, in particular iron, a process referred to as **nutrient immunity**. Iron is bound by the porphyrin heme which itself is locked up in the blood oxygen transport protein hemoglobin. Hemoglobin itself is safeguarded in a cellular vault, the red blood cell, which is kept together by a membrane bilayer. To access this iron, bacteria must secrete toxins to lyse the red blood cell, other proteins that bind or degrade the hemoglobin to release the heme, and receptors that transport the heme so that this too can be degraded inside the bacterium, thereby freeing the iron. Free iron released in the extracellular milieu is bound by tiny molecular chelators termed siderophores that are secreted by bacteria when they sense they do not have enough iron. The affinity of the siderophore for free iron is so great that its dissociation cannot be readily measured. None of this comes easy, so the host's ability to sequester the iron is still a substantial growth-limiting factor. For this reason, many bacteria, even if they get this far, simply cannot grow well in blood. Without the ability to make more of the invaders, the phagocytic cells of the blood find them easy pickings.

Like sanctions on a rogue state, nutrient immunity is meant to suppress bacterial growth, and it is by far a major limitation to bacterial advancement once in this environment. But the very best of bacterial pathogens find clever ways to get what they need, and even flourish in these nutrient-restricted environments. If growth cannot be prevented, it is the blood, the gateway to bacterial nutrient heaven, which takes the challenge of being the last great stand against invasion. This last phase of engagement originates in the analysis occurring in the lymphoid command centers such as the Peyer's patches that are localized through the body. The tonsils in your throat, the spleen in your abdomen, and the appendix all serve in a similar manner; they house a waiting army of specialized soldiers and generals that are called to action when the most serious of breaches has occurred. This final fighting force differs from the innate system in its specificity and its endurance. Termed the **adaptive immune system**, it is the topic of our next chapter. The microbe hunter must appreciate that at the most simple level, when all the complexity of the host-pathogen interaction is distilled to its smallest unit, it is the bacterial invader's ability to evade and in some cases destroy the host's immune response and counter response that is the root of all infectious diseases. A high level of understanding that moves beyond mere appreciation is absolutely necessary for combating the most skilled bacterial evaders, most of which do not have vaccines for their prevention or antibiotics because of resistance.

Summary of Key Concepts

1. Bacterial pathogens are kept out of the host through physical, chemical, and cellular barriers.
2. Physical barriers include thick layers of mucus or dead cells, chemical barriers include secreted molecules that may directly harm the bacteria or signal to the immune system, while cellular barriers include well-formed epithelium packed to limit diffusion from apical to basolateral areas.

Suggested Reading

3. The host responds to invading bacteria via the secretion of chemical alarms that recruit professional phagocytic cells to the infection.
4. Phagocytosed bacteria are encapsulated in a vesicular structure designed to digest them; antigens released from this process are presented to immune cells in specialized lymphoid centers located throughout the body.
5. Additional bacterial sensing mechanisms include surface and cytoplasmic epithelial receptors that translate the signal into a change in gene expression. These new proteins are designed to respond to the threat.
6. Breaching of barriers leads to infiltration of bacteria into the blood where additional immunological precautions either prevent bacterial growth or kill bacteria directly.

❓ Expand Your Knowledge

1. As new Assistant Professor and Lecturer at a small liberal arts College, you are assigned to be the Course Director of Introductory Microbiology. You wish to highlight the challenges bacterial pathogens face as they transverse the skin and mucosal barriers. Make four Power Point Slides that clearly demonstrates the layers of defenses against bacteria of these two surfaces. Give a mock lecture to a group of friends or your classmates.
2. Fast forward to the ▶ Chaps. 7 and 10 on bacterial adhesins and toxins. Read these chapters. Make a table that lists all the innate immune responses discussed in this Chapter and then a counter table of some of the known bacterial factors or mechanisms that counter these responses. Then make a third column and rank order in this column what you believe are the most justified avenues for future therapeutic intervention to counter these bacterial counter responses to the innate immune system.
3. A wealthy benefactor has issued a Request for Applications (RFA) with the following title: "Call for New Ideas on the Molecular Basis of Colon Cancer." You believe some colon cancers may have a bacterial origin, that is, the presence of a certain species of bacteria in the intestine, and their access to a stem cell niche in the intestinal crypts, over time, increases the risk of developing colonic polyps. Write a 1-page Specific Aims document with a Rationale, Background, Relevant Data, Hypothesis, and two Specific Aims that addresses how a colonizing species of human intestinal bacteria gain access to this niche.

Notes

1 = We will learn later that the spaces between cells, called gap junctions, can serve as tunnels by which bacteria move between and sometimes through an epithelial layer. Pathogenic bacteria can make proteases that specifically degrade these gap junction proteins.

2 = A symbiosis is a union between two organisms for which both receive a mutual benefit from the association. For example, some microbes of the intestine make certain vitamins that a human needs. In return for the production of these vitamins, the host provides a warm, moist, and relatively safe place to live. In other cases, there may be no symbiosis. Instead, the bacterium may have evolved to become less virulent, trading its ability to cause disease for the chance at living in close association with the host.

3 = The lymphoid command centers will often house a high density of T- and B-cells, the major players in the adaptive immune system. The dendritic and M-cells, antigen in hand, will present these foreign particles to these cells. If they have previously seen these antigens, they can quickly mobilize, enter the systemic circulation, and be deposited in the intestine ready to directly engage the invaders. T-cells can not only kill bacteria directly, but they also serve as important generals in directing where the firepower should be targeted. They may also tell other cells to play a larger role in the fight while down-modulating others. B-cells have the select function of secreting antibodies that neutralize bacterial processes. At mucosal surfaces, these antibodies are of the IgA isotype, which represent a more localized secretion. IgA will also bind tightly to the mucus and bring them into close contact with embedded bacteria. The coming Chapter discusses these points in more detail.

Suggested Reading

Artis D, Spits H (2015) The biology of innate lymphoid cells. Nature 517:293–301. https://doi.org/10.1038/nature14189

Berends ET, Kuipers A, Ravesloot MM, Urbanus RT, Rooijakkers SH (2014) Bacteria under stress by complement and coagulation. FEMS Microbiol Rev 38:1146–1171. https://doi.org/10.1111/1574-6976.12080

Flannagan RS, Jaumouillé V, Grinstein S (2012) The cell biology of phagocytosis. Annu Rev Pathol 7:61–98. https://doi.org/10.1146/annurev-pathol-011811-132445

Ganz T (2003) Defensins: antimicrobial peptides of innate immunity. Nat Rev Immunol 3:710–720. https://doi.org/10.1038/nri1180

4

Gao W, Xiong Y, Li Q, Yang H (2017) Inhibition of toll-like receptor signaling as a promising therapy for inflammatory diseases: a journey from molecular to nano therapeutics. Front Physiol 8:508. https://doi.org/10.3389/fphys.2017.00508

Iwasaki A, Medzhitov R (2015) Control of adaptive immunity by the innate immune system. Nat Immunol 16:343–353. https://doi.org/10.1038/ni.3123

Lázaro-Díez M et al (2017) Human neutrophils phagocytose and kill Acinetobacter baumannii and A. pittii. Sci Rep 7:4571. https://doi.org/10.1038/s41598-017-04870-8

Lv Y et al (2014) Antimicrobial properties and membrane-active mechanism of a potential α-helical antimicrobial derived from cathelicidin PMAP-36. PLoS One 9:e86364. https://doi.org/10.1371/journal.pone.0086364

Pasparakis M, Haase I, Nestle FO (2014) Mechanisms regulating skin immunity and inflammation. Nat Rev Immunol 14:289–301. https://doi.org/10.1038/nri3646

Perez-Lopez A, Behnsen J, Nuccio SP, Raffatellu M (2016) Mucosal immunity to pathogenic intestinal bacteria. Nat Rev Immunol 16:135–148. https://doi.org/10.1038/nri.2015.17

Peterson LW, Artis D (2014) Intestinal epithelial cells: regulators of barrier function and immune homeostasis. Nat Rev Immunol 14:141–153. https://doi.org/10.1038/nri3608

Sonesson A et al (2017) Identification of bacterial biofilm and the Staphylococcus aureus derived protease, staphopain, on the skin surface of patients with atopic dermatitis. Sci Rep 7:8689. https://doi.org/10.1038/s41598-017-08046-2

Van Kessel KP, Bestebroer J, van Strijp JA (2014) Neutrophil-mediated phagocytosis of staphylococcus aureus. Front Immunol 5:467. https://doi.org/10.3389/fimmu.2014.00467

Zhou X et al (2014) Remodeling of the intestinal brush border underlies adhesion and virulence of an enteric pathogen. MBio 5. https://doi.org/10.1128/mBio.01639-14

Zipfel PF, Hallström T, Riesbeck K (2013) Human complement control and complement evasion by pathogenic microbes--tipping the balance. Mol Immunol 56:152–160. https://doi.org/10.1016/j.molimm.2013.05.222

Adaptive Immunological Defenses Against Bacterial Attack

© Springer Nature Switzerland AG 2019
A. W. Maresso, *Bacterial Virulence*, https://doi.org/10.1007/978-3-030-20464-8_5

Learning Goals

In this chapter, we discuss how the innate immune response approached in ▶ Chap. 4 transitions into the long-term adaptive immune response that attempts to contain the bacterial attack. This includes addressing the mechanism by which antibody and cell-based antibacterial measures are generated and sustained as well as a discussion of the way in which such a response is regulated. The basic structure and function of the antibody is framed in the context of the multifaceted ways the body uses these molecules to restrict bacterial expansion. At the conclusion of this chapter, the reader will be able to understand how the body's immune response is effective at exploiting vulnerabilities in bacterial virulence mechanism for the long-term protection of the host.

5.1 Introduction

Imagine a device that could inactive any weapon. Imagine it did not matter what mechanics constituted the functionality of the weapon; this device could take any of a trillion possible forms and wedge its way into a critical component of the weapon's function to block that function. Imagine the device also has memory; once it learns how to disable the weapon, upon exposure to the weapon a second time, the response is faster and more intense. The size of the weapon is not a factor either; if it has a smaller part that makes it work, the device exploits that functionality. The number of weapons also does not matter; the device is capable of producing millions of inactivating responses at once, and can sustain them indefinitely. The device itself is practically indestructible, resistant to heat, salt, contrasting pH, water, drying and so on.

We just described an antibody. Antibodies, or more accurately primitive versions of them, were created by nature hundreds of millions of years ago, likely when the first multicellular groups of bacteria learned that some proteins can protect the group from invasion. The process by which antibodies are made is called acquired immunity. The antibody is the signature molecule, the star of the show, for the **adaptive immune system**. The adaptive system in some ways is everything the innate response isn't. Whereas the innate response is a first responder to the battle, the adaptive system is there to win the war. Here, the microbe hunter will learn how knowledge in this area can inform the future development of useful therapeutics.

5.2 Specialty of the Adaptive Immune Response

There are three main ways in which the adaptive response differs from the innate response, and these ways represent a good way to begin the discussion. First, as its name implies, the adaptive system is designed to be malleable. This malleability allows the system to rapidly adjust to changing circumstances. Biology is an organized way to use energy to constrain the expansion of entropy. But all organisms make decisions based on environmental cues. Pathogenic bacteria are some of the best adapters on the planet, quickly pivoting gene expression to adjust to conditions of their hosts. The host must be equally if not more adaptable in response. Not only must various aspects of immunity be coordinated to kill the invader, the assault must also be stopped when the war is over. The adaptive immune system is unlike any other organ system in that not only can it direct a highly focused response to a single molecule produced by one strain of bacteria, it can turn off this response to not forsake its own tissues with collateral damage.

Second, the adaptive response is highly specific. The innate immune system – the walls, the missiles, the soldiers sent in for the kill – are more or less universal responses to any invading bacterium. The adaptive immune response, however, is laser focused. It assesses vulnerabilities in the specific bacterial strain performing the attack and then reverse engineers a response targeting these vulnerabilities. Such a response may be so specific to a component of one strain of bacteria it may not be effective against a closely related strain of the same species. Each response by the adaptive immune system is unique to the pathogen, the pathogen's virulence factors, and, as we will come to learn, a particular molecular feature of the virulence factors that are necessary for function.

Third, the adaptive immune system is in it for the long run. One of its primary strengths is its ability to outlast the will of the invading bacterial army. To continuously replenish specific commandos for each battle, to initiate a systemic response that activates other portions of the body to get ready for a fight, and to also remember the tactics used by the invader (and exploit them) for not only the current war but the next, is a testament to the creative powers of evolution. It is this latter point, that of immunological memory, that is a unique adaptation unlike any other bodily system. Long after the war is over and the bacterial invaders repelled, the adaptive immune system will store away the information of a pathogen's weaknesses. If, years later, another invasion is attempted, this knowledge can be quickly pushed to the forefront to mount an even more swift and deadly response to the bacterial usurper. All the collective information from all previous battles and wars are stored in this way. Should another invasion be attempted, the intruder will need to devise a new way to be successful. If not, the onslaught of the specific response that follows is almost certain to maintain a defense of the body and the health of the host. It is this latter point that is the success behind the concept of vaccination.

5.3 Cells of Adaptive Immunity

The adaptive immune response consists of two main functional arms; the humoral arm and the cellular arm. The **humoral** arm refers to the production of antibodies by **B-cells**, the great disabling weapon we spoke of above. The name comes from early studies that indicated there was some anti-bacterial activity in fluids, which was considered one of the four bodily humors.

Indeed, antibodies circulate the body in blood and have access to all tissues and fluids, even the spinal fluid in privileged sites like the brain. The second component, the **cellular** arm, refers to the cells that either produce the antibodies or otherwise regulate the long-term response to a particular pathogen. The latter constitutes mostly antigen presenting cells and **T-cells**. The T-cells are the primary effector cell of the adaptive response. They not only coordinate the military campaign against the invader, they also directly engage pathogens. Our discussion begins with the cellular arm.

How does one make a standing army of host cells read to kill a specific pathogen in a moment's notice? Just like with any soldier, the process starts with training, or, as Immunologists refer to it, "education." Training instills in the soldier discipline, punctuality, and absolute obedience to orders from officers. So too are the soldiers of the adaptive immune system, the soldiers being the T-cells. T-cells are so named because they mature in the **thymus** (T), a lymphoid organ located under your sternum near to the heart. Born in the bone marrow from hematopoietic stem cells, T-lymphocytes (called immature thymocytes) migrate from the marrow to blood and deposit in the thymus. There, they undergo **T-cell education** whereby they are "taught" to distinguish friend from foe. Epithelial cells in the thymus display a specialized receptor termed the **major histocompatibility complex**, or **MHC**. The MHC is a central molecule in immunological adaptation and recognition. Most cells of the body make an MHC receptor in one form or another and display this molecule on their surface. You may recall that antigen presenting cells, such as dendritic cells and macrophages, phagocytose bacteria or their components and digest them into smaller peptides. These peptides, or antigens, represent the physical evidence, the smoking gun, that the body is under attack. In the thymus, as the T-cells mature, they interact with epithelial cells displaying one of the MHC receptors via their own specialized receptor termed the **T-cell receptor**, or TCR.

If the T-cell binds through its T-cell receptor to MHC, it passes the first step in its education. The body wants T-cell soldiers that are capable of recognizing MHC. If the T-cell could not do this, it would be utterly useless, as such a cell would not even be capable of fighting in any directed manner. This is because at some point, bacterial antigen will be displayed on the MHC. If the T-cell receptor has no ability to complex to the MHC, it will not be able to recognize that the antigen is present, and thus fail to respond to it in the future. But the selection of fighters is a slippery slope. You want the right type of fighters, more specifically, ones that don't fight oneself, *i.e.* host cells. This can be compared to the military being instructed to avoid at all costs civilian or friendly casualties. Collateral damage accumulated during the war for the body is costly to health. Not only is acute inflammation likely to make one feel ill, the long-term consequences of attacking oneself can also be debilitating, and at the worst end, deadly. To educate fighters to kill only foreign intruders, the T-cell undergoes a second test in the thymus. All those that recognize MHC are then passed through cells that display MHC with self-antigen, that is, a little peptide taken from our bodies' proteins (self) that are displayed on the MHC surface for presentation to the T-cell. If the TCR of the T-cell binds too tightly to the MHC with self-antigen, it is instructed to die. This ensures the T-cell will not be reactive to peptides derived from your own bodily proteins. Of all the young new recruits hopeful of becoming a T-cell soldier, only about 5% will survive this process. The rest will have been deemed either too passive (did not recognize MHC at all) or too aggressive (recognized MHC too well) for the war effort. Without this strict **positive selection**, there would no immune response at all. With this strict **negative selection**, T-cell soldiers would induce **autoimmunity** (the immune system attacking oneself), a condition that can lead to conditions such as arthritis, multiple sclerosis, and lupus. The maturation of T-cells is illustrated in ◘ Fig. 5.1.

Out of the Box

It is now possible for T-cells to be taken from patients, stimulated in culture with any antigen of choice, the T-cells reactive to that antigen expanded and isolated, and then placed back into a patient. In fact, this is a budding method for the treatment of cancer, so called T-cell therapy. In theory, such a concept should be applicable to any disease where T-cells may be helpful in restoring health, including bacterial infections. In particular, for chronic bacterial infections that are often refractory to antibiotics or other approaches, partly because the antibiotic cannot penetrate the tissue or area where the infection is localized, T-cells stimulated against such antigens may allow for a precise response in tough-to-reach places. In addition, T-cells made in this nature against antigens from intracellular bacteria may lead to eradication of host cells harboring these stealthy combatants.

5.4 The Selective and Killer T-Cell

The T-cell, having been educated in the rules of war, are now ready for their post and are placed on assignment. They leave the thymus and circulate throughout the body, eventually landing in **lymphoid centers** (◘ Fig. 5.2) such as the lymph nodes or more specialized tissue command centers such as the Peyer's patches in the gastrointestinal tract. At the command center is where the innate and adaptive immune systems will intersect so as to activate the latter. Antigen presenting cells coming back from the battle front will be carrying bacterial antigens they have phagocytosed (see ▶ Chap. 4). In the presenting cell cytoplasm, the phagocytosed components will be digested into smaller peptides. These peptides, usually between 8 and 25 amino acids in length, are loaded onto the MHC receptors. This occurs in the endoplasmic reticulum of the cytoplasm. The endoplasmic reticulum will fuse with the antigen presenting cell membrane, thereby allowing the MHC plus its bound peptide/antigen to be exposed to the extracellular environment. Antigen presenting cells with MHC-peptide will

5

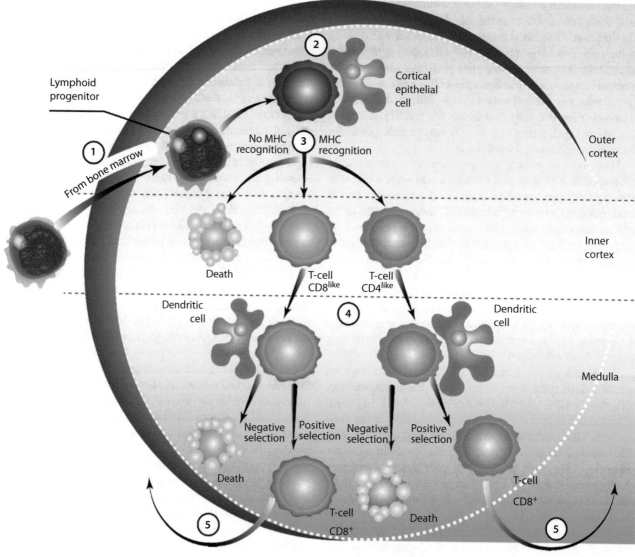

Fig. 5.1   Maturation of T-cells. Immature T-cells enter the thymus after birth from progenitor cells in the bone marrow. In the outer cortext of the thymus they interact with epithelial cells that express MHC receptors. Lack of ligation of a T-cell via its T-cell receptor with MHC results in death of the T-cell. T-cells that bind the MHC move on to the medulla where they encounter dendritic cells presenting MHC with self-antigen. Those that react with self-antigen die whereas those that do not move into the circulation to search for antigen presenting cells with MHC loaded with bacterial antigens

Fig. 5.2   Immune cell coordination. Shown is a germinal center of B-cells, T-cells, macrophages, in a popliteal lymph node. The congregation of each cell type in a concentrated area in the presence of antigen maximizes coordination of antigen-stimulated B- and T-cells. (Adapted from Niesner et al (see *suggested readings*) under a creative commons license with immune cells now labeled. (▶ https://creativecommons.org/licenses/by/4.0/))

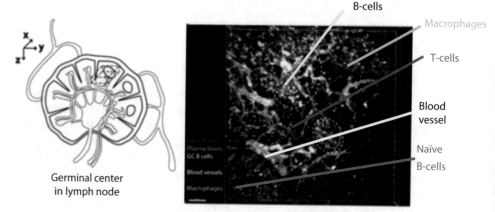

Germinal center
in lymph node

migrate into the lymphoid center and present the antigen to a T-cell. The T-cell at this point is likely to be **antigenically naïve**; that is, it will not have seen a non-self bacterial antigen in the context of MHC. Upon the presentation of the MHC and its bound antigen to the T-cell, the T-cell becomes activated to recognize that specific antigen. This functional link occurs through the binding of the MHC-antigen complex by the T-cell receptor. The MHC-antigen-TCR triple complex sets in motion a series of downstream signaling events to activate the T-cell. In a kind of double check of the process, other receptors on the antigen presenting cell engage a second receptor on the T-cell – it is the presence of both these signals that result in activation.

Once the T-cell becomes activated via the stimulation of the TCR by the APC's presentation of antigen, the T-cell can leave the lymphoid center and enter the circulation. It is now on a mission to seek and destroy any bacteria that have the exact peptide (antigen) that was presented to it by the APC. Here we see firsthand the specificity of this process. The combination of selecting against autoreactive T-cells in the thymus by educating them about self-peptides and the APC presenting a foreign antigen from the bacterial invader directly to the T-cell ensures that the fully trained and now ready T-cell soldier will only attack bacterial cells that display that antigen. Should that T-cell not find any bacteria with this match, perhaps because the defenses of the innate immune system held, the activated T-cell will return to a lymphoid center and wait. Having been educated and trained to kill a certain type of bacterium, it is far too valuable to just let die. Upon restimulation of the T-cell with the same antigen by an APC at a later time, the T-cell can quickly mobilize to engage the bacterial invader. One can imagine that having a reservoir of many T-cells ready to respond to antigens of all types and varieties is a very efficient way to direct a specific response should another attack come.

5.5 Main Types of T-Cells

There are two main T-cell types that are important for the adaptive immune response against bacterial pathogens. The first is the **cytotoxic T lymphocyte** (CTL), also called the CD8+ because it expresses the receptor CD8 (a feature that defines them as a CTL after maturation in the thymus). The CTL does exactly as its name implies; hunts down and kills foreign invaders. The unique feature of the CTL though is that it can kill bacterial cells that are hiding in host cells. A good example is that of the infection of host cells by *Mycobacterium tuberculosis* (Mtb). As we have discussed already, Mtb prefers to grow and persist inside the cells of the lung. We learn of the advantages of living in your cells in ▶ Chap. 8; but for the time being, let us assume here the reason why Mtb enters host cells is to hide. Inside a host cell, the MtB believes it will not be detected. After all, we just learned that T-cells are educated to ignore host cells and their antigens to avoid autoimmunity. It would thus seem that T-cells will not find the Mtb and the pathogen can go about its dirty work without fear of harm. This is true for many viruses. Viruses provide the primary

pathogen infected host cells that are recognized by CTLs. All viruses are obligate intracellular pathogens; they can only replicate in the host cytoplasm using host machinery that they hijack for this purpose. CTLs recognize these virally-infected cells because the host cell is able to present in some cases viral peptides on its MHC receptor and display this MHC-peptide complex on the surface of the infected cell.

The host uses a very similar mechanism to tell T-cells that it is infected with intracellular bacteria. By displaying peptides on MHC and localizing this complex to the surface (in this case, a non-self Mtb peptide), the CTL will recognize this foreign antigen, especially if it has previously been presented to the T-cell by APCs in lymphoid centers. The CTL knows that although the host lung cell is self, it is currently being used as a Trojan horse to infiltrate the body. The MHC complexed to foreign peptide tells the T-cell "Infected - Kill Me!" This is achieved via **granulysin**, an enzyme stored in granules inside the T-cell that are released into the extracellular environment upon ligation of the TCR with MHC presenting antigen-peptide. Granulysin bombards the membrane of the infected host cell, lysing it, which releases the cytosolic contents including the intracellular bacterium. Now exposed, the bacterium is also killed by granulysin or is phagocytosed by resident macrophages that chemotax to the area. This in turn generates more antigen presenting cells harboring MHC with Mtb antigens which in turn can be used to educate more T-cells.

The second type of broadly defined T cell is the **T-helper lymphocyte**, or THC, also known as a CD4+ cell because it expresses the CD4 receptor (which defines them as a helper cell after maturation in the thymus). The T-helper cell does what its name implies; it helps other immune cells for the ultimate purpose of amplifying the attack. More specifically, the T-helper cell relays knowledge between the antigen presenting cells at the front line (which have acquired bacterial antigens) and the cells of the body that make the ultra-coveted inactivating weapon. Remember that foreign bacterial antigens represent critical intelligence in the war effort. This would be equivalent to acquiring a piece of an opposing army's technology, say a control panel of a stealth drone or a casing of a long-range missile, in hopes of using such knowledge to jam the control panel or design armory to penetrate the casing. Most bacterial virulence factors are proteins and thus composed of amino acids. These amino acids are arranged in a way that gives the virulence factor some structure and some function. The factors are digested into the 8-25 amino acid peptides. Antigen presenting cells via surface MHC-antigen complexes relay this information to the T-helper cell, which then relays this information to another immune cell. This begins the process of analyzing the components of the virulence factor so that construction of the inactivating weapon can begin. So critical is this to producing an effective immune response that the process of learning how to exploit bacterial vulnerabilities occurs in its own little factory – secret, and heavily guarded. In this way, the THC accelerates the immune response by activating other immune cells to work against the bacterium. These other cells are described below.

5

5.6 The B-Cell

The United States government is known to have a secret military installment in the Nevada desert. Known as Area 51, it plays out in American movies and media as a place where the military is conducting revolutionary weapons testing. In the war effort against bacteria, the human body contains its own Area 51 – the spleen. The spleen and lymph nodes are silos of immune maturation and function, kept apart from other organ systems and out of the reach of direct attack by pathogenic bacteria. In these silos occurs the assembly of the inactivating device, and it begins with the **B-lymphocyte** or **B-cell**. The B-cell journey starts from obscure to hero in the bone marrow through **hematopoiesis**, or the process of making new immune cells. These new cells, referred to as naïve B-cells because they have not yet seen antigen, then migrate to either the spleen or lymph nodes, two lymphoid organs highly organized to maximize the production of specific and effective B-cells. There they wait, patiently and quietly, for antigen, either delivered directly by an APC or via the flow of lymph fluid, which carries with it all the enemy debris generated from the encounter with the innate immune system (◻ Fig. 5.3). On the surface of these B-cells is the **B-cell receptor** or **BCR**. The BCR is the precursor to a secreted **antibody** and its most distal portion, extending out from the surface of the B-cell, can bind antigen. The successful binding of antigen by the BCR results in the internalization and processing of the antigen and display on the B-cell version of an MHC. If a T-helper via its TCR has previously seen this antigen, it will complex with the B-cell MHC. This is a critical second signal confirming the antigen is real. The B-cells will experience signals to maturate and proliferate, which leads to more B-cells that recognize the antigen and an amplification of the inactivating weaponry. The general mechanism of antigen processing and presentation to B- and T-cells is illustrated in ◻ Fig. 5.4.

At this point, the expanded B-cell population will undergo one of three possible fates. Some will leave area 51 and enter the systemic circulation to become an antibody-secreting **plasma cell**. A plasma cell is a B-cell that releases its BCR from the surface. The released BCR is effectively an antibody specific to the bacterial antigen it first encountered in the lymphoid organs. These released antibodies do not have the highest affinity for the antigen but they are a way for the body to quickly ensure at least some antibody is circulated in response to the first stages of invasion. A second group of these B-cells will stay put and become **memory cells**. Their function is to remember (hence the name) the bacterial antigen that first led to their stimulation and thus maintain a stable population of B-cells with a BCR that matches said antigen for a later activation event. Antibody-secreting plasma cells that left Area 51 are short-lived; should more be needed at a later time, memory B-cells can answer the call.

The third population of B-cells moves into a highly secure facility of the spleen to be genetically engineered to make even better antibodies, a process termed **somatic hypermutation**. The name itself is worthy of a science fiction film but make no mistake, it's an amazingly clever process. When all cells of the body divide, the DNA must be duplicated without any errors. An error changes the code, a change in the code is a mutation. Mutations can be deleterious. If for example they occur in an important protein, when that protein is made, the protein may no longer function. This can lead to abnormal cell physiology and ultimately translate into a disease. There are many human diseases that are the direct result of mutation but certainly the most prominent is cancer. The reason mistakes are made in copying the DNA is that the enzyme that does this, DNA polymerase, is not perfect. Although

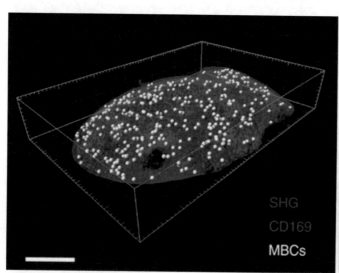

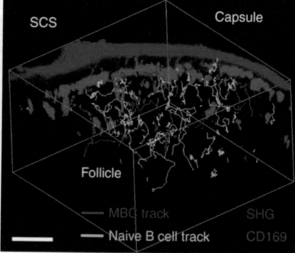

◻ **Fig. 5.3** Antigen presentation to memory B-cells. *Left panel,* intravital two-photon microscopy reveals macrophage (pink) interactions with memory B-cells (white) in murine lymph nodes during active antigen presentation. *Right panel*, tracking the movements of B-cells as they scan for antigen-presenting macrophages. Red = memory B-cells, Green = naïve B-cells, Pink = macrophages. (Adapted from Phan et al (see *suggested readings*) under a creative commons license. (► https://creativecommons.org/licenses/by/4.0/))

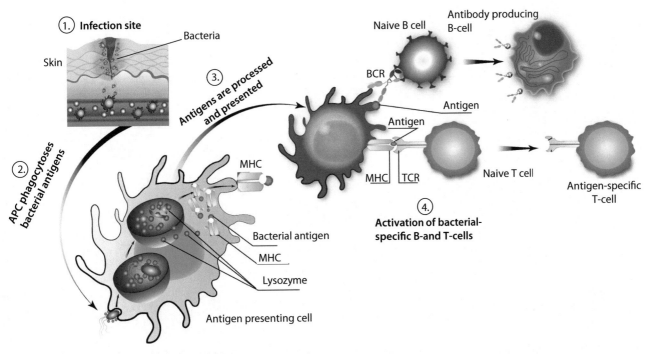

Fig. 5.4 The phagocytosis of bacteria and the presentation of their antigens. Invading bacteria are phagocytosed by antigen presenting cells and digested in phagolysosomes. Bacterial peptides are loaded onto MHC molecules and displayed on the APC surface. APCs present antigens to B- and T-cells expressing B-cell and T-cell receptors, respectively, which, in the presence of other regulatory factors and signals, are stimulated to become antibody-producing (B-cells) or regulatory/cytotoxic T-cells that are now primed and specific for bacterial antigens

infrequent, it sometimes makes a mistake (or fails to recognize it has made a mistake and does not repair it – a process termed proofreading). In somatic hypermutation, the B-cell polymerase makes mistakes at 100,000 to one million times the frequency as other polymerases in other cells. It does so in one particular region of the B-cell DNA that encodes the very tip of the antibody, the region that happens to bind the bacterial antigen. As a result of this error process in this region, the DNA that encodes the tip of the antibody is called the **hypervariable region**. The protein product of this region is called the variable fragment. If enough mutations are made, some of them will actually result in antibodies (as membrane bound BCRs at this stage) that have a higher affinity for the antigen than the original BCR. It is important to recognize that the mutations occur in one region of the code that when translated makes the variable fragment. This area of the DNA code is usually designated the VDJ region. It undergoes a shuffling of the DNA, in almost infinite combinations, such that novel codes are generated. This code then combines with a more constant region of the DNA to produce, when translated, the full antibody (one fragment of the antibody, the tip that recognizes the antigen, being variable and the other fragment, the base being constant – see below). The entire process is called VDJ recombination and is illustrated in ◘ Fig. 5.5.

Once new B-cells with new BCRs are made, they pass through a field of antigen presenting cells that display all the antigens acquired from the battle front. Only the B-cells with the highest affinity, the result of somatic hypermutation, undergo expansion or survival signals. These B-cells are

again either made into memory cells or plasma cells. The plasma cells again leave the lymphoid center and become fully-fledged antibody-secreting cells via the release of their now exquisitely evolved BCR into the systemic circulation. The diversity of antibodies created from millions of possible antigens, some antibodies evolved to contain affinities stronger than most known protein-protein interactions, leads to an arsenal of freely circulating antibodies that seek and bind the very virulence factors bacteria need for invasion.

Antibodies are amazing little proteins. They are often designated by the letter "Y" with two extra outstretched arms, a short-hand notation that connotes their overall structure at the molecular level. The stem of the "Y" is referred to as the **fragment crystallizable/constant** region, or **Fc** for short[1]. The arms of the "Y" are termed the **fragment antigen-binding** region, or **Fab** for short. The Fab arms are the portion of the antibody that binds the bacterial proteins or antigens. The specific region of the bacterial protein that the Fab binds is called an epitope. The epitope will be the same 8–25 amino acids that was originally used to select for high-affinity B-cells in the lymphoid tissue. As such, each Fab can be quite variable in its local structure and amino acid composition so as to be a good fit for the bacterial epitope. It is the Fab portion that confers the binding specificity of each antibody. The Fc or stem region is not variable; it is constant and for good reason. While the Fab arms of the antibody grab onto their bacterial epitopes with high affinity, the Fc stem protrudes outward and can serve as a recognition site for phagocytic cells. Hold that thought for now, we will return to it shortly.

5

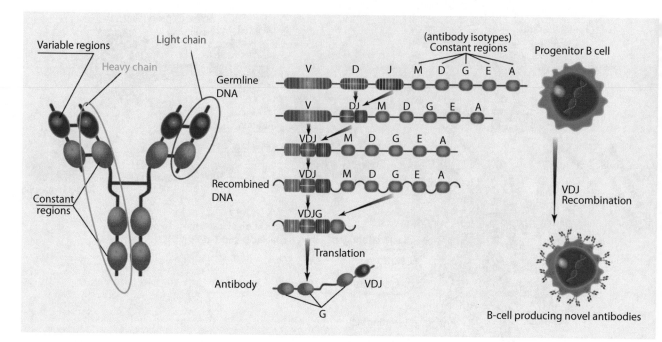

Fig. 5.5 The making of antibodies. B-cells undergo genetic recombination of the V, D, and J variable regions of DNA to make highly diverse antibodies in a process termed somatic hypermutation. After recombination, the constant regions are joined to the newly recombined variable regions and the new gene transcribed and translated into a novel antibody. Note that the constant regions specify the isotype of the antibody (M, D, G, E, and A)

5.7 The Amazing Antibody

This leads us to the ways in which antibodies are effective. There are three main ways this can happen. The first is by disarming bacterial weapons – **antibody-based neutralization**. Remember that antibodies will recognize small peptides produced by dissolution of the engulfed bacterium. These regions of the protein antibodies recognize are called **epitopes**. Most epitopes recognized by B-cells are located on bacterial proteins. Proteins are the action molecules of living systems, and most virulence factors are proteins. These virulence factors can also be processed by antigen-presenting cells into peptide antigens and used to make antibodies, as described above. Let us say the virulence factor is a secreted protein toxin and that this toxin enters host epithelial cells after binding to a host receptor. Upon entering the host cell, the protein toxin's enzymatic activity modifies the host cytoskeletal protein actin, leading to actin's depolymerization and collapse of host cell architecture (this is an actual strategy used by many bacteria that we will discuss in ▶ Chap. 10). The cell rounds, loses its connections with neighboring cells, and makes a tunnel that allows entry to underlying tissues. During the processing of this toxin into antigens yielding antibody-recognizing epitopes, one or more of the generated antibodies might just bind the same region of the toxin that interfaces the host receptor. Since antibodies bind with very tight affinity to their epitopes, the antibody-toxin interaction may very well prevent the toxin-receptor interaction, and thus prevent its entry into the host cell. Chemically, the name for this is **steric**

hinderance – no two molecules can occupy the same space at the same time. One must be hindered from that space. Here, we see the antibody has prevented the bacterium from using its own weaponry to break down a critical barrier, all by neutralizing a key function needed for toxin activity. This is why vaccination against bacteria that cause diphtheria, pertussis, and tetanus is successful. These diseases are largely the result of a single toxin produced by these bacteria; vaccination with the inactivated toxin leads to antibodies that neutralize the toxin's activity.

Antibodies work in many ways to inhibit virulence factors. They can bind bacterial adhesins and prevent the adhesin from interacting with the host. Antibodies can neutralize bacterial proteases, which protects the integrity of host tissues and prevents the release of nutrients bacteria consume. Antibodies can bind to the proteins that constitute the flagellar motor, stopping bacterial movement. Just about any protein activity, enzymatic or otherwise, can be inhibited by the binding of an antibody; and since this effect is not limited to a single virulence factor, the entire arsenal of surface or secreted virulence factors, as long as they are accessible by free floating antibodies, is fair game for direct inactivation.

The second mechanism by which antibodies antagonize bacterial advances is via a process termed **opsonophagocytosis**. An **opson** is the name given to an antigen that has been bound by an antibody, but in this case, it leads to deposition of the antibody on the bacterial surface. We have already learned that macrophages recognize PAMPs on the surface of bacteria via their TLRs, and this recognition leads

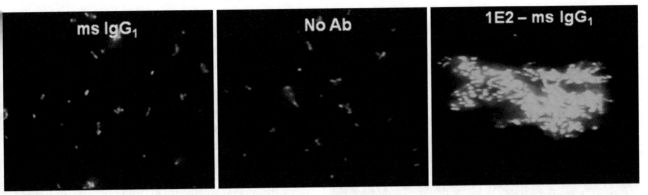

Fig. 5.6 Agglutination activity of antibody. In this experiment, *Streptococcus pneumoniae* (a cause of lung infections and meningitis, here fluorescently labeled) was incubated with either an isotype control antibody (left), no antibody (middle), or antibody reactive to *S. pneumoniae* (right). In this particular case, the *S. pneumoniae* antibody induces agglutination of the bacteria. (Adapted from Pirofski et al (see *suggested readings*) under a creative commons license. (▶ https://creativecommons.org/licenses/by-nc-sa/3.0))

to phagocytosis of the pathogen. PAMPs are a good way to tell foreign from self, but bacteria also have ways to disguise their PAMPs to avoid recognition. If antibody binds to the bacterial surface, it removes any ambiguity that this is "enemy." Since antibodies can be generated against thousands perhaps millions of different bacterial surface epitopes, it makes it difficult for bacteria to escape detection because conceivably any surface protein may serve as a docking site for circulating antibody. The Fc portion of the antibody stem is also sticky with other stems. Thus, if many antibodies bind the bacterial surface, they can aggregate with other stem portions and glue bacterial cells together. This is called **agglutination**. The limited mobility not only restricts their war advance, the larger glom of bacteria is more likely to be recognized by macrophages and killed (**Fig. 5.6**). Because each arm of the "Y" can ligate its own epitope, antibodies can also aggregate individual virulence factors. This concentrates them which also promotes phagocytosis. The neutralizing and opsonophagocytic activity are most commonly used against extracellular bacteria or secreted virulence factors.

5.8 Antibodies that Kill

A third mechanism by which antibodies confer anti-bacterial immunity is during **antibody dependent cell mediated cytotoxicity** (ADCC). ADCC is similar to opsonophagocytosis except that the killing mechanism occurs via the release of granzymes from natural killer or other T-cells. This mechanism can occur directly on extracellular bacteria but it is commonly employed by the immune system to kill host cells infected with intracellular bacteria. Antigens from the bacterium are displayed on the surface of the infected cell. These antigens are bound by circulating antibody. When enough antibody has bound the infected host cell surface, the Fc regions serve as a docking site for **natural killer (NK) cells**, a specialized immune cell that recognizes these surface-bound antibody complexes. The close association of the NK cell and the infected host cell

promotes the local release of granzymes, which disrupt the host cell membrane. Phagocytes sweep in and finish the job by killing any released pathogen. Several bacteria that cause diarrhea, notably shigella and salmonella, invade host cells as a way to stealthily avoid the immune response. ADCC is an important defense against their infection.

The final mechanism by which antibodies stop bacterial advances may be the most creative of all. This mechanism, referred to as **classical complement activation**, links the production of antibodies by the acquired immune system with toxic blood proteins of the innate immune system. Complement-mediated killing of bacteria was one of the earliest observations of the anti-bacterial effects of blood in the beginning of the nineteenth century. When the red and white blood cells are removed from blood, the resulting substance (serum), when added to live bacteria, can directly kill these bacteria. This was a striking finding at the time, as it was already known that white blood cells kill bacteria. The killing in the presence of serum suggested the factor was not a cell but some type of substance. It was initially named "alexin" but later renamed "complement" because the substance complemented the activity of blood in an antibacterial fashion. We now know that complement is a protein complex, upwards of twenty at a time, that directly acts on bacterial cells.

The complement system is a textbook example of how multiple distinct proteins can assemble into a nanomachine. In this case, the machine is a laser-guided missile system. When antibody binds to an antigen on the bacterial surface, the stem or Fc region acts as a "mark" or docking site for a blood protein complex known as **C1qrs**. The more antibodies that bind, the stronger the association of C1qrs with the bacterial surface. Binding induces changes in the structure of C1qrs that facilitates its enzymatic activity, which results in the cleavage of two other blood proteins, C2 and C4. Two of the proteins that result from this cleavage, C2b and C4b, have affinity for each other and form a second enzyme, **C3 convertase**. As its name implies, C3 convertase converts a third serum protein C3 into two components, of which the

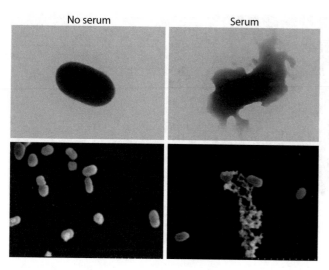

No serum **Serum**

❑ **Fig. 5.7** Killing activity of serum. *Edwardsiella tarda*, a pathogen of reptiles, fish, and mammals, was treated with serum (right panels) or not (left panels). Notice the obliteration of the cells with serum, an effect that is likely due to complement. Of note, this was a genetically modified strain of *E. tarda* made sensitive to killing by serum. (Adapted from Sun et al (see *suggested readings*) under a creative commons license. (▶ https://creativecommons.org/licenses/by/4.0/))

b component C3b links to C3 convertase to form a second convertase, termed C5 convertase. C5 convertase cleaves C5 into two components, again a and b, and the b form termed C5b lands on the bacterial surface. There, it serves as a docking site for several other C-like proteins that assemble together into a giant pore called the **membrane attack complex (MAC)**. Doing exactly what its name implies, the MAC inserts into the bacterial membrane as a cylindrical complex, thereby depolarizing the membrane and eventually killing the bacterial cell (❑ Fig. 5.7). In this analogy, the antibody serves as the laser, marking the exact spot on the enemy where the guided missile (MAC) should land. ❑ Figure 5.8 illustrates the anti-bacterial properties of antibodies.

The adaptive immune system employs a memory-generating system that produces antibodies that inactivate key bacterial virulence strategies. In addition, antibody leads to the direct killing of bacterial cells by cytotoxic immune cells that recognize antibody on the surface, or bacterial antigen. T and B cells are the workhorses of this response and undergo education in the art of war in privileged immune lymphoid tissues that act as command centers for a coordinated, and measured, attack.

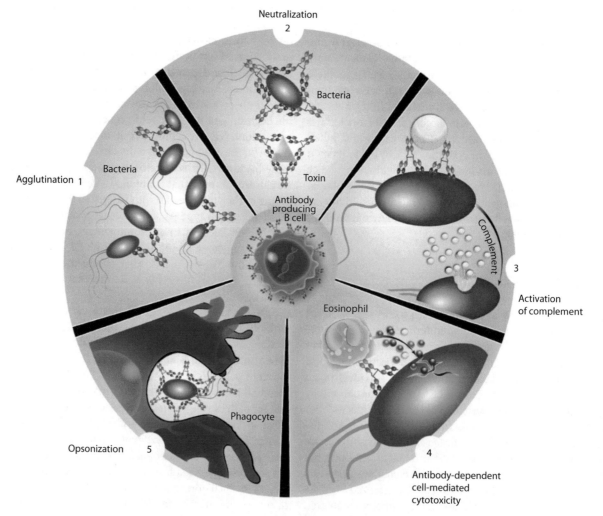

❑ **Fig. 5.8** The many beneficial functions of antibodies. From the neutralization of bacterial toxins to stimulation of the destruction of bacterial membranes, antibodies are the body's most effective and diverse anti-bacterial molecules

Summary of Key Concepts

1. Versatility, specificity, and persistence are the hallmark characteristics of the adaptive immune response.
2. The dominant two cells of the adaptive immune response are T-cells and B-cells. Whereas T-cells regulate the response and kill infected host cells, B-cells produce antibodies directed against bacterial antigens.
3. These cell populations are educated in immunological organs to react to bacterial antigens and not host.
4. A specific rearrangement of the host DNA leads to countless types of antibodies that react with specific bacterial antigens. Antibodies can inhibit the function of bacterial proteins or directly stimulate their killing.

300 amino acids in length and could be processed into *non-overlapping* peptide antigens for MHC display, how many different T- and B-cells would be needed to display a single MHC against each of these peptides? Talk about whether there is an upper limit for what the immune system can reasonably "remember."

Note

1 = This region of the antibody is also termed the heavy chain because of its electrophoretic mobility on an SDS-PAGE gel, a system used to separate proteins according to their size. Functionally, one may think of this region as constant since its amino acid content has little bearing on the antibodies' overall specificity for its antigen.

Expand Your Knowledge

1. As a scientist for the Center for Disease Control in the U.S., you are sent to the Guam to investigate a very fatal disease spreading amongst villagers that live near a tropical forest. Blood samples from patients indicate the presence of a new species of bacteria, a large rod-shaped organism with a thick cell wall and disproportionate levels of teichoic acid compared to other Gram-positive bacteria. The teichoic acid looks like bead studs emanating from the surface of the peptidoglycan. The organism is resistant to all types of mammalian blood, including from patient's sera that have survived the infection when cultured in the presence of their white blood cells. Animals vaccinated with killed bacteria of this species and challenged with live organisms are not protected from the infection. Provide an explanation as to how this new bacterium may be resisting the host's immune system to become the killer it is.
2. Read a scientific review about VDJ recombination. Describe the molecular mechanism of this process to a lay friend or colleague in terms they would understand. Then discuss how this very life-giving process can also give way to the formation of a leukemia.
3. Use Pubmed and Genbank to determine the approximate size of an *E. coli* genome. Determine the average number of distinct proteins encoded by this genome and estimate the fraction displayed on the bacterial surface or secreted. Then multiply this number by all the known distinct species of bacteria that can cause an infection in humans. If each of these proteins from each of these species was about

Suggested Reading

Basso K, Dalla-Favera R (2015) Germinal centres and B cell lymphomagenesis. Nat Rev Immunol 15:172–184. https://doi.org/10.1038/nri3814

Garcia BL, Zwarthoff SA, Rooijakkers SH, Geisbrecht BV (2016) Novel evasion mechanisms of the classical complement pathway. J Immunol 197:2051–2060. https://doi.org/10.4049/jimmunol.1600863

Kumar BV, Connors TJ, Farber DL (2018) Human T cell development, localization, and function throughout life. Immunity 48:202–213. https://doi.org/10.1016/j.immuni.2018.01.007

Kurd N, Robey EA (2016) T-cell selection in the thymus: a spatial and temporal perspective. Immunol Rev 271:114–126. https://doi.org/10.1111/imr.12398

Li MF, Sun L (2018) Sip2: a serum-induced protein that is essential to serum survival, acid resistance, intracellular replication, and host infection. Front Microbiol 9:1084. https://doi.org/10.3389/fmicb.2018.01084

Moran I et al (2018) Memory B cells are reactivated in subcapsular proliferative foci of lymph nodes. Nat Commun 9:3372. https://doi.org/10.1038/s41467-018-05772-7

Nutt SL, Hodgkin PD, Tarlinton DM, Corcoran LM (2015) The generation of antibody-secreting plasma cells. Nat Rev Immunol 15:160–171. https://doi.org/10.1038/nri3795

Rajewsky K (1996) Clonal selection and learning in the antibody system. Nature 381:751–758. https://doi.org/10.1038/381751a0

Rakhymzhan A et al (2017) Synergistic strategy for multicolor two-photon microscopy: application to the analysis of germinal center reactions in vivo. Sci Rep 7:7101. https://doi.org/10.1038/s41598-017-07165-0

Schatz DG, Ji Y (2011) Recombination centres and the orchestration of V(D)J recombination. Nat Rev Immunol 11:251–263. https://doi.org/10.1038/nri2941

Yano M, Gohil S, Coleman JR, Manix C, Pirofski LA (2011) Antibodies to Streptococcus pneumoniae capsular polysaccharide enhance pneumococcal quorum sensing. MBio 2. https://doi.org/10.1128/mBio.00176-11

The Mutagenic Tetrasect

© Springer Nature Switzerland AG 2019
A. W. Maresso, *Bacterial Virulence*, https://doi.org/10.1007/978-3-030-20464-8_6

Learning Goals

Perhaps the most fearsome attribute that pathogenic bacteria possess is their ability to change. More specifically, to undergo one of four main mutagenic mechanisms that, when occurring at a high enough frequency in a population of billions or more of cells, generates the rare variant that can become the next dominant clone. The acquisition of new virulence factors, the resistance to antibiotics, and the escape from vaccination, all derive from the powers of these mutagenic forces. In this chapter, the reader will be exposed to the underlying mechanisms of mutagenesis, the ways bacteria mix and match their genomes to generate pathogenic varieties, and other cellular processes that control virulence at genomic and post-genomic levels.

6.1 Introduction

What is the greatest predator of humans? Some would say sharks – they kill about 100 people a year worldwide. Others might say tigers – there are approximately 1000 fatalities due to large cats annually. Attacks from bears and wolves are harder to pin down but it is unlikely total deaths from these animals are much higher than large cats. All of these beasts invoke fear that is unmistakable. If you are swimming in the open ocean or hiking through dense jungle where these animals are endemic, you are likely to have them on your mind. But considering that there are nearly eight billion people in the world today, one can reasonably conclude that the fear is unfounded. You are, statistically speaking, not likely to be killed by a shark or tiger or any other animal for that matter in your lifetime. You are unlikely to know anyone that has been killed such an animal. More people are accidently electrocuted in a year in the U.S. than are killed by wild animals. As a species, most of us have long foregone the hunter-gatherer type of existence that would have put us in harm's way. Now, the comfort of a village or city and home with roof and door offer more dangers than wild animals.

The above description does not mean human beings are not preyed upon. We are. There is one form of life that reigns in this context, but goes unnoticed as a predator because, well, it can't be seen like a shark or tiger. The visual impact is simply nullified by its invisible form. Nevertheless, pathogenic bacteria kill five to eight million people a year, a number that is likely much lower than the actual burden because record keeping globally is poor. No single animal, natural disaster, or war takes more human lives on a consistent basis than do infectious microorganisms, especially bacteria. In fact, up to a third of world-wide deaths may in some way be related to infection of some type. There is good reason why bacteria would evolve to prey upon *H. sapiens*. Think about the nearly limitless supply of nutrients your blood and tissues will provide to bacteria in the weeks to months after you die. Even when still alive and confronted with the immune system and nutrient sequestration, bacteria still can multiply to high levels in your tissues. It is readily established that the causative agent of anthrax disease, *Bacillus anthracis*, can grow to levels approaching 10^{10} organisms per 1 ml of blood. Not inconceivable is it that those ten billion organisms in that drop of blood originated from a single cell whose progeny used the vast nutrients available to grow and divide.[1] On a mass basis, a single human being has, on average, 6^{17} more mass than a single bacterial cell. This is a lot of mass, in the form of critical amino acids, lipids, sugars, and metals, for a bacterium to tap into to make many progeny. In essence, your body is a smorgasbord of goodies, and if you are dead, these goodies are free. It is doubtful your first worry when swimming in the ocean or walking a forest at night is bacteria, but given the numbers, it probably should be.

Not only are bacteria the greatest predator of *H. sapiens*, they are also its most ravenous scavenger. Prior to the days of embalming or otherwise preserving our dead, all human beings that have ever died in the open countryside where temperatures were above freezing have been consumed inside-out by bacteria. The gut microbes as well as those on our skin and other crevices must spread when their living host dies. The breakdown and fermentation of the dying host accelerates the decaying process, thereby providing nutrients for bacterial blooms. The expansion of the abdomen of a dead elephant in the hot savannah countryside or the floating ballooned whale in the open ocean, made by the gases bacteria produce as they metabolize and grow, is an example of the consumptive power of bacteria. They are nature's cleansing agents, their hunger shaping entire ecosystems, path-makers for new life to take its place, only to grow biomass and eventually be consumed again.

Stopping the bacterial predation on unsuspecting humans has not been an easy task, but great strides have been made in the past hundred years by *H. sapiens*. We have to address them here because in doing so it sets the discussion for why bacteria are such successful disease-causing agents. An appreciation for the underlying mechanisms of their pathogenicity as a way of life is essential knowledge for all successful microbe hunters.

6.2 The Trinity of Anti-bacterial Technology

There are three main technological inventions that have dramatically reduced the worldwide mortality from bacterial diseases (▢ Fig. 6.1). The first is **civil engineering**. Water purification and food processing facilities, as well as human waste treatment plants and basic plumbing, decrease the risk of ingestion of deadly gastrointestinal bacteria. As such, common life-threatening diseases such as dysentery (shigella), salmonellosis (salmonella), and cholera (vibrio), for the most part, are infrequent in the developed world. The air we breathe is safer as well. Ventilation is another engineering feat that decreases risk from the air. HVAC systems are a common mechanical feature of closed quarters, and some are designed to either capture particles or direct the air external to the facility. Such practices can protect against bacterial infections like tuberculosis and pneumonia. Face masks on health care personnel decreases transmission in hospitals

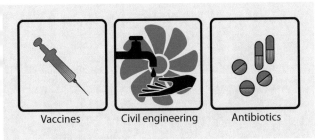

Fig. 6.1 The trinity of antibacterial technology. Vaccines, civil engineering, and antibiotics have had a substantial impact on decreasing the worldwide mortality to bacterial infections

and clinics, as do sterile gloves and instruments. As a result, the number of infections caused by bacteria one "catches" from the outside, that is the environment, has precipitously dropped in the preceding ten decades.

The second major technological advance that has led to a world-wide decrease in deaths from bacterial infection is **vaccination**. Diptheria, tetanus, and pertussis, all caused by bacterial infections, are completely preventable with a vaccine given during childhood. Including measles vaccination, this practice alone is estimated by the World Health Organization to save between two and three million lives each year. Other vaccines that are not a part of the normal childhood regime but are recommended for select populations or under certain circumstances have also been helpful in decreasing mortality. This includes the meningococcal vaccine for students living in college dormitories or in areas where the outbreaks are common, the cholera vaccine for those travelling to areas endemic with the disease, and a vaccine for tuberculosis which, albeit not universally protective, might offer enough protection to lower mortality and achieve so-called herd immunity.[2] We talk more of vaccine in ▶ Chap. 16.

The third major technological advance is the discovery of **antibiotics**, beginning with Alexander Fleming's finding, after a summer away from the laboratory, that a mold growing on his petri dish had killed the surrounding staphylococcal colonies. The widespread synthesis and mass production of penicillin in 1942 generated a booming industrial sector focused on small molecule chemical synthesis. Nowadays, upwards of 100 different antibiotics can be used in patients suspected of having a bacterial infection, and seven major chemical classes have been uncovered. Penicillin itself may have saved the lives of greater than 80 million people since its inception. The Center for Disease Control of the United States estimates 4 out of 5 Americans take at least one antibiotic regime a year. Added to everything from livestock and agriculture to soaps and toys, perhaps unnecessarily, these diverse chemicals complete the technological trinity that keep bacteria at bay. Antibiotics, like civil engineering and vaccination, have become a permanent feature of modern society. We cover antibiotics in ▶ Chap. 15.

Yet still, in one of the most technologically developed nations in the world, the United States, where the antibacterial trinity is maximized, there were over one million cases of bacterial sepsis last year (2018). How can this be?

Children are vaccinated early. If they get sick from a bacterial invader, they can be given antibiotics, and, for the most part, their water and food is free of the bacteria that in the past could have taken their life.

The simple answer is that the paradigm for the underlying causes of bacterial infections has changed. Whereas developed nations face less of a threat from bacteria from our outside environment – the physical space immediately around us – we have nearly forgotten about the ones that live in and on us. These bacteria, especially adapted to their human hosts, have evolved clever ways to circumvent the immune system. This makes vaccination against these species more challenging; and, since they live on our skin, in our noses, our lungs, and perhaps, most importantly, our gastrointestinal tract, they are unlikely to be cleared by civil engineering approaches alone. We can't bleach our intestines. What about antibiotics? In some cases, they have become obsolete, with strains resistant to their effects emerging on a nearly constant basis. It would seem that the trinity of antibacterial technology – engineering, vaccination, and antibiotics – has reached the point of diminishing returns. The trinity gets us far, but making an additional dramatic impact in reducing morbidity or mortality from bacterial infections will require us to understand why and how bacteria overcome these approaches.

6.3 Mechanisms of DNA Change and Exchange

6.3.1 *De Novo* Mutation

The key to this understanding is mutability. Simply stated, because of their ability to mutate, bacteria are the most adaptable living lifeform on Planet Earth. This mutability, which confers the potential for adaptation to a challenging environment, allows them to overcome the obstacles we have created against them. This is especially true for pathogens that are a part of our microbiome, as well as those associated with animals that live in close association with humans.

We can identify four main ways in which bacteria can change or mutate – referred to here as the **mutagenic tetrasect** (▭ Fig. 6.2) because, essentially, it is the intersection of these four processes that often leads to the generation of new "superbugs." The evolution of virulent strains, the selection of strains that colonize the human host, overcoming vaccines, survival in man-made environments, and the resistance to chemical antibiotics, can, in essence, be explained by the happenings and occurrences of these four mutagenic mechanisms.

The first is **de novo** mutation. That is, mutation that occurs by an error in the copying of the DNA code during the production of progeny. Three main types of *de novo* mutations are recognized. There are *deletions*. These occur when one or more bases of DNA are excised and nothing put in their place. There are *insertions*. These occur when one or more bases are added between two bases in an already

◼ Fig. 6.2 The mutagenic tetrasect. The mutagenic tetrasect consists of *de novo* mutation, transformation, conjugation, and transduction. Each of these means of acquiring new DNA content contributes to the spread and virulence of pathogenic bacteria

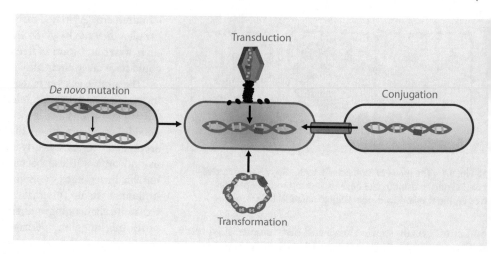

existing code. Both *deletions* and *insertions*, if occurring in the transcribed region of a gene, can alter the reading frame of that gene, leading to a truncated or completely scrambled polypeptide. Often, such changes are catastrophic for the protein, and if inherited, the gene and organism itself. If these mutations occur in the promoter region of the gene, they may alter expression. Finally, there are *substitutions*. When a substitution occurs, one of the bases is substituted with another, different base, without changing the total number of linear bases in the code. The reading frame is preserved, but the change may result in the placement of a different amino acid at that position in the expressed polypeptide.

The enzyme that copies DNA is termed DNA polymerase. DNA polymerase has a defined fidelity – it is highly accurate for the most part but does occasionally make mistakes and insert the wrong base. These mistakes are either not in a gene coding region, are in a gene but are silent (*i.e.* do to the fact that several different codons can encode for the same amino acid), are in a gene but are corrected by a built in proofreading system or other repair processes, or are in a gene but have a negative effect on that gene's overall function (when translated into a protein). So, in general, *de novo* mutation may be quite detrimental to the bacterial cell.

But some *de novo* mutations are beneficial, a good thing for the bacterium, but a problem for us. The best example of this is resistance to antibiotics. A single mutation in the enzyme that encodes β-lactamase, the enzyme that degrades penicillin, can make it refractory to inhibition with the antibiotic clavulanic acid. If the lactamase is not inhibited, it can degrade the penicillin and this will make the bacterium resistant to treatment with penicillin. Thousands of mutations of this type, all conferring some level of resistance to antibiotics, have been described in the scientific literature. Many of these mutations arose as an accident, and, because bacteria divide so rapidly, they are selected for survival because that mutation conferred an advantage in an environment rich in antibiotics. Those strains that lacked the mutation were less fit and die off. *De novo* mutation can also select for strains in measurable, real-world time frames. If one is taking antibiotics, if antibiotics are pumped into our livestock or agriculture, or

used in household items, etc., resistant variants can be readily enriched and become the dominant players in an environment saturated with these practices. Since the strain cannot be killed with antibiotics, the ability to defeat the drugs we throw at them also promote their virulence.

6.3.2 Gene Transfer, Laterally

The second way bacteria can evolve is through horizontal (sometimes termed "lateral") gene transfer. There are three main mechanisms described. The first is **transformation**. This is the process by which the cell acquires entire chunks of DNA, often in the form of a replication-competent, circular plasmid. These plasmids or DNA elements may have been released from dead or dying bacterial cells in the surrounding neighborhood. Cells that can take in DNA like this are said to be **competent**. Competency refers to the process by which bacterial cells naturally acquire large pieces of free DNA. Not all bacteria can do this, but many can, including those that live in the gastrointestinal tract of mammals. The acquisition of plasmids can provide a momentous selective advantage to bacteria. Plasmids range in size from very small (a couple of kilobase pairs with only one, two or three open reading frames) to quite large (hundreds of kilobases harboring a hundred or more genes). Using the above example of a β-lactamase, a bacterium that lacks this gene will be highly susceptible to β-lactam antibiotics such as penicillin. However, the β-lactamase gene is often encoded on mobile plasmids; a bacterium that acquires a plasmid containing one, when suddenly exposed to antibiotics, will certainly have a selective advantage over those that do not. The benefit of acquiring a plasmid is that entire genes can be attained at once and quickly. It may have taken millions of years for that gene to have evolved separately on its own. Through transformation, bacterial cells can skip this arduous process and acquire immediate versatility by harnessing genomic content that has already been invented. Transformation is a powerful mutagenic force.

Plasmids can transfer more than genes that confer resistance to antibiotics. In many cases, a sizable fraction of the genes encoded on the plasmid, may in some way, enhance the virulence of its bacterial carrier, or may be responsible for most, if not all, the virulence. For example, the causative agent of anthrax (*B. anthracis*) somehow acquired two large, approximately 100-gene each, plasmids. One of these plasmids encodes a protective capsule that resists the host immune system. The other encodes for anthrax toxin, which disables the host immune system. The loss of both plasmids renders bacilli avirulent. Since the infection and extensive replication of bacilli in vertebrates is an absolute necessity to continue its life-cycle, these plasmids clearly enhance its survivability and environmental dissemination. Often times, entire **pathogenicity islands**, or clusters of virulence factors that enhance virulence, are encoded on plasmids, and their shuffling between bacterial hosts is a way to quickly acquire new sets of virulence systems that would otherwise take a long time to independently evolve. Plasmids encode all types of virulence factors, including toxins, adhesins, secretion systems, and nutrient uptake systems.

The third mechanism by which bacteria can evolve to be virulent is through **conjugation**. Conjugation is the process by which one live bacterium delivers DNA directly to a recipient bacterium via a **conjugative filament**. It is often described as the prokaryotic version of sex. The conjugative filament resembles a long cylindrical rod, similar to a pilus, that connects the donor to the recipient. Pili are discussed in the next chapter. After pairing, DNA is transferred through the rod into the recipient cell in a linear fashion. The recipient can then either keep the DNA as a free existing extrachromosomal plasmid or integrate the DNA into the bacterial chromosome.

The fourth and final means by which bacteria can change their genome is through **transduction**. As amazing a predator as bacteria are, they themselves are also the victim of predation. The predators of bacteria are viruses called bacteriophage ("bacteria eating"). Phage are quite possibly the most numerous self-replicating entity on Earth. A 1 with 31 zeroes following it inhabit our oceans, lakes, ponds, forests, soil, and even atmosphere. Upon infection of a suitable bacterial host, they deliver their nucleic acid into the bacterial cytoplasm. The phage DNA has two fates. It either directs the synthesis of new phage that are assembled on the spot in the cytoplasm, or it integrates into the bacterial genome. The former is called a **lytic phage** infection while the latter is referred to as **lysogeny**. Lysogenized viral DNA can lay dormant for many generations until a trigger, usually a cell stress, induces it to be excised and code for the assembly of a virion. Discovered in 1952 by Joshua Lederberg and team, transduction was used to identify DNA as the "transforming principle", *i.e.* the material that directed the cell to be a cell. This event revolutionized biomedical science because it meant that DNA was the unit of heredity. The point here is that when new phage are made in the bacterial cytoplasm, the viral nucleic acid is packaged into the head of the virus. Sometimes, bacterial DNA gets accidentally packaged as well, so that when the virus infects a new bacterial host, that bacterial DNA is brought into the cytoplasm of the recipient cell. If the DNA confers an advantage to the new cell, it may be retained.

6.4 Virulence Strategies Based on Genomic Alterations

6.4.1 Gain and Loss of Genes

These four means to mutation (*de novo* changes, transformation, conjugation, and transduction) are the overarching ways the mutagenic tetrasect commands the evolution of virulence. Under each of these global processes lie any of a dozen different molecular mechanisms that induce change, often involving more than one of these themes. For instance, transformation, conjugation, and transduction can lead to the gain or loss of a gene. **Additive evolution** is where bacteria gain a gene and retain that gene if natural selection determines it is beneficial to the fitness of the bacterium. A good example of additive evolution is the acquisition of a protein toxin. Several bacterial species were made more virulent by acquiring a toxin. In some cases, the toxin is so important for disease that its deletion results in a strain that is avirulent. The successful childhood vaccination programs against pertussis, diphtheria, and tetanus are good examples of primarily toxigenic diseases that can be eliminated if the vaccine against them includes their toxins as antigens. ◘ Figure 6.3 illustrates the many ways the genome of a bacterial pathogen can be modified.

Quite the opposite, reductive evolution results in greater fitness when a gene or genes are lost. Some bacteria, particularly prominent human pathogens such as *M. tuberculosis* or various rickettsia species, have established themselves as stable pathogens with extremely small genomes. They are both **obligate intracellular** bacteria and thus *must* infect host cells to survive. The shedding of excess genetic elements (or the rejection of a growing genome) has clearly been beneficial; their niche is so restricted that they have become experts at occupying it, including using host nutrients and host functions that they usurp as their own. By losing key biosynthetic elements that would make nutrients they can simply take from the host, for example, they save the energy and burden of having to carry these pathways themselves. Resources and energy can be directed elsewhere, perhaps towards evolving systems that avoid or detoxify phagolysosomes, which are needed to survive in such a hostile place. Think of a soldier moving quietly amongst enemy territory. The lighter, swifter, and quieter that he is, the more likely his success. A soldier with fifty pounds of clunky and heavy gear might be detected. A basic theme here is that if the host can provide the function, there may not be a need for the invading bacterium to have evolved it by themselves.. These bacteria have streamlined their genome for maximal efficiency.

6

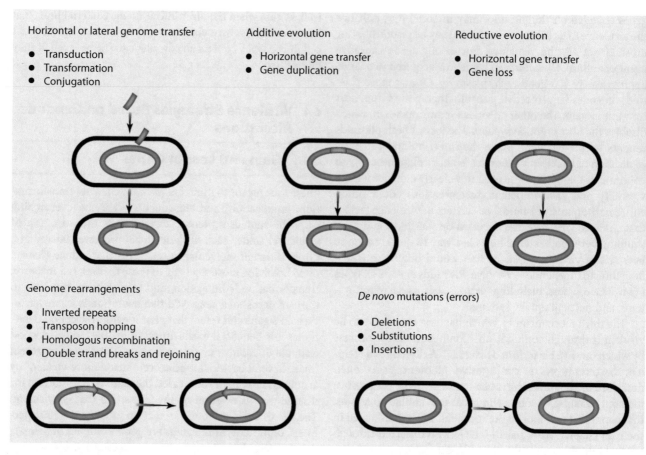

Fig. 6.3 Genome modifications that alter the virulence of pathogenic bacteria. Additive and reduction evolution generate bacterial genomes that are streamlined to be efficient for survival in specific niches. Significant genome modifications include those mediated by horizontal gene transfer, including transduction, transformation, and conjugation. A level below these are genome rearrangements and include inversions, mobile transposons, DNA breaks/rejoining, and homologous recombination. The simplest types of mutations include deletions, substitutions, and insertions

6.4.2 Phase Variation

Additive and reductive evolution represent the extremes of the manipulation of gene content. There are far more subtle systems in place to change virulence, including regulatory mechanisms that control the expression levels of genes. One of these ways is called **phase variation** and it represents a type of molecular switch that bacteria use to toggle genes on or off ("phase on or off"). This control can be very advantageous to bacteria. One might imagine a situation whereby an important protein on the bacterial surface might be harmful to the bacterium if the immune system can recognize it as a prominent antigen. Turning the expression of the gene off for a part of the infection (perhaps when it is less needed) and then turning it back on at another point in the infection when most needed ensures virulence is specialized for the situation at hand. Binary systems such as this confer a rapid ability to adapt, and adaptability is the hallmark of a bacterium's survivability. Some of the most significant elements involved in virulence and discussed throughout this work are regulated by phase variation, including adhesive factors such as pili and fimbriae, outer membrane proteins important for nutrient uptake, flagella for bacterial movement, the capsule,

and the production of lipopolysaccharide, the latter to avoid recognition by the immune system.

Phase variation leads to a number of genomic changes that are very important for pathogenesis. Broadly speaking, there are two distinct types of phase changes at the genomic level; those that lead to a change in the DNA code (**genomic modification**) and those that do not (**epigenomic modification**). Both are inheritable and in many cases reversible. It is these properties that allow for adaptation on a single cell basis. They are powerful drivers of virulence.

Phase variation that leads to a change in the DNA code (genomic modification) is quite diverse. One type is **DNA inversion**. During this mechanism, the DNA around the promoter of a gene is actually inverted in its 5 to 3 prime orientation. The inversion of the DNA alters the activity of the promoter. In most cases, an inversion event turns the promoter "off." This is mediated by a specialized enzyme termed a **recombinase**; it recombines the DNA in a way that leads to that DNA being inverted. Often, the recombinase is part of a larger multi-gene element and specifically acts on the genes in that element. The classic example of this is the regulation of the Fim pilus, a common system present in many Gram-negative bacterial pathogens, including *E. coli* and

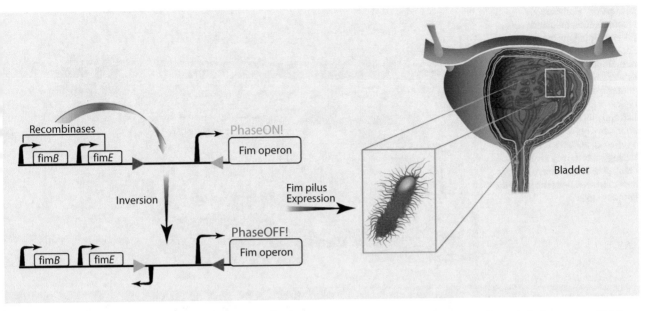

Fig. 6.4 Phase variation of pili tip proteins. One way to disguise an important surface protein from the immune system is to compartmentalize its expression. Uropathogenic *E. coli*, a subset of extraintestinal pathogenic *E. coli*, adjusts the expression of the pilus tip protein FimH via the inversion of a DNA element that includes its promoter. This is mediated by two Fim recombinases encoded upstream of the FimH, whose activity inverts the promoter leading to gene repression

salmonella. The pilus is a long fimbrial structure that extends from the bacterial surface; the end of this long tentacle can bind to receptors on host tissues or cells. The tip is also a highly immunogenic antigen that may be recognized by specialized mucosal cells that aid in antigen processing. Upstream of one of the pilus assembly proteins is an invertible DNA element that encodes the promoter for the gene in question. This element can be recognized by the recombinase which will invert the arrangement of the DNA in the exact opposite direction inactivating the production of the pilus protein. By controlling when this event occurs, the expression of the pilus fimbriae is controlled. Since antigen processing cells are present in the intestine but less so in the bladder, it is thought this may allow *E. coli* to avoid antigen presentation in the intestine but then turn the pilus on when needed to stick to the bladder cells during urinary tract infection. This concept is illustrated in Fig. 6.4.

Another phase variation mechanism that results in genomic modification is **homologous recombination**. In this mechanism, two very similar sequences of DNA within the same genome can base pair together. Another type of recombinase facilitates a "crossover event" where one strand invades the physical space of the other and vice versa resulting in a seamless swapping of the two sequences at the two genomic locations. The elegance of this system is on full display in *N. gonorrhea* and the regulation of one of its pilus tip proteins. Because the tip protein contains the part that touches host cells, having the ability to change its structure depending on its need to bind or hide from immune recognition is important. Using homologous recombination, the main pilus protein can swap out various N-terminal portions of its tip using several transcriptionally silent genes located elsewhere on the genome. When these N-terminal segments are fused to the main frame of the pilus via this mechanism, it results in a pilus different than the original (Fig. 6.5). It is believed this can result in up to a million different variants, certainly enough diversity to confuse the host immune system.

The last phase variation mechanism that results in genomic modification includes **slipped-strand mispairing** (SSM). This modification of the DNA only occurs during replication or repair of the bacterial genome. It occurs when repeat sequences in the genome "confuse" the DNA polymerase such that a single nucleotide is slipped into or out of the replicated DNA, resulting in a single base change. If this occurs in the area of a gene's promoter or open reading frame, it can have a dramatic impact on the production of that gene.

Finally, for adaptations that do not involve a change in the DNA code, but which can affect the expression of virulence genes, we turn to **epigenomic modification**. Here, the DNA is chemically modified, the chemical moiety in this case a methyl group and the process of modifying the DNA termed **methylation**. Methylation is performed by a specific enzyme called a methyltransferase. The methyltransferase will add a methyl group to the promoter of a gene. This represents a bulky modification such that the normal transcription factor that activates the production of the message of the gene is blocked from doing so, usually through physical interference. The result is the suppression of the expression of that gene. A good example of this is the Pap adhesin in *E. coli*. By methylating the promoter of this element, Pap becomes transcriptionally silent (not expressed). It is presumed that shutting the gene down in this way, which can be controlled by regulating the production of the methyltransferase, allows the bacterium to turn off expression when it is advantageous to do so (Fig. 6.6).

6

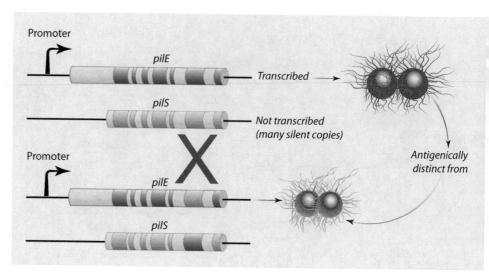

■ **Fig. 6.5** Homologous recombination mediating new pili elements. One mechanism of DNA rearrangement is through homologous recombination of similar DNA sequences. In *N. gonorrhea*, exchange of a small region of DNA between the genes pilE and pilS leads to new arrangements of pili that are antigenically distinct. This strategy, which may result in many possible combinations of new pili, helps neisseria avoid the immune system

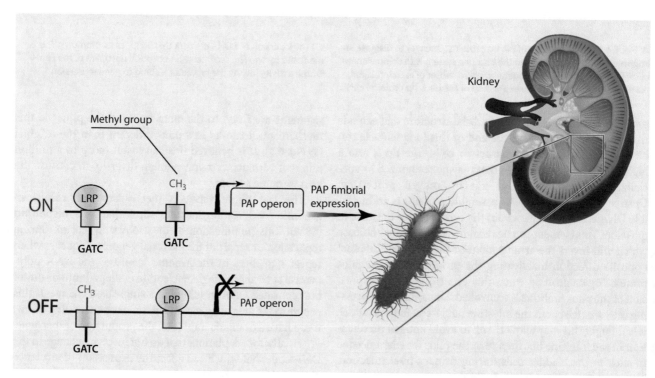

■ **Fig. 6.6** Modification of pili expression through epigenetic mechanisms. The PAP pilus (see ▶ Chap. 7) is controlled by methylation of its promoter. In the phase ON position, the Lrp protein prevents methylation by Dam methylase of an adenine residue in the first GATC sequence of the promoter, thereby maintaining its ability to be transcribed. However, upon methylation of the first GATC sequence after binding of Lrp to the second, transcription is repressed and the PAP pilus is not made. This fimbrial system is known to be important for infection of uropathogenic *E. coli* of the kidney

6.4.3 Duplication and Redundancy

Phase variation is understudied as a mechanism of variance of virulence. But its impact is one of the main reasons why traditional therapeutic measures developed against such bacteria, especially vaccines, have largely been unsuccessful. There are other ways the modification of the genome alters virulence. This includes **gene duplication**. Sometimes, the presence of two genes of similar function is better than just a single copy of that gene. Although duplication may occur from a gene the bacterium already harbors, similar or related genes can also be acquired from exogenous sources using the mechanisms described above. Gene duplication leads to what is sometimes called **functional redundancy**, namely, that although the actual DNA sequence might be quite variant, especially as more and more time passes following the duplication event, the overall function is still highly conserved. Genes that differ by as much as 70% at the DNA level can still be nearly identical functionally, especially if highly important amino acids or domains remain conserved. In general, gene duplication can serve two main purposes, which are not mutually exclusive. First, two may be better than one. If a bacterial pathogen finds itself in an environment in the host where nutrients may be plentiful, then having two genetically different but functionally redundant transporters both working full-speed to import the nutrient may increase the replication rate of the pathogen. Since it is often growth versus how well the immune system can kill, this can be seen as an advantage. Second, during this replication, a gene may become damaged (phage-mediated excision, *de-novo* mutation, *etc*). Having two copies that are functionally redundant ensures at least some of this basic property will be present. Using the surface transporters here as an example, it is not uncommon for bacterial pathogens to have half a dozen related transporters for a similar or family of structurally related ligands.

Out of the Box
Homo Errorless

Thinking about the biology of bacteria, particularly their replicative rate and evolution, can stimulate insights into the biology of other organisms, particularly those much more complex. This is especially true when pondering the topics of mutation, selection, evolution, and disease. Bacteria are single-celled organisms, but their fundamental biology still adheres to the laws of evolutionary change, as all cells do. Sometimes one can see a bit clearer because of their simplicity, without the more complex phenomena that define eukaryotes mudding the water. Because bacteria replicate in real-time, because their generation can be 20 min instead of 20 years, one can follow how the mutations they acquire make them better adapted to the environment in which they currently find themselves. If one had the objective of say preventing bacterial resistance to antibiotics, one might suggest that a strategy that stops bacteria from acquiring mutations during their division would eliminate *de novo* adaptation to antibiotics. This is not too difficult a premise to defend. We know some resistance occurs with such changes, so assuming horizontal gene transfer is not occurring, it must be true that preventing mutations will prevent resistance. It is simply one cell to two to a million and all the accumulated mutations in between, and selection for a rare change that resists the antibiotic, followed by clonal expansion, that drives the phenotype.

Now imagine, for the sake of argument, one replaced bacterial cells with cells of your own body. It need not matter the type of cell; all of them are governed by the same natural laws. As your own cells replicate, just like in bacteria, they acquire mutations. The right combination of these mutations, built up with each successive replication, and ongoing for the trillion cells in your body, will also lead to a cell that is more fit than the rest. Perhaps it divides faster (thus more progeny are produced with time) or perhaps it is more efficient in acquiring nutrients than the others, or more so, perhaps it finds ways to avoid its own timed suicide or recognition by the immune system. Like a bacterial cell acquiring a mutation that destroys the antibiotics makes it more fit in their presence, this eukaryotic cell will expand and grow and dominate the population inside of you.

This is cancer.

Of course, it is a very rare event. But, there are enough mutations occurring in just enough cells that, over one's lifetime, a unique combination of mutations arises that produces a more fit lineage. Much like a bacterial population undergoing selection in the face of antibiotic pressure, driven of course by mutation, cancer cells use acquired mutations to outgrow their normal cellular niche.

Whereas there are many mechanisms by which mutations can be created (see this chapter for examples), there seems to be only two ways to *induce* a mutation in a eukaryotic cell. The first way is by living in an imperfect, and rather damaging, environment. These include all possible mutagens. Examples are ultraviolet light, cigarette smoke, asbestos, and even viruses and bacteria. They indirectly or directly induce changes in your DNA. Environmentally induced mutagenesis includes single or multi-base substitutions, insertions or deletions or other rearrangements including inversions and misplacements in other regions of the genome. Your cells understand that the environment can do this and have built a repair system, termed the mismatch repair system (MMR), that recognizes these mutations and corrects them. It's not perfect though and some slip by, being inherited by the daughter cell when the parent divides. With enough misses, these mutations grow in number.

There is one other way you can acquire mutations. You make mistakes. These are not induced by the environment. They come from within. Just like in bacteria, your DNA polymerase, as it makes a single copy of DNA, will make an error every 10 or 100 million bases synthesized. Just as with mutations induced by the environment, you have evolved compensatory mechanisms to correct these errors. DNA polymerase too has a proof-reading function. Thus, even though for every three billion bases per replicative event you can acquire about 30 mutations, you don't. Some of these mistakes are noticed, and polymerase corrects them itself or the MMR finishes the job.

But not all of them. Over time, with thousands upon thousands of replications, these mutations accumulate in daughter cells. The right mutations in combination with other mutations in the right cells yields cancer.

But what if you could avoid mutations all together? What if every time you replicated your DNA, there were no errors? What if when the environment induced mutations in your DNA, the MMR system fixed it every time? If your DNA was always replicated with complete fidelity and every environmental insult was fixed, would you ever get cancer? Since mutations acquired over time lead to altered proteins (and even their altered expression, up or down), and since proteins are the machines of all cellular life, the more amino acid changes a protein has, the more likely these proteins will perform their job less optimally. If most proteins in some way are impacted functionally by these changes, and these changes accrue with time, the organism, and all its integrated parts, will also become less efficient and functional with time. So, in many ways, it would seem that this concept would also be the primary driver of aging.

Where the real problem occurs is when these mutations occur in the cells that beget all other cells – the stem cells. When they acquire *de novo* mutations via error, or induced mutations via the environment, every cell they produce will have these mutations. They become a continuous source of mutated cells. It would seem that it is the stem cells that must be protected … or enhanced.

How? If the main enzyme and accessory subunits for DNA polymerase and MMR for example were engineered in the laboratory to be a little more efficient at catching and repairing mistakes, in theory, there would be less mutations per replicative event and less mutations induced by the environment. Look no further than bacteria for the suggestion this can be achieved. Molecular biology companies sell an engineered DNA polymerase from a bacterium that makes high fidelity PCR products. We already know that if the polymerase makes more errors than usual, and MMR itself is mutated and less capable, animals (including humans) with these changes acquire cancer more readily. It would thus seem that doing the opposite, making these enzymes better, would decrease the mutation rate. This may lead to less cancer and prolonged life. It stands to reason then that engineered enzymes that never allowed a single mutation to occur in all stem cell populations in a human would never develop cancer and, just perhaps, never age.

If we begin to accept that we can use tools of molecular biology to "edit" deleterious germline mutations, already being attempted for inherited mutations, it is not too much of a stretch to argue that all new human embryos should be constructed with enhanced copies of the genes that code for these highly fidel repair enzymes. It simply would become standard practice for everyone prior to implantation and birth. Because of the inherent complexity of all cancers, again, arising from mutations in unique combinations, it would also seem that each treatment for them would need to be tailored to that cancer. In fact, T-cell therapy is just this. But if one could simply prevent mutations from forming in the first place, no treatment would be needed. The cure would not be treatment, it would be prevention. In some ways, this parallels what we have accomplished with modern vaccination programs against bacteria, another lesson learned from bacteria that applies to other diseases. The only difference here is you are preventing the disease by replacing the wild-type copies of the fidelity and repair enzymes in the embryo. They then do their job for life. Even a marginal improvement of each of their activity, when additive, might bring down the mutation rate below the average number of mutations needed to start cancer in all cells, and prolong life considerably.

Of course, this argument merely stresses the importance of learning from bacteria to understand higher eukaryotes. It says nothing about the ethics of the concept. Whether or not you want to live another 500 years is another debate.

6.5   Regulation of Virulence

Bacterial cells have sensing systems. These systems are located in their surface membranes. The signal is received by a protein at the membrane and transduced to proteins inside the cell. These transducers then may themselves alter gene expression or recruit another protein to do so. The signal that these systems respond to can be quite diverse. Truthfully, the microbe hunter knows very little about such signals and how they trigger bacterial sensing systems (at least from the standpoint of the interaction on the bacteria surface), but some signals are known and rather obvious. These include temperature, pH, osmolarity, membrane stress, and small solutes that may be present in the host environment. What may be unique about pathogenic bacteria is they sense the signals that are specific for "host" and can tell them from a myriad of other "environmental" signals that are not host. Temperature is a good example. A healthy human body maintains an internal temperature of 37 degrees F. When moving from a colder environment to one that holds this temperature, a pathogenic bacterium knows that it must prepare for its new environment of being in a host.

6.5.1   Components … Two

How do bacteria do this? The most prevalent mechanism is the **two-component system**. The name gives away its form; they are indeed composed to two components, linked to one another, and with each component serving an important but distinct function. The first component is the **sensor kinase**. It often resides in the membrane of the bacterial cell. More specifically, it is a histidine kinase. We know from the elegant lessons of mammalian cell biology studies that kinases transfer signals via chemistry. The chemistry in this case is a phosphate group transferred from the kinase to a recipient protein. This recipient may then transfer that signal further down the line (like a baton relay race) or may adopt a function induced by the modification at which point the signal would have been converted into an output of some type. A two-component system works the same way. The histidine kinase, being localized to the membrane, will bind the chemical stimuli, and undergo some type of conformational change (the presence of the ligand being transmitted via structural changes down the polypeptide mainframe to the histidine kinase domain where it induces its own autophosphoryation on the histidine residue). The second component, termed the **response regulator**, will then receive the phosphate group from the sensor domain in the form of the phosphorylation of an aspartic acid in its receiver domain. This is a key step. Often times, it is the phosphorylation of this residue that turns the response regulator into an actionable protein. Many response regulators are transcription factors themselves. Their phosphorylation will change their affinity for DNA, either making it stronger or weakening it. Depending on whether binding is an activator of the start of transcription or as a repressor of it, the net effect is the turning on or off of a gene or set of genes. If these genes happen to be toxins, or adhesins, or nutrient transporters, for example, the original chemical signal has been successfully converted into a bacterial response that directly influences the virulence potential of the bacterium. An example of a two component system is illustrated in ▫ Fig. 6.7.

Two-component regulatory systems are not restricted to transitions to a pathogenic state. Indeed, most of the greater than 5000 such systems identified in the sequenced genomes of bacteria are likely to have a main function independent of mammalian hosts. This includes environmental sensing in other ecological niches of non-pathogens, such as lakes, rivers, streams, the soil, on plants, and rocks and so forth. There are clear examples though of their involvement in pathogenesis, probably more so than is known about the signals that

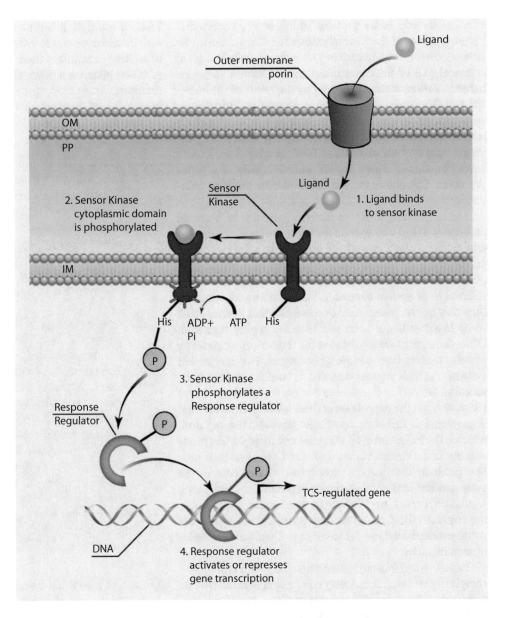

■ **Fig. 6.7** Bacterial two-component systems. The bacterial TCS is a versatile way to rapidly respond to changing conditions. A sensor kinase in the inner membrane binds a ligand in the periplasm, an event converted into a chemical signal with the phosphorylation of the cytoplasmic domain of the sensor kinase. This signal is then transferred to a response regulator which may directly or indirectly effect gene expression

stimulate their phosphor-relay cascades. Host signals that activate these systems include metals (discussed in ► Chap. 11), the afore mentioned temperature, dissolved gases, and pH (especially if low as may be encountered in a maturing phagolysosome). There are dozens of reports that link the engineered deletion of such systems to defects in virulence in animal models or host cell lines. Less clear is the reason for such attenuation, although some include reduction in the ability of bacteria to invade host cells (► Chap. 8), production of flagella and adhesins (► Chap. 7), modification of surface polysaccharides including LPS and capsule structure, and nutrient uptake (► Chap. 11).

6.5.2 Central Regulators and Regulons

Another way the genome can be modified to aid in virulence is by building in regulatory toggles. The host environment is very complex and may change on a moment's notice. These changes can be deadly to a growing bacterium. The ability to quickly regulate entire clusters of genes after sensing these changes provides a substantial fitness advantage. It is not surprising then that for most major human pathogens where this topic has been studied we find **central regulators** of virulence. These regulators are of course proteins, cytosolic in that, and often are transcriptional enhancers or repressors. Sometimes, they can be both. The central modulator does exactly what its name implies; it modulates the state of the cell by effecting transcription of key genes after it has received a stimulus. The stimulus can be specific for the environment it is in and, depending on the nature of the stimulus, the modulator will go down one path or another. Often, these modulators are **allosterically** regulated. That is, the stimulus may be a small molecule ligand (a nucleotide, an amino acid, a sugar etc.) that binds to the modulator and alters its function, usually by effecting its affinity for DNA. Here we see that by simply binding or not binding the ligand one can directly control what the modulator does. Other allosteric

6

effectors include entire proteins (think of a complex that becomes activated upon complexation) and even post-translational covalent modifications (phosphorylation is a good example). All of these can direct the modulator to toggle between various states depending on the needs of the bacterial cell. These modulators often recognize specific signals embedded in the DNA of the bacterium, sort of an airstrip instructing them as to the genes they should bind. These platforms, usually short stretches of DNA ranging from 5 to 20 bases, are almost always located in the vicinity of a gene's promoter. This allows for great control over the gene transcription.

Lastly, one might expect that the genomes of bacterial pathogens would also encode for integrated systems or protein machine complexes whose function as a unit would be greater than would otherwise be possible for a single gene product to accomplish alone. This type of nucleation can be referred to as **system assembly**. Such systems are complex; they may be composed of 20 or more different proteins that come together like a Lego set. They are highly regulated. Often times, they are regulated at the transcriptional level by proteins that respond to some type of signal. Two component systems and their cognate transducers (which are often transcription factors) and central regulators (as outlined above) are most often the puppeteers of these systems. The unit that is regulated is called, appropriately enough, the **regulon**, which is the collection of all the genes and their protein products under the control of that regulator. Genes and their protein products that partake directly in the virulence of the pathogen are termed a **virulence regulon**. In most cases, regulation occurs by binding to the regulon's promoter, thereby activating or repressing gene transcription. The pathogenicity islands we discussed in ▶ Chap. 2 are examples of such regulons.

Regulons can include system assemblies with remarkable complexity and elegance. A very good example is the type III secretion system used by a number of Gram-negative bacteria to inject effector proteins into host cells (secretion systems are discussed more in ▶ Chap. 9). The Yersinia system, which looks like a syringe and needle extending from the bacterial surface, may transport up to 20 different bacterial effector proteins into the host milieu or directly into the host cytoplasm. The base of the system is anchored to the bacterial membrane, therefore giving it stability. The cytosolic side engages the outgoing effectors to be secreted using specialized chemistry to solve the problem of protein folding during and after transport. The needle portion delivers the effector across a host space that may be damaging to the bacterial effector, thereby protecting it during transit. This also ensures that the effector gets to where it is supposed to go and does not diffuse away, which would be inefficient. The tip of the needle uses additional chemistry to make a hole in the host cell. Finally, the effector gets into the host cell and carries out an enzymatic function that will benefit the bacterium and disable the host. Once assembled, the amount of effectors injected can be controlled, as well as the order of injection.

Thus, if multiple different effectors each having a specific activity and mission are delivered, they can be delivered in an order that maximizes their effectiveness. The bacterial flagella and pilus, each of which aid in virulence, are additional examples. Assembled nanomachines like these are weapons; knowledge of their assembly and mechanistic functions is critical to disabling them.

Summary of Key Points

1. Natural selection chooses the traits that are most likely to lead to survival of the organisms. Since survival increases the chances one will have progeny, those traits which enhance survival are also likely to be inherited by progeny.
2. Bacteria undergo mutagenesis at astounding rates, driven by the four main mutagenic mechanisms of *de novo* mutation, transformation, conjugation, and transduction.
3. These mutagenic mechanisms work against our attempts to control bacteria, including treatment with antibiotics and prevention with vaccines.
4. Virulence can be a regulated process. Virulence factors such as toxins, secretion systems, and adhesins are often found as part of pathogenicity islands. These islands can be exchanged by horizontal gene transfer. Virulence factor expression can be turned on or off through the many processes associated with genomic rearrangements.
5. Virulence can be regulated by protein toggles that act as transcription factors that sense the metabolic and environmental state of the bacterium and its host.

❓ Expand Your Knowledge

1. The director of a public health department in a small college town is investigating an outbreak of *Neisseria mengitiditis* in the college dormitory. Upon culturing the organism in Luria Broth and injection into a murine host, no virulence is observed. Another member of the unit, down the hall, is investigating the effect of lead on neuronal development and notices one day the culture media contaminated with neisseria. All the neurons are killed in a few hours. Isolation of this strain and injection into the murine hosts results in death of half of the experimental animals. Isolated strains from the half that do not die do not kill neurons. Sequencing of both strains reveals a single change of 10 bases in the promoter of what looks like an operon. Provide an explanation as to what may be happening.
2. A commonly sold intestinal probiotic strain, attainable over the internet and with claims it prevents colitis, is found associated with colitis after two dozen cases are reported to the Center

for Disease Control. Sequencing of the strain found in patient samples demonstrates it differs from the strain the company is selling in two seven base pair regions upstream from a putative restriction endonuclease system. These two elements are only found in a series of sequenced phages that were isolated from a patient with severe colitis 15 years previously. Provide an explanation as to what may be happening in patients taking the probiotic.

3. An emerging disease task force is commissioned by the World Health Organization to offer recommendations and predictions as to what may drive the evolution of virulence in bacteria as humanity encroaches further onto the environment. As part of the commission, you are asked to write a one-thousand word essay on the balance between the evolution of bacterial virulence in a human host versus its maintenance as an asymptomatic carrier. In this essay, touch upon why virulence may or may not be beneficial to the bacterial progeny that result from the infection.

Notes

1 = Studies of monkeys that have inhaled anthrax-causing spores suggest that a low infectious dose (1–10 spores) can trigger anthrax disease. There are also reports that the spores themselves may lie dormant for weeks or months after inhaled, at which point a single spore may germinate and begin the infection.

2 = Herd immunity is the concept that every member of the population need not be vaccinated for the group as a whole to have near complete prevention of the disease. By reducing the number of carriers in a population, with either incomplete vaccination of the entire population or mass vaccination with a vaccine that is partially protective, the overall rates of person to person transmission is reduced, thereby cutting down on the number of people that contract the infection.

Suggested Reading

Didelot X, Walker AS, Peto TE, Crook DW, Wilson DJ (2016) Within-host evolution of bacterial pathogens. Nat Rev Microbiol 14:150–162. https://doi.org/10.1038/nrmicro.2015.13

Hacker J, Kaper JB (2000) Pathogenicity islands and the evolution of microbes. Annu Rev Microbiol 54:641–679. https://doi.org/10.1146/annurev.micro.54.1.641

Juhas M (2015) Horizontal gene transfer in human pathogens. Crit Rev Microbiol 41:101–108. https://doi.org/10.3109/1040841X.2013.804031

Johnson TJ, Nolan LK (2009) Pathogenomics of the virulence plasmids of Escherichia coli. Microbiol Mol Biol Rev 73:750–774. https://doi.org/10.1128/MMBR.00015-09

Lane MC, Mobley HL (2007) Role of P-fimbrial-mediated adherence in pyelonephritis and persistence of uropathogenic Escherichia coli (UPEC) in the mammalian kidney. Kidney Int 72:19–25. https://doi.org/10.1038/sj.ki.5002230

Stock AM, Robinson VL, Goudreau PN (2000) Two-component signal transduction. Annu Rev Biochem 69:183–215. https://doi.org/10.1146/annurev.biochem.69.1.183

van der Woude MW, Bäumler AJ (2004) Phase and antigenic variation in bacteria. Clin Microbiol Rev 17:581–611, table of contents. https://doi.org/10.1128/CMR.17.3.581-611.2004

Bacterial Bindance: Adhesins and Their Engagement to Host

© Springer Nature Switzerland AG 2019
A. W. Maresso, *Bacterial Virulence*, https://doi.org/10.1007/978-3-030-20464-8_7

Learning Goals

In this chapter, the student will be introduced to the fundamental molecular unit of bacterial adherence, the adhesin. The interaction of bacteria with its host is framed in the context of the benefits of these interactions to bacterial survival as well as the long and short term consequences in relation to infection and disease. The organization and function of several classes of adhesins are outlined, as is their engagement of specific host ligands in the context of importance to pathogenesis. The reader will understand the diversity of strategies bacteria use to bind their host and the vulnerabilities the microbe hunter may exploit to prevent such interactions.

7.1 Introduction

Touch is fundamental to the emotional wellness of a human being. It is the difference between what is perceived as real and what is not, it is the present versus what has or has not yet happened, or what is close and what is distant. It is a state of being, if you will, allowing you to frame your current ethereal existence relative to the environment and the objects and people around you.

Such is true with bacteria. For bacteria, touch means a foothold, a landing pad, a signal that this area, this niche, might be a suitable place to live, or a hostile, caustic place where there will be challenges. It means either beginning a programmed process of adaptation to take advantage of its predicament through the utilization of resources, or a path of general inaptitude patiently waiting for conditions to change.

From the host's standpoint, the touch of a bacterium usually signals danger; be prepared and recruit friends. If it's a bacterial pathogen, and the right combination of pathogen associated molecular patterns (PAMPs) are present, touch can only really mean one thing – a possible attack or invasion. Bacterial bindance may be the point of first engagement between these two opposed beings. It is the first step towards aggression from both sides. Bacteria bind to their host and the host responds, in turn the bacteria adjust to this response and so forth. This continuous dance, in tight, intimate quarters sways back and forth until in one way or another the union is broken and the outcome either favors the pathogen or the host.

7.1.1 Adherence

When we speak of touch between bacteria and host cells, bacteria and the extracellular matrix, or bacteria and other host components, albeit those in blood or some other medium, what we really mean is **adherence**. This is the term Microbiologists use to describe the interaction of the bacterium's molecules on its surface with that of the molecules of the host. As such, the bacterial molecules that interface with the host are globally referred to as **adhesins**, a play off the word adherence. The host component that the adhesin binds is sometimes termed the **receptor** (if fixed and relatively immobile) or the **ligand** (often used in context of a more free, perhaps even diffusible, substance). The adhesin and the receptor can be as diverse as the bacterium and host themselves; proteins, lipids, sugars, and sometimes various combinations of them, form these interactions, and from both sides. Because of this diversity, no two mechanisms of adherence seem to be the same, and no two bacteria, even between closely related species, seem to use the same adhesins and mechanisms to stick to their unsuspecting host. Even within a single species, and a given strain of that species, there can be multiple adhesins and mechanisms of adherence. Most times, the word adhesion refers to a gene-encoded protein polypeptide with a binding domain that has specificity towards a host molecule, commonly a carbohydrate or a glycoprotein. The host molecule is often located on the surface of a host cell or embedded in the matrix laid down between host cells.

It may then be obvious that one strategy to prevent bacteria from invading our territory would be to prevent attachment. Indeed, small molecule inhibitors of bacterial adhesins are in development as potential antibacterial agents. There are also vaccines targeting adherence factors that have been experimentally demonstrated to be protective in animal models of infections, and some which have been entered into clinical trials. None of these approaches have received government clearance to be routinely used in the clinic yet, despite very promising results in the lab. There are many reasons why this may be true, but perhaps the most prominent of them is that Microbiologists have only scratched the surface in understanding the importance of these adhesins for various stages of the infectious process; and with so many adhesins between different species and even within the same strain, which ones should we pick? Let's foray into this area so the microbe hunter knows where we stand on the topic of bacterial adhesins as they pertain to their interactions with mammalian cells.

7.2 The Function and Consequences of Bacterial Adherence

The functional and advantageous reasons for why a pathogenic bacterium would evolve to adhere to host tissues are numerous. The first functional advantage, from the pathogen's point of view, is that adherence allows for **acute colonization**. Bacteria use adherence mechanisms as a type of catch-net. This type of adherence is one that promotes the association of the bacterium with host tissues or niches so that short-lived binding allows for just enough time to quickly utilize new resources and reproduce. A good example of this are ingested bacteria that express sticky adhesins which facilitate the association with the mucosa during transit through the intestinal tract. The bacteria that are causes of acute diarrhea, often acquired from contaminated food or water, including the pathogens that cause cholera, salmonel-

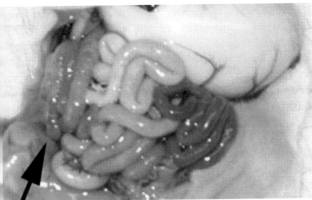
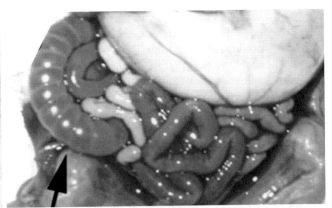

No *V. cholerae*

V. cholerae

Fig. 7.1 The excretion of pathogenic bacteria. Some pathogenic bacteria use the host as an incubator to make more progeny, of whose excretion is controlled by the bacteria themselves. Shown here is the cecum (equivalent to the large intestine of humans) of infant rabbits with (right) or without (left) infection by *V. cholerae*, an intestinal pathogen that induces massive diarrhea in its unfortunate victims. The swollen cecum on the right is due to excess fluid filling the cavity which will eventually result in diarrhea. (Adapted from Waldor et al (see *suggested readings*) under a creative commons license. (► https://creativecommons.org/licenses/by-nc-sa/3.0))

losis, and dysentery (to name a few), all are known to express adhesins that promote their capture by the many different environments of the very long (by bacterial standards) digestive system. This includes the mucosa of the mouth and esophagus, the stomach, and the four segments of the intestine. Collectively, these tissues express a diverse array of molecules, including high levels of mucus, that act as a catch-net for bacteria. Here, adherence slows the excretion of the pathogen from the body, likely allowing for it to utilize nutrients in these environments. It can also replicate. The final act is a coordinated and directed attempt to induce diarrhea in the host, and even disrupt its own adherence, in order to be shed at high numbers into the environment, where it will contaminate the soil or water (▢ Fig. 7.1). The next unsuspecting host then ingests the bacterium, and the process repeats.

A second advantage of adherence for bacteria is **invasion**. This can mean invasion of a mucosal barrier or invasion of host cells. The invasion of host cells is a complicated series of molecular events whereby the pathogen rides normal host uptake pathways to gain entry into the host cell cytoplasm, or forcefully alters cell processes for the same outcome. ► Chapter 8 is dedicated to the presentation of these events. For now, suffice it to say that adherence provides the footing for which this activity is initiated. The adhesins that make contact with the host may trigger rearrangements of the host cell's actin network, a process that promotes entry. Pathogenic bacteria will also bind to surface proteins that are linked to the host cell's architecture. One example is fibronectin and the binding to integrin. Upon integrin ligation with a bacterial adhesin, the host complex becomes activated and recruits more integrins. A threshold is reached, leading to signaling proteins being recruited which eventually activate actin networks that form a coordinated entry system that engulfs the bacterial cell. In this mechanism, adhesion stimulates

invasion. The host cell is often powerless to stop it. Without these factors, bacteria whose life-cycle involves the inhabitation of host cells cannot survive.

A third advantage adherence may bring to the bacterial invader is **transient combat**. Adhesins allow the bacterium to get close enough to the host cell membrane so the bacterium can provide a lethal thrust of weaponry. The contact is so close that specialized injection systems can penetrate the membrane and pump toxins or effectors into the host cytoplasm. As we will see in ► Chapters 9 and 10, these secretion systems and toxins effectively disrupt host cell metabolism, often reprogramming the cell to either intake the bacterium, cripple its defenses, or kill it outright, especially if it is a part of the immune system. Toxins delivered by specialized contact-dependent secretion systems require adherence as a first step. Framed in this manner, adherence may help the bacterium get a head start for the fight to come.

A final important advantage of adherence is long-term colonization and the finding of an **ecological niche** bacteria can call home (▢ Fig. 7.2). Although presented as enemy throughout this volume, a portrayal that is accurate given the damage they can do to the human body, many bacteria are just looking for a comfortable place to survive. A notable feature of many of the pathobionts that comprise our microbiome is the presence of many different adhesive systems in the same species. Staphylococcus and streptococcus, two stable colonizers of our skin, contain a dozen different surface proteins that help bind epithelial cells. *E. coli*, which colonizes the GI tract, makes so many distinct adhesive structures, each with their own shape and function, it has been difficult to determine which ones are the most important; and, they can be important to bind specific tissues as well, perhaps at different stages in the infection process. For example, colonization of the urinary bladder epithelium may be distinct from that of the intestinal tract.

An important consideration too is that the experimental knockout of one adhesin rarely results in the complete ablation of host cell association. Thus, a theme repeated many times over in this work is that **functional redundancy** is a common pathogenic strategy. Having separately encoded (even quite different structure) factors that perform a similar, sometimes overlapping function, helps ensure survival in the face of host-mediated neutralization of one of these factors. A range of similar and diverse adhesins may simply help the bacterium cope with a changing host environment in a preferred ecological niche. In summary, some of the benefits, from the bacterial standpoint, of adherence are illustrated in ◘ Fig. 7.3.

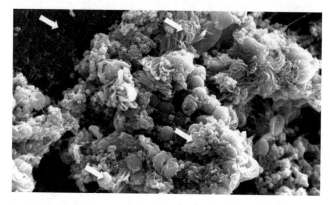

◘ **Fig. 7.2** Chronic bacterial colonization. Mucosal surfaces may be sites of chronic colonization by pathogenic bacteria. Shown here is an electron micrograph of the nasal passages of mice that have been infected with *Streptococcus pneumoniae*, which colonizes a significant fraction of human adults and is a common cause of community-associated pneumonia. In this image, the arrows indicate clusters of bacterial cells (little grape-like structures, larger leukocytes, and matrix type material consistent with the formation of biofilms. (Adapted from Orihuela et al (see *suggested readings*) under a creative commons license. (▶ https://creativecommons.org/licenses/by-nc-sa/3.0))

Adherence is not a unidirectional event. Bacterial adherence may also prepare the host. In this regard, one alternative outcome of adherence is inflammation. We learned from ▶ Chap. 5 that the host harbors surface proteins termed toll-like receptors that respond to bacterial PAMPs. Some adhesins are direct ligands for toll-like receptors, providing the direct signal that leads to downstream activation of inflammatory pathways. Microarray studies suggest that when a pathogenic bacterium adheres to host cells, it changes the expression (either up or down) of hundreds to thousands of host genes. Many of these genes are linked to inflammation. You can think of adherence as breaking a trip-wire and therefore activating a host alarm. These gene changes often prepare the host cell, as well as neighboring cells. Cells of the immune system may be recruited, barriers may be strengthened, and antibacterial molecules made. Although adhesins themselves are rarely considered to be directly toxic to cells, the immune response they invoke can certainly be. Thus, in addition to the basic aiding of bacterial directives, from the standpoint of the stimulation of inflammation, adherence is an important part of pathogenesis.

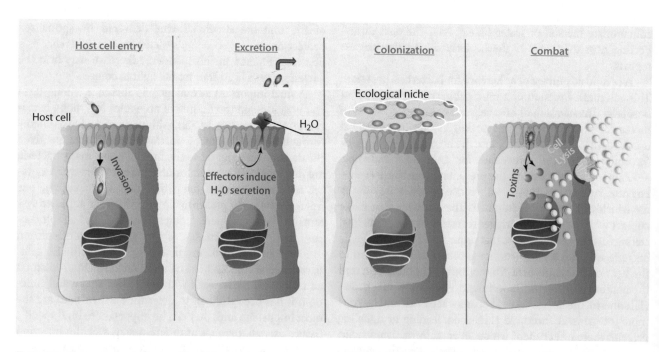

◘ **Fig. 7.3** Some reasons bacteria adhere to host cells. Adhesins are important contributors to bacterial infections because they often represent the first formal engagement of the bacterium with host cells or tissues. Adhesins aid in the entry or invasion of bacteria into host cells, their acute or transient colonization (which provides an opportunity to quickly acquire nutrients, reproduce, and then exit), their long-term or chronic colonization, and to enhance their ability to win a fight via the delivery of toxins or effectors.

7.3 Types of Adhesins (Gram-Negative Pili)

A structural and functional discussion of adhesins must first make the distinction between **adhesive appendages** and **adhesive molecules**. An adhesive appendage is a highly ordered, multimeric grouping of at least two different surface proteins whose association often forms a visible bacterial organelle (by microscopy). Included in this classification are **pili** and filamented **fimbriae**. The tips of these structures often contain the actual adhesin, which binds a host receptor, but the entire structure is needed for full functionality. An adhesive molecule, on the other hand, is a stand-alone surface protein, most often attached to the outer membrane or cell wall, that does not form an extracellular organelle but whose intrinsic structure facilitates binding to a host receptor. Each has advantages for certain niches and functions, and each has drawbacks that make it susceptible to attack by the host. An adhesive appendage such as a pilus may span two or more cell lengths from the bacterial surface like giant, waving tentacles. This is "adherence from afar." As long as one of those tentacles can stick to a surface, the bacterium can latch on to that surface even though they are not physically interacting on a cell-cell basis. There may be repulsive charges that prevent the intimate association of both cells as well, or other surface components that are inhibitory or harmful to bacteria. Long appendages can get around these obstacles to adherence. Pili are particularly strong. They resist shear forces, fluctuations in the chemistry and composition of the surrounding environment, and degradation by proteases. But their long filaments also makes them vulnerable to recognition by the immune system. Furthermore, they are potentially limited in specificity by their tip protein,

which may be the most important determinant of binding specificity. Non-appendage adhesins, which exist as an individual unit or a short, smaller multimer, may avoid the immune system by being tucked away in the outer membrane or cell wall. In addition, the preponderance of different adhesins encoded in the genome of pathogenic bacteria that do not form pili, often with different ligands they bind, confers upon the bacterial cell the ability to bind different surfaces and colonize different niches. To interact with their receptor via these adhesins, however, the bacterium and host cell or tissue must be in close contact, which can trigger the innate immune trip-wire.

7.3.1 P Is for Pili

Fimbriae were first observed in the 1940s from studies with bacteriophage, which sometimes use them as receptors. Eighty years of work since then has revealed several adhesive forms that can be delineated on the basis of their structure, function, and gene content. One of the first structurally characterized pili was that of the type 1 or p (pyelonephritis associated pili – pap) pilus, circa the late 1960s. The **P pili** are found in members of the Enterobacteriaceae, in particular *E. coli* (◻ Fig. 7.4). The P pili are very similar to another pilus adhesive structure termed the **type I pilus**. Whereas the type I pilus is rather ubiquitous and chromosomally encoded, the P pili are associated with a pathogenicity island that includes some protein toxins and, as such, are not found in all bacteria. In this sense, they are within our definition of a virulence factor. This is especially true since P pili are associated with the binding and colonization of the urinary tract. The proto-

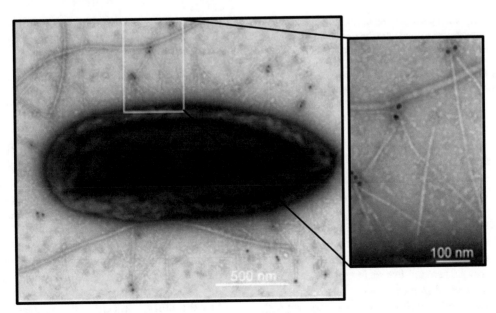

◻ **Fig. 7.4** Type I pili of *E. coli*. In this electron micrograph, the type 1 pili are observed as lighter (and smaller) filament-like structures against the dark grey backdrop of the image (see the enlarged inset). The pilus tip is shown being labeled with an anti-FimH primary antibody followed by a gold-labeled secondary antibody that binds the primary label (the dense gold particles appear as dark spots – see inset). Notice these dark spots localize to the tip of the pilus, the expected localization of FimH. (Adapted from Fleckenstein et al (see *suggested readings*) under a creative commons license. (► https://creativecommons.org/licenses/by/4.0/))

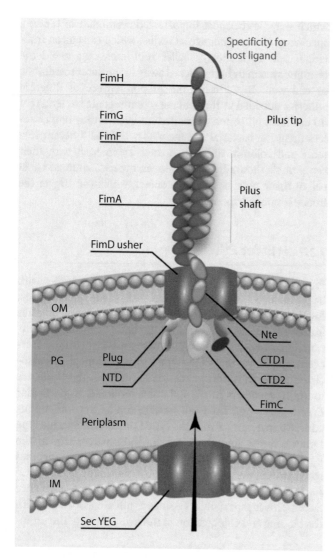

Fig. 7.5 Type I. The type 1 pili are arranged as an ordered assembly of repeating pilin subunits that extend from the bacterial surface and culminate with a tip protein that confers host ligand specificity. Pilus proteins are secreted across the inner membrane by the Sec system (see ▶ Chap. 9) and the outer membrane with the assistance of periplasmic chaperones and membrane localized usher proteins. Shown is the system as studied in *E. coli*.

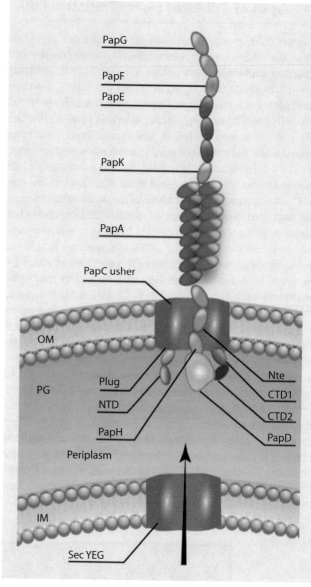

Fig. 7.6 P-pili. The p-pili, like type 1 systems, are also formed via the action of periplasmic chaperones and usher proteins that deliver the unit monomers to the growing pilus shaft. Shown is the system as observed in *E. coli*.

type p pilus is the **PAP system** whereas the prototype type 1 pilus is the **Fim system**. Both have similar features and are considered here together (☐ Figs. 7.5 and 7.6).

The type I or p-type pili are encoded in an operon or genetic cluster that encompasses many genes (11 is common). The pilus structure is about 7 nm thick and consists of hundreds to thousands of pilin subunits that can stretch up to 2 microns[1] in length. Each gene in the multi-gene system performs a specific duty. There are five main components, each part either being involved in assembly of the structure or a part of the structure itself (and thus makes direct contact with the host). The mechanism of their assembly is a testament to the marvels of biological organization. It begins with the production of the main pilus shaft, which are often referred to as pilin subunits. These subunits have a number of conserved

structural features that can be divided into different classes. Each class is organized by the width and length of the pilus. This means that similar structural appendages (overall morphology and size) determines the grouping. The subunits are transcribed in the cytoplasm of the bacterial cell and then exported as unfolded polypeptides through the sec secretion system. We learn more of secretion systems in ▶ Chap. 9; the sec secretion system, a commonly employed secretion apparatus of many extracellularly destined proteins, is thus of central importance in diseases caused by bacteria.

Once the pilin subunit enters the periplasm, it encounters a protein termed a **chaperone**. As its name implies, the chaperone will guide the pilin to its proper location, gently assisting in its folding while doing so. The chaperone likely also protects the subunit from proteases. The chaperone may be specific for its cognate subunit, recognizing this subunit by a conserved structural feature not present in other exported periplasmic proteins. The chaperone-subunit complex then recognizes another conserved protein encoded in the system – the **usher**. The usher is a β-barrel protein whose three dimensional structure resembles that of other outer membrane proteins in bacteria. Composed of a hydrophobic region that embeds in the outer membrane, it oligomerizes upon itself to form a cylindrical pore[2]. The chaperone essentially hands off the pre-formed subunit to the usher which next threads an assembly of the subunits through the pore and on to the external surface of the cell. The addition of each subunit on the periplasmic side at the usher mouth extends the growing pilus from the surface by a mechanism called donor strand complementation. Once external, the pilus becomes helical with each pilin subunit rotating slightly along the shaft, a total of about 3–4 subunits completing one full rotation. At the tip of the pilus is the tip adhesin, which differs from the subunits of the shaft in having two domains. One domain is dedicated to association with the shaft subunits while the other domain confers ligand-binding specificity for the interaction with host components, which for pilus proteins is usually some type of carbohydrate. It is believed that the order of assembly, *i.e.* pilus tip adhesin first

then pilus subunits that comprise the shaft second, occurs through the affinity of the chaperone-subunit for its cognate usher with the tip protein having the highest affinity. The process concludes with the addition of a base subunit that anchors the pilus to the membrane. Collectively, this is termed the **chaperone-usher pathway** of pilus biogenesis.

Whereas the structure itself is of the utmost importance, it is the pilus tip protein that confers the actual adhesion and specificity for host cells or tissues. In the case of P or type 1 pili, the tip proteins are PapG and FimH, respectively. Both sit at the tip of the appendage, presumably waving in the solution searching for a ligand. In this case, the ligands are glycosylated surface receptors present on the urinary tract epithelium, and perhaps similar ligands in the intestinal tract, the home-source of many of the bacteria that carry P or type 1 pili. Here we see how the specificity of the tip protein can confer **tropism** of the bacterium to a specific bodily tissue. Tropism is the term used to describe why certain pathogenic bacteria infect certain tissues or hosts. Essentially, it boils down to the adherence and other colonization factors encoded in their genome. Often, the degree of the infection or disease will be determined by the complement of accessory virulence factors that accompany these tropic determinants.

Out of the Box

Tropism and Disease: Stochastic Events or Disease Partners?
What is the relationship between a bacterial pathogen's tropism for a cell or tissue, which is largely dependent on its ability to adhere to said cell or tissue, and the downstream pathophysiology that results when the infection is in full swing? Another way to put it, if bacteria did not have a specific tropism, that is, they did not discriminate one tissue or cell from another, would an infection even begin? The state of the art in this area is that whereas we have much knowledge about the mechanisms by which bacteria bind to the host, and understand at even the atomic level how many adhesins work, we do not really appreciate how these factors have evolved to target the tissues they direct them to, and whether this is even the most optimal path to establishment of a niche. Perhaps bacteria just want to find a peaceful place to carry out their lives, reproduce, and move on. Virulence might be in this

setting accidental, or even provoked, with the immune system aiming to clear the bacterium and bacterium aiming to fight back and stay alive. When is the balance between colonization without disease and colonization with disease lost, and what factors tilt the scales? Temporal factors also contribute. Colonization or association may precede virulence, but perhaps downstream virulence is already in place and colonization or association is the icing on the cake. The host also matters. Mucosal surfaces, for instance, are not the same between two people, being largely constructed by one's genetic make-up. We know several human genes lead to differential states of protein and mucin glycosylation. Since the glycome is a target for bacterial adhesins, this implies that both sides of the equation – the bacterial adhesin and the host mucosal surface – determine the binding, tropism, colonization, and susceptibility to infection.

From a practical perspective, the type 1 fimbriae facilitates adherence to mannosylated proteins on the surface of the urinary epithelium of the bladder and is necessary for invasion of bladder cells. As such, this is a major mechanism in the causality of urinary tract infections, a disease that inflicts nearly eight million people a year in the U.S. alone. Groups of bacteria that invade the urinary epithelium are termed **intracellular bacteria communities** (IBCs) – ◘ Fig. 7.7. It is believed entry into the urinary epithelium prevents the bacteria from being excreted with the outgoing urine. From a clinical standpoint, these communities also are protected from antibiotics and thus makes them difficult to treat. Chronic infections in UTI are very common and if left untreated can lead to **urosepsis**, a condition whereby the bacteria enter the blood and go systemic. Here we see how

the assembly of the type 1 pilus allows for a key adaptation to the host's normal process of excretion, avoidance of clinically administered antibiotics, and the potential for long-term and serious infections. We discuss sepsis in ▶ Chap. 14.

7.3.2 Alternates, Bacterial "Legs" and Bacterial "Glue"

The secretion of pilin subunits into the periplasm, where they are folded and assembled with the aid of a chaperone, is a theme played out by other pilus systems that resemble in form and function the P or type 1 systems but whose genes are seemingly unrelated. This includes the **CS1 pili**, found in *E. coli*. Comprised of only about four genes, the major (CooA)

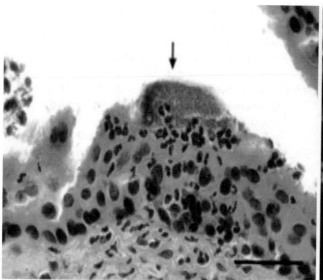
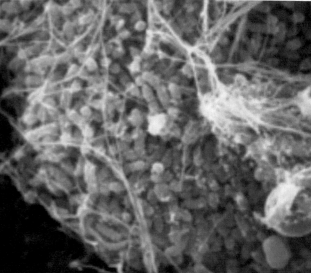

Fig. 7.7 Intracellular bacterial communities. Transmission electron microscopy of urine from a patient suffering from cystitis (a urinary tract infection of the bladder – right panel) demonstrates balls of *E. coli* cells wrapped in fibrous material. Uropathogenic *E. coli* such as this are known to adhere to and invade the bladder epithelium in a pili-dependent manner. The histological stain on the left shows a human uropathogenic *E. coli* strain that has formed a large intracellular bacterial community (purple area indicated with the arrow) in the murine bladder epithelium. Note: the large purple blebs are host nuclei. (Adapted from Hultgren et al (see *suggested readings*) under a creative commons license. (▶ https://creativecommons.org/licenses/by/4.0/))

and minor (CooD) pilin subunits are secreted by the sec system into the periplasm. There, a chaperone (CooB) that is unrelated to the chaperones of P and type I pili binds the pilins and catalyzes their assembly. An outer membrane channel (CooC) facilitates the transit of the pilin structure to the surface of the cell. Because the chaperones for these pathways are distinct from that of the chaperone-usher pathway, this pathway has been termed the **alternate chaperone pathway**.

Bacteria are remarkable in their ability to evolve similar structures yet by seemingly different evolutionary trajectories. Case in point, the **type IV pili** which, like P or type I pili, also form fimbrial appendages albeit by different mechanisms and genes. Type IV pili are larger with a ~ 6 nm diameter and length that can be up to five times or more the length of the bacterial cell itself (■ Fig. 7.8). The prototype system is the Pil system, highly prevalent in the pathogenic neisseria and pseudomonas species. Upwards of 40 genes may be involved in the assembly of type IV pili with several highly conserved components. These pili are divided into type IVa pili, which encompass pili from neisseria and pseudomonas species, and type IVb pili from enteric bacteria that cause diarrhea, including escherichia, salmonella, and vibrio species. The type IVb pilus of enteric bacteria is very long – up to 15–20 μm and necessary for colonization of the gastrointestinal tract. In one pathotype of diarrheagenic *E. coli*, *enteropathogenic E. coli* (EPEC), the type IVb pilus is named the **bundle forming pilus (BFP)**, which form twine-like aggregates that continuously stack on each other. The aggregative nature of the BCP is thought to drive the formation of EPEC microcolonies in the GI epithelium. In the causative agent of cholera, *V. cholerae*, the type IVb pilus is termed the **toxin co-regulated pilus** or TCP. It too is long, mediates microcolony formation

and without it *V. cholerae* is weakly able to colonize the GI tract. Here, we see how pilus structures promote an aggregative state that facilitates their retention in the intestine.

The subunits of the type IV pilus shaft are referred to as pilins. Immature forms of pilins, termed pre-pilins, are co-translationally synthesized/secreted across the inner membrane via the sec secretion system. As they are threaded, an N-terminal positively charged leader sequence is recognized by a **pre-pilin peptidase** localized to the inner membrane. Cleavage of this leader sequence by the pre-pilin peptidase somehow facilitates the assembly of the now mature pilin subunits into the fiber. As the fiber grows, in a process dependent on the use of ATP, the fiber is extended through an outer membrane protein that oligomerizes into a gated, doughnut-shaped pore (■ Fig. 7.9).

The type IV pilus is amazing, moonlighting between multiple important functions for the bacterial cell. The type IV pilus also participates in twitching motility, a type of bacterial "walking" by which pili anchor themselves to the underlying substratum and pull themselves along, sort of like a starfish on the seabed. Because no one receptor is believed to be involved in this activity, the pilus tip is promiscuous in binding cognate host ligands. Interacting with all types of surfaces, host extracellular matrix components, cells, and even other bacteria themselves, the diversity of ligands ensures movement will continue. This latter function is especially important. We learned in ▶ Chap. 6 about the importance of the transfer of horizontal genes in the evolution of pathogenesis, including conjugation as a mechanism to transfer DNA between bacterial cells. The type IV pilus facilitates the conjugation between bacterial cells where DNA is transferred through the shaft of the structure. Being a large

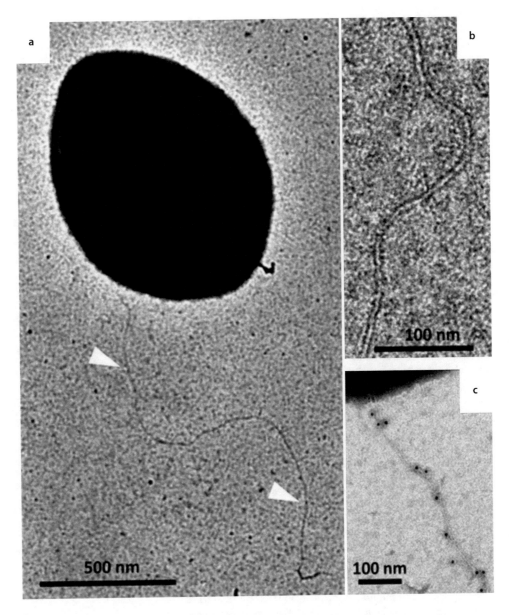

Fig. 7.8 Type IV pili. **a** Shown is an electron micrograph of a single *S. pneumoniae* bacterial cell with a very long pili (arrows). **b** A closer view of a long pilus. **c** Immunogold labeling (dots) of one of the pilin shaft subunits. These pili are involved in the conjugative transfer of DNA between streptococci. (Adapted from Fronzes et al (see *suggested readings*) under a creative commons license. (▶ https://creativecommons.org/licenses/by/4.0/))

unit, it is easy to imagine the type IV pilus a target for the immune system; indeed, vaccination with pili subunits does provide protection against disease in experimental models of infection. We learned of antigenic variation and how this confuses the immune system by providing diverse epitopes. The type IV pilus is one of those structures that undergoes phase variation via the swapping of active pili genes with dormant ones lying elsewhere on the chromosome. This presumably allows the pilus to adopt a number of different molecular structures to ensure it is not recognized or neutralized by the host immune system.

The highly ordered process by which type 1 and 4 pili assemble is in contrast to the building of what are called **curli** (▶ Fig. 7.10). Curli are the bacterial pathogen's version of crazy glue – they bind, and quickly, to whatever they touch. Technically described as adhesive amyloids, curli have the notable property of directing their own self-assembly, starting at the base and building outwards, on the extracellular side of the outer membrane. They are assembled by what is referred to as the extracellular **nucleation-precipitation pathway** whereby a filamentous structure builds from the repeated precipitation of an insoluble fibril protein on an extracellularly localized nucleating factor. The prototype is the Csg system commonly found in enteric pathogens such as *E. coli* and salmonella. There are four main components. CsgD seems to function to activate the expression of the system, including the production of the two factors that make up the filament, CsgA and CsgB. CsgA and B are secreted by the sec secretion system outside the cell. CsgA is initially soluble but is thought to become insoluble upon contact with CsgB localized on the outer membrane. The aggregative properties of unfolded CsgA cause it to precipitate on itself with CsgB directing the extension of continuously precipitated monomers into a regularly ordered array that extends out from the cell. A fourth component, CsgG, is an outer membrane protein that stabilizes the entire A/B filament, likely acting as a base by which CsgB can anchor the growing filament.

7

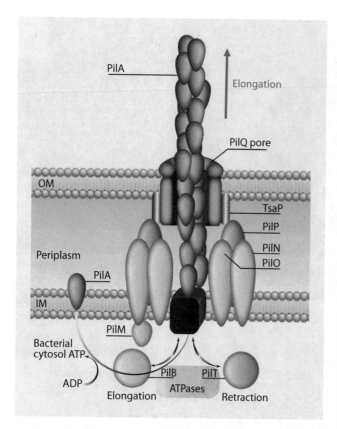

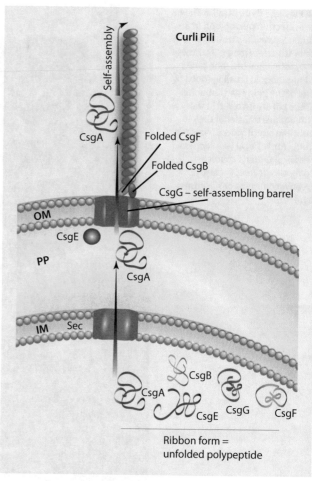

◼ **Fig. 7.9** Organization of type IV pili. The formation of the type IV pilus is an orchestrated process involving the secretion and assembly of pilin subunits in the periplasm and their extension through the outer membrane PilQ pore as the entire structure is pushed outward. An elongation factor (pilB) and retraction factor (PilT) govern the net formation of the filament in an ATP-dependent manner. The drawing is modeled after studies of the type IV pilus from *Neisseria meningitidis*.

◼ **Fig. 7.10** Curli fibrils. Self-aggregating curli proteins constitute the nucleation-precipitation pili pathway. Sec secreted Csg proteins, in particular CsgA, are recognized by the self-assembling barrel protein CsgG and exported to the extracellular surface. There, they self-nucleate into an extended structure (shown here being straight but in nature is usually highly tangled and irregular), here modeled after studies of *E. coli*.

7.4 Gram-Positive Pili

The importance of pili for Gram-positive bacteria resembles what we have already touched upon for Gram-negatives. They contribute to colonization and adherence to their host and the establishment of a host niche. Pili are used by *Streptococcus pneumoniae*, a cause of pneumonia, to colonize the respiratory tract by adhering to lung epithelial cells. The cause of "strep throat", *Streptococcus pyogenes* (group A strep), a common childhood infection often confused with the flu, uses pili to adhere to the cells of the tonsils. Pili from enterococcus and streptococcus are important for the formation of biofilms. The receptor for several Gram-positive tip proteins is the abundant extracellular matrix proteins collagen and fibronectin.

Where Gram-positive pili differ from their Gram-negative counterparts is in their structure and mechanism of assembly. As we will see, the pilin subunits of Gram-positive bacteria are not linked by non-covalent interactions. Instead, they are attached by covalent bounds. This makes them stronger as well. The covalent link maybe be partially explained by a different set of assembly challenges. The Gram-positive outer most layer is not a fluid membrane in

motion. It is a thick and immobile cell wall, the peptidoglycan and its primary role is as a structural scaffold for the cell. We learned about the cell wall in ▶ Chap. 2, but here we discuss how Gram-positive bacteria use their cell wall to anchor proteins that mediate the binding of the cell to its target host niche. For more than 50 years, it was thought that Gram-positive bacteria do not form surface appendages like pili. Then, Yanagawa and colleagues reported in 1968 fibers extending from the surface of corynebacterium sp. It would take another 30 years or so before the mechanism of their formation and anchoring was uncovered with the discovery of the enzyme **sortase**. This enzyme does exactly what its name implies; it sorts proteins destined to be displayed on the surface to the cell wall.

Many proteins destined for the covalent attachment to the cell wall contain four main features. The first is an N-terminal signal peptide that directs their secretion through the lone membrane. The others include a C-terminal five amino acid "signal" that is recognized by the sortase,

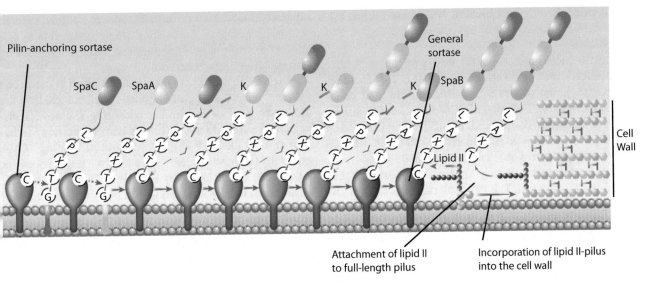

Fig. 7.11 Sortase pili in Gram-positive bacteria. Gram-positive bacteria face different challenges in the formation of pili on their surface due to the presence of the cell wall. The enzyme responsible for attaching proteins to the cell wall is sortase. A specific pilin sortase recognizes pilin subunits and polymerizes their extension through continuous sorting reactions at the five amino acid sorting signal. After the pilus has reached a certain length, the final linkage is carried out by the normal sortase enzyme (sortase A) that transfers the final pilin subunit before attack by lipid II, the cell wall precursor unit. Lipid-II linked pili are then attached to the cell wall via normal cell wall biosynthesis reactions.

followed by a hydrophobic stretch of amino acids and finally a string of basic residues on the C terminus. Sortase recognizes the five amino acid signal (the canonical sequence is LPXTG with X being any amino acid) and cleaves between the T (threonine) and the G (glycine). For a brief moment, the sortase is covalently linked to the glycine of the cell wall protein until a cell wall component, lipid II, reacts with the threonine thereby removing the C-terminus of the cell wall protein from sortase and linking the N-terminus of the cell wall protein to lipid II. Since lipid II is a normal part of the cell wall biosynthetic pathway, when it gets incorporated into the growing cell wall, the now attached protein goes with it.

Many Gram-positive adhesins are anchored to the cell wall in this manner, including Yanagawa's pili. Known as the **sortase pili anchoring system** (Spa), the prototype example of this occurs in the pathogen that causes diphtheria, *Corynebacterium diphtheria*. In this case, the pilin subunits are sortase substrates that harbor the C-terminal three-part sorting signal. A sortase (designated sortase C to differentiate it from three other sortases that do not anchor pili) recognizes the pilin subunit SpaC via its sorting signal and cleaves between the T and G. In non-piliated anchor proteins, this linkage would normally be resolved by the attack from lipid II. But instead of lipid II, the sortase-SpaC linkage is resolved by a lysine residue of another pilin subunit, that of SpaA. SpaC remains at the tip but the pilus is grown by essentially repeating this attack of sortase intermediates by SpaA, continuously, until the final pilin subunit, that of SpaB, terminates the elongation process. How the cell knows to end the filament at a rather defined length is not well understood, but what is known is that SpaB attacks after itself being cleaved by the another sortase, the housekeeping sortase – sortase A. When lipid II chemically reacts with the sortase A-SpaB intermediate, the entire pilus gets incorporated into the cell wall like any other anchored protein (◘ Fig. 7.11). Adhesive pilus structures, and the mechanism of their surface display, has now been recognized in several different Gram-positive pathogens, including bacillus and streptococcus species.

7.5 Non-pilus Adhesins

7.5.1 MSCRAMMS

Non-filamentous adhesins do not form pili, appendages, fibrils, or filaments of any kind. Instead, they are deposited on the bacterial surface as an individual protein (or an oligomeric complex composed of the same protein) with one domain as surface anchor and another domain willing to engage an extracellular host ligand. Whereas pili, by virtue of their long length (sometimes as long as several times the length of the bacterial cell themselves - ~ 1 micron or 1000 nanometers) make for adherence "from afar", other adhesins seem to function as such spanning no more than the length of a single unit of itself (~ 10 nanometers). Since we just discussed sortase and Gram-positive bacteria, it seems relevant to now introduce **Microbial Surface Components Recognizing Adhesive Matrix Molecules** (or MSCRAMMS), which may be the most widely recognized non-filament adhesins in Gram-positive bacteria. MSCRAMMs are anchored to the surface of the cell wall of Gram-positive bacteria by the same chemical mechanism described for the base pilin subunit of pili. Namely, resolution of a sortase-linked intermediate via attack by lipid II which then results in the incorporation of the protein into the cell wall. As such,

MSCRAMMs harbor the canonical N-terminal sorting signal of LPXTG (or variant of it), hydrophobic region, and polybasic tail.

MSCRAMMs are notable for their preference to bind **extracellular matrix components** (ECM). This includes fibronectin (most common), elastin, laminin, and collagen, to name a few. Targeting of ECMs by microbial adhesins is a common theme and rightfully so; they bring bacteria into close proximity to cells, sometimes between cells (avoiding detection), and are highly decorated with ligands bacteria love, mostly sugars. Fibronectin is preferred in this case as it is a key molecule that bridges the strong network of ECM components, such as fibrin and collagen, to the bacterium itself. Being a heavily glycosylated protein, it is often the glycosylated portion that the microbial adhesins recognize.

The most well studied MSCRAMMs are the homologs of fibronectin binding proteins (FnbA) that are found in the staphylococcal and streptococcal species. This prototype adhesin contains a signal peptide that directs its secretion, repeating regions whose function are still unknown, several fibronectin binding regions, and finally the N-terminal sorting signal. The mechanism by which these MSCRAMMs bind fibronectin is still being explored, but it is interesting to note that almost all humans sampled have circulating antibodies to FnbA and some of them even enhance the ability of MSCRAMMs to bind to fibronectin. Why then do people still get infections, and sometimes deadly ones, with these bacteria? Scientists have used specialized optical technologies to determine that the region of FnbA that binds fibronectin may actually be somewhat disordered. In addition, FnbA binds fibronectin that circulates in the blood and likely does so as soon as it is available on the bacterial surface. Here we see two strategies of how human-adapted bacteria avoid the deactivating antibodies discussed in earlier chapters. Not only might the MSCRAMM order its fibronectin binding region upon binding this ligand (thus any circulating antibodies against it will not fit properly), but it also keeps the interface hidden from the immune system by cloaking itself through binding of a human ECM protein. This is just another example of how adhesins can implore functionality that enhances bacteria survival.

The MSCRAMMs have now been described in more than a dozen human pathogens. Although not all of them have the same structural or cell surface anchoring features (Gram-negative bacteria do not anchor proteins via sortase mechanisms), they likely all share the feature of binding ECMs, especially fibronectin. Here we see what we might refer to as a universal target for many bacteria – ECMs – and their exploitation by MSCRAMMs and in many different types of infections. Similar features are observed in the mycobacteria that causes tuberculosis, campylobacter species that cause diarrhea, and even porphyromonas that contribute to tooth decay and dental cavities. Other MSCRAMMs recognize factors in blood, such as complement. ◘ Figure 7.12 provides a structural view of an MSCRAMM.

7.5.2 Autotransporters

There are other bacterial adhesins of importance. Three additional groups or families for Gram-negative bacteria are now discussed. One of the first such families of proteins characterized in this manner were the **trimeric autotransporter adhesins** (TAA) – ◘ Fig. 7.13. Their name stems from a fascinating molecular capacity to transport themselves, without another factor, through the outer membrane while orienting themselves to engage host ligands. The polypeptide is first synthesized in the bacterial cytoplasm and transported through the sec secretion system. In the periplasm, a C-terminal domain called the transporter domain forms into a β-barrel structure and inserts into the outer membrane. Next, the N-terminal domain, the passenger domain, enters the pore and exits on the exterior of the membrane while still covalently linked to the membrane-embedded transporter pore. The passenger domain is the ligand binding domain. In

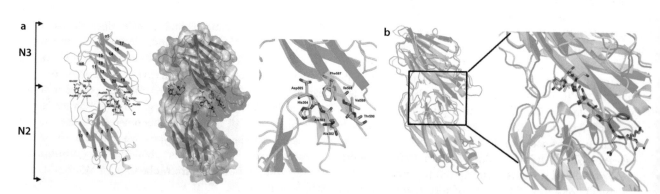

◘ **Fig. 7.12** Molecular structure of an MSCRAMM. **a** A three-dimensional ribbon structure (far left) and surface charge density (middle) representation of the crystal structure of the *S. aureus* serine aspartate repeat protein E (SdrE) MSCRAMM is shown. The image to the right of panel A. zooms in on the interface between domains N3 and N3 and highlights the residues that line this groove. **b** The structure of SdrE is superimposed on the known structure of another MSCRAMM protein (Bbp) bound to a peptide fragment from fibrinogen (between N3 and N2), the blood glycoprotein that contributes to blood clotting and wound healing and thus can serve as an attachment point for bacteria pathogens. (Adapted from Wang et al (see suggested readings) under a creative commons license. (► https://creativecommons.org/licenses/by/4.0/))

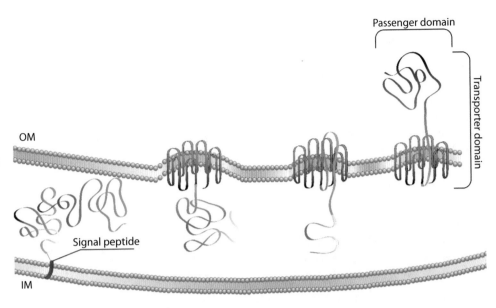

Fig. 7.13 Autotransporter adhesins. In this simplified diagram, an autotransporter is shown first being secreted across the inner membrane via its N-terminal signal peptide (recognized by the sec translocon – see ▶ Chap. 9), making its way across the periplasm, and then auto-inserted into the outer membrane by its β-barrel-forming transporter domain. It is then believed the passenger domain inserts into the barrel and folds on the surface of the cell where it can interact with host ligands

Passenger domain

Transporter domain

OM

Signal peptide

IM

the best studied example of this molecule, that of YadA from yersinia species, the ligands for the passenger domain are components of the extracellular matrix, such as collagen.

7.5.3 Afa and MAM

There are also adhesins that lie somewhere between an individual sole arbitrator of adhesion (such as an outer membrane protein) and a bonafide appendage-like structure (such as a type I pilus). This includes the **afimbrial adhesins (afa)**, also called the Dr. adhesins because of early studies which demonstrated they bind to the Dr blood group antigens and promote red blood cell agglutination. These adhesins are made by bacteria that cause urinary tract infections. Some are stand-alone adhesins; others form into smaller, thin fimbrillar structures. They are **homopolymeric**, which means their association into structures consists of essentially one repeating unit but whose gene is a part of a multi-gene network, some of which may be accessory factors that aid in the assembly and/or localization of the adhesin itself. One key functional feature of afa adhesins is their preference to bind integrins. Integrins are intimately linked to the host cell's cytoskeletal signaling pathways and architecture. Afa adhesins may facilitate the remodeling of this architecture to promote the entry of bacteria into the cell.

Another group of afimbril adhesins are the **multivalent adhesion molecules (MAMs)**. Mams are distinguished by a series of internal repeating units termed mammalian cell entry (MCE) domains that, as their name implies, promote the entry of bacteria into the host cell. They are widespread in commensal and pathogenic enteric bacteria but similar sequences are found in certain species of Gram-positives (as well as mycobacterial species). Their ligand seems to be fibronectin, particularly glycosylated residues, but they are quite unique in also binding to lipids, including phosphatidic acid, which is a rarity amongst adhesive ligands found in bacteria.

7.6 Anti-adhesive Approaches

The seemingly critical role of adherence as one of the first steps in a bacterial infection underscores why an investigation into their operational mechanisms is an important undertaking. Without the ability to adhere to host tissues, the pathogen cannot colonize or invade. Being free-floating in the blood exposes it to circulating macrophages, complement, and antibodies. With much knowledge concerning the types of adhesins bacteria possess, and insights into their role during disease causation, one would expect the formation and approval of adhesin-based vaccines for all major types of bacterial infections. There are not any, so why?

The first attempts to use pili as vaccines began in the 1970s and, incidentally, revealed very quickly some of the obstacles ahead. Although antibodies were generated against these pili, and they decreased adherence to host cells, the ability to change the pili via antigenic variation allowed the bacterial cells to bypass some antibody responses, or lower the response all together. Redundancy is a problem too; some *E. coli* encode for a dozen or more different adhesins, pili or other appendage-like structures. Knocking one out may reduce adherence but others can often fill the void. From a production standpoint, considering the unique chemistry of each adhesin and the likely different methods needed to attain highly purified material, it may not be a viable approach to construct a vaccine from many different adhesins. Some adhesins are also differentially expressed, that is, the protein product is made under a defined set of environmental conditions. We learned above about how MSCRAMMs may mask the fibronectin binding interface until it encounters the ligand. These stealth measures of cloaking the adhesin keeps the immune system from detecting it. Thus, the evolutionary pressure that has driven some of these adhesins to conceal critical epitopes, or make them less antigenic, is another obstacle. Horizontal gene transfer or mutation (see the mutagenic tetrasect in ▶ Chap. 6) also pose problems. A good example is the human experimental vaccine against the plague (caused by the Gram-negative bacterium *Yersina pestis*), which is effective as a pathogen because of the presence of the F1 pilus antigen in circulating strains. However, in strains that have lost F1, the vaccine is ineffective. Dr. and type IV pilus antigens have demonstrated efficacy against *E. coli* and *P. aeruginosa* infections in experimental animals, and mannose analogues have been developed that prevent type 1 pili tip proteins from adhering to glycosylated receptors. Thus, there are new approaches on the horizon. The microbe hunter will have to consider these in the context of the obstacles that have presented in the past.

Summary of Key Concepts

1. Bacterial adherence to its host is often a precursor to the establishment of an infection. Adherence benefits the bacterium by providing acute or chronic establishment of a local niche, access to nutrients, or facilitates the delivery of toxins or effectors.
2. Bacterial adherence is mediated by surface molecules termed adhesins. Often proteins, they allow for the association with host cells, the extracellular matrix, or other components, often via specific receptors.
3. There are many types of adhesive structures, including those that form filaments such as pili. Pili are long structures composed of repeating units whose tip can ligate a host receptor. Afimbrial adhesins are non-filamentous surface proteins.
4. Adhesins are often virulence factors and targets for chemical inhibition or vaccine development. However, their ability to avoid detection of the immune system, often redundant binding roles, and other specialized functions can present formidable challenges the microbe hunter must overcome.

❓ Expand Your Knowledge

1. You are studying the adherence of *Streptococcus pyogenes* to human pharyngeal cells. Patient sera from those previously infected with a virulent strain completely abrogates the binding of this pathogen to these cells when added in the culture media. Read a technical report about column chromatography and propose a method by which you can identify the adhesive component from the surface of *Streptococcus* that binds the pharyngeal cells. How can you use this adhesin to protect children against these infections?

2. A strange, chronic type of pneumonia is occurring in primates housed in a major city zoo. The zoo keepers and dignitaries are concerned the primates, a valuable asset and large crowd draw, will succumb to the disease. You isolate the bacterium which, after sequencing, seems to be most related to klebsiella species, but certainly is a new pathotype. Your studies show:

(a) The bacterium does not adhere to lung epithelial cells in tissue culture in the lab.
(b) The bacterium does adhere to the lungs of Rhesus Macaques (histological analysis after animal necropsy and tissue fixation) but only on the first day of infection.
(c) After day 2, no bacteria adhere to the lung. Instead, they are easily washed away and the washes are full of a strange filament-type structure.
(d) The filament, when injected into mice, leads to severe asthma and autoimmunity in the lung.

Provide an explanation, molecularly and physiologically, as to what may be happening in the primates.

3. Read one review and one primary manuscript concerning the secretion and assembly of the Type I pilus in *E. coli*. From memory, draw and label each step in the process of secretion and assembly.

Notes

1 = A micron is short for micrometer, one one-thousandth of a millimeter.

2 = Oligomers are non-covalent molecular complexes that typically consist of two, three or four repeating units. These units can be identical, at which point the oligomer is a homo-oligomer, or they can be distinct molecules, where they are termed hetero-oligomers. Of note, the term is usually applied to protein complexes.

Suggested Reading

Blanchette-Cain K et al (2013) Streptococcus pneumoniae biofilm formation is strain dependent, multifactorial, and associated with reduced invasiveness and immunoreactivity during colonization. MBio 4:e00745–e00713. https://doi.org/10.1128/mBio.00745-13

Croxen MA, Finlay BB (2010) Molecular mechanisms of Escherichia coli pathogenicity. Nat Rev Microbiol 8:26–38. https://doi.org/10.1038/nrmicro2265

Hendrickx AP, Budzik JM, Oh SY, Schneewind O (2011) Architects at the bacterial surface - sortases and the assembly of pili with isopeptide bonds. Nat Rev Microbiol 9:166–176. https://doi.org/10.1038/nrmicro2520

Hospenthal MK, Costa TRD, Waksman G (2017) A comprehensive guide to pilus biogenesis in Gram-negative bacteria. Nat Rev Microbiol 15:365–379. https://doi.org/10.1038/nrmicro.2017.40

Joh D, Wann ER, Kreikemeyer B, Speziale P, Höök M (1999) Role of fibronectin-binding MSCRAMMs in bacterial adherence and entry into mammalian cells. Matrix Biol 18:211–223

Kline KA, Fälker S, Dahlberg S, Normark S, Henriques-Normark B (2009) Bacterial adhesins in host-microbe interactions. Cell Host Microbe 5:580–592. https://doi.org/10.1016/j.chom.2009.05.011

Laurenceau R et al (2013) A type IV pilus mediates DNA binding during natural transformation in Streptococcus pneumoniae. PLoS Pathog 9:e1003473. https://doi.org/10.1371/journal.ppat.1003473

Luo M et al (2017) Crystal Structure of an Invasivity-Associated Domain of SdrE in S. aureus. PLoS One 12:e0168814. https://doi.org/10.1371/journal.pone.0168814

Ritchie JM, Rui H, Bronson RT, Waldor MK (2010) Back to the future: studying cholera pathogenesis using infant rabbits. MBio 1. https://doi.org/10.1128/mBio.00047-10

Rosen DA, Hooton TM, Stamm WE, Humphrey PA, Hultgren SJ (2007) Detection of intracellular bacterial communities in human urinary tract infection. PLoS Med 4:e329. https://doi.org/10.1371/journal.pmed.0040329

Sanchez BC, Chang C, Wu C, Tran B, Ton-That H (2017) Electron Transport Chain Is Biochemically Linked to Pilus Assembly Required for Polymicrobial Interactions and Biofilm Formation in the Gram-Positive Actinobacterium. MBio 8. https://doi.org/10.1128/mBio.00399-17

Sheikh A et al (2017) Highly conserved type 1 pili promote enterotoxigenic E. coli pathogen-host interactions. PLoS Negl Trop Dis 11:e0005586. https://doi.org/10.1371/journal.pntd.0005586

Soto GE, Hultgren SJ (1999) Bacterial adhesins: common themes and variations in architecture and assembly. J Bacteriol 181:1059–1071

Bacterial Invasion of the Host Cell

© Springer Nature Switzerland AG 2019
A. W. Maresso, *Bacterial Virulence*, https://doi.org/10.1007/978-3-030-20464-8_8

Learning Goals

In this chapter, the learner will be introduced to the concept that pathogenic bacteria invade host cells. This invasion is not only a mechanism to safeguard bacterial survival, it is often a precursor to disease for the host. The benefits of host cell entry for the invading pathogen are discussed, as is the host response to invasion. The mechanisms pathogenic bacteria use to subvert these host responses are framed in terms of promoting the intracellular survival, and lifestyle, of the bacterium and examples are used from prominent human intracellular bacteria to highlight this interplay. After this chapter, the learner will be able to explain the molecular processes that lead to bacterial uptake and survival, including key steps that might be exploited for therapy.

8.1 Introduction

In 1994, the United States Federal Bureau of Investigation (F.B.I.) arrested Aldrich Ames after a multi-year sting into his role in espionage against America. Ames was a 20-plus year Central Intelligence Agency (C.I.A.) veteran whose projects dealt with worldwide U.S. interests. His activities took place during the time of the Cold War, an intense period in American and Russian history that pitted the two nations for economic, strategic, and military control on the world stage. During this time, both countries had hundreds if not thousands of spies and informants, many of them in complete anonymity as to their purpose. Falling on hard economic times, and seduced by the realization he could become rich quick, Ames began a 10-year clandestine campaign to provide critical information to the Russians about U.S. C.I.A. operatives that were supplying the U.S. intelligence about Russian plans. The operation was a landmark success for the Russians. In addition to a wealth of sensitive and classified information they attained, it also resulted in the identification of at least ten secret agency operatives working for the U.S. to secure Russian information. After getting this information, the Russian authorities executed most of them. Through Ames, the Russians infiltrated the most sophisticated and secretive intelligence agency in the world, and at the height of the Cold War. A single underground mole, unbeknownst to such a great spy agency, dealt a momentous blow to this agency's integrity and standing.

Pathogenic bacteria engage in clandestine operations as well. Faced with the daunting challenge of having to survive the host immune system and all its sophisticated weaponry, becoming a microbial mole just might be as effective a strategy as any. The way bacteria engage in espionage is by rowing straight into the heart of darkness itself – *the host cell*. This is called **bacterial invasion**. It may be a brilliant strategy. Inside a host cell, the bacterial antigens that might be processed by antigen presenting cells or bound by antibody are hidden. In that host cell, the harmful shrapnel of inflammation and the membrane piercing properties of antimicrobial peptides or complement have no effect. They cannot even access the bacterium. The special ops cells of the immune system – they

have no juridiction. Most phagocytic cells and killer T-cells are instructed not to attack their own citizens. This means intracellular bacteria are also protected from the most deadly reach of the immune law.

The cellular invasion of host cells is an ancient process. Our own mitochondria are believed to once have been bacteria themselves, or at least an ancestor of the modern day prokaryote. The theory of **endosymbiosis** holds that early cells were invaded, or they otherwise acquired, smaller respiring prokaryotes which resulted in a beneficial relationship for both cells. The incoming cell could use the larger cell for protection and other metabolic needs. The acquiring cell could diversify its energy production by using high-energy ATP generated from respiration of the smaller cell to increase its building potential. Over millions of years the functions became specialized, resulting in such an effective symbiosis that one could not live without the other. Now, our cells use the energy generated by mitochondria to power our health and balance. Thus, there is evolutionary precedence for the benefits an invasive phenotype may confer. In this chapter, we consider this topic in the context of bacteria that use invasion as a pathogenic strategy.

8.2 The Advantages of Invasion for the Bacterial Cell

The first step in the invasion of mammalian cells by bacteria is adherence. We tackled adherence in ▶ Chap. 7. In some cases, the bacterium itself directly reprograms the host cells to do its bidding. In other cases, the host cell uses normal engulfment mechanisms such as phagocytosis to take up the bacterium (of course with the intention to destroy it). In this latter example, the bacterium avoids the completion of its own killing by disarming one or more of the key steps in that process. This is discussed in ▶ Sect. 8.4 below.

Any understanding of bacterial invasion must first consider why it is worth the risk for microbes to even attempt to enter mammalian cells. We investigate here why the evolutionary payoff for such risk-takers might be justified. We focus on each concept separately but the microbe hunter should note they are probably not mutually exclusive.

8.2.1 Stealth

The first is what we may call **immunological stealth**. Intracellular bacteria are rarely recognized by the surveilling immune system. Their antigens are cloaked under the guise of "self". By avoiding detection, the strong cellular and inflammatory responses that in most cases would lead to their death are not initiated. As mentioned above, antibodies bind to bacterial antigens and may either inhibit their function or promote the opsonophagocytosis by a macrophage. If bacterial antigens are tucked away inside cells, antibodies cannot bind them. Phagocytic cells will gloss right over a pathogen if masked by self-antigens, and so will T-cells, especially if the host cell does not display the bacterial antigens on its surface. Complement cannot initiate the membrane attack complex on the surface of hidden bacterial membranes, and antimicrobial peptides are also blocked. Entrapment in mucus, neutrophil nets, and other antibacterial catches are also avoided.

It is not as though immunological stealth is flawless. The host has counter-evolved molecular alarms to detect intracellular bacteria. **Nod-like receptors** (NLDs) are host proteins that recognize bacterial surface structures. The NOD1 protein recognizes meso-diaminopimelic acid, a component of the Gram-negative cell wall. The NOD2 proteins recognize muramyl dipeptide, a component of the Gram-positive cell wall. Other NODs recognize additional bacterial products including nucleic acid or toxins, both of which may be released when a bacterium enters the cell. The recognition of bacterial **pathogen associated molecular patterns** (or PAMPs), a term introduced earlier in this volume, is fundamental to stimulating the downstream changes in protein function and gene expression that accelerates the immune response. This includes downstream signaling events leading to the formation of the **inflammasome**. The inflammasome is a collection of host proteins that function as a large multimeric complex that initiate two important events in the response to intracellular bacteria. The first is the release of inflammatory cytokines. These cytokines ramp-up inflammation for the purpose of drawing other immune cells to the area. The cells, which may include dendritic cells or professional phagocytes, function to kill bacteria and process their antigens (see ▶ Chaps. 4 and 5 on immunity). Activation of the inflammasome also leads to a purposeful cell death termed **pyroptosis** ("death by fire"). In contrast to apoptosis, whereby the cell undergoes a quiet programmed cell death without the objective of inducing inflammation, pyroptosis is noisy and generates more inflammation after the cell swells and eventually bursts. The fire that pyroptosis lights is purposeful. By drawing attention to the infection site, more immune cells are recruited to help contain the infection.

8.2.2 Nutritional Abundance

A second reason bacteria invade host cells is because they are hungry. The concentration of nutrients that bacteria like, including metals, amino acids, and sugars, are often higher in host cells than the surrounding tissues and fluids; and, potentially, because of the diverse metabolic reactions needed for cells to thrive, the plethora of different substances bacteria are exposed to is also greater. Thus, bacteria sometimes invade for **nutritional abundance**. There is evidence the supply of food is also constant. Whereas your blood can fluctuate between extreme highs and lows between meal satiation and fasting, cells try to keep the intracellular concentration of useful metabolites steady. The dependence of intracellular bacteria on host nutrients is also evidenced by the noticeable reduction in biosynthetic capacity of these bacteria. Indeed, some bacteria cannot grow at all unless they parasitize their

host. Thus, in addition to escaping many of the systemic immune surveillance mechanisms, the host cytosol is a nutritionally privileged area that pathogenic bacteria can use as a specialized niche for their health and growth.

8.2.3 Dissemination

A third reason pathogenic bacteria invade is what we can creatively term **Trojan horse dissemination**. Macrophages, dendritic cells and polymorphonuclear cells such as neutrophils are mobile, phagocytic cells that move in and out of tissues. Hitching a ride in them is a clever way for bacteria to move around the body undetected. Salmonella hijacks intestinal macrophages, which then traffic to the blood. If they exit these cells, salmonella can disseminate to other parts of the body. Alveolar macrophages may harbor latent mycobacteria for long periods of time, all while moving wherever these immune cells traffic. The paradigmatic model for the initiation of anthrax disease is that *Bacillus anthracis* spores are phagocytosed by lung macrophages which then travel to the mediastinal lymph nodes. There, the spores germinate into vegetative cells and kill their unsuspecting host carrier, which allows them to exit and disseminate. Antigen sampling M-cells in the intestine are the site of shigella and salmonella infection, sometimes leading to the death of the M-cell and an open gate for further invasion. This strategy, using the body's most elite warriors as Trojan Horses, is an elegant mechanism to gain access to the deepest caverns in the host fortress.

Finally, for some bacteria, including the mycobacterial pathogens of the lung, this state of intracellular stealth can last for years, a strategy termed **latency**. This is the process by which the bacterium lays dormant in a state of low metabolic activity until the conditions are just right to take advantage of the change in environment, so-called **reactivation**. For other bacteria, the avoidance of the immune system is more transient. Listerial species are a good example. After it avoids cellular digestion, it replicates in the host cytoplasm and quickly propels itself through and out of the host cell, sometimes straight into the next cell, where the process of growth and advancement can be repeated. For the most part, latency is a way for the bacterium to find a comfortable niche and just persist. A form of parasitism, latency is particularly problematic for antibiotic treatment which often requires metabolically active bacteria for full inhibitory properties. Waiting for the right moment, perhaps for nutrients or a depression in the immune system, the latent bacterium can decide when and where to best emerge. Some of the benefits of invasion from the pathogen's perspective are illustrated in ☐ Fig. 8.1.

8.3 Mechanisms of Bacterial Invasion

Researchers that study bacterial invasion have classified the ways they enter host cells. The distinguishing features are based on morphological changes and downstream molecular

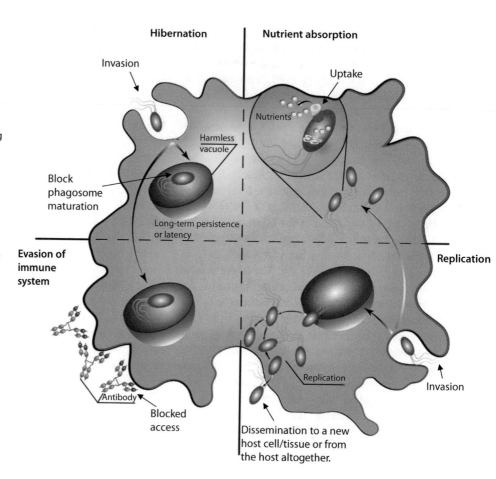

Fig. 8.1 The benefits of the invasion of host cells for pathogenic bacteria. Shown are some of the reasons entering host cells can benefit bacteria pathogens. They include using the host cell as a safe ecological niche for long-term persistence (hibernation or latency), avoiding the immune system including detection by antibodies or phagocytes (immunological stealth), greater access to key metabolites and building blocks (nutrient absorption), and use of these nutrients to grow, divide, and eventually disseminate to other areas of the host or exit the host altogether

signaling in host cells. We start with the **zipper mechanism**, so named because it results in the massive re-construction of actin filaments that resemble the two sides of an open zipper that flank the bacterium to be engulfed. Of course, the first step is adherence. Contact between the bacterium surface ligand and the host cell receptors triggers signaling events that distort the local architecture of the membrane. This structure is sometimes referred to as a cup. Early stages resemble what happens during the process of phagocytosis. The lips of the cup begin to extend around the bound bacterium, the lips fuse, and the bacterium becomes enclosed.

The cause of listeriosis and Far-East Scarlett Fever, *Listeria monocytogenes* and *Yersinia pseudotuberculosis*, respectively, are masters of zipper invasion. These pathogens first secrete a protein named **invasin** (▣ Fig. 8.2). Invasin binds proteins that participate in everyday host-to-host interactions, the β-1-integrins, using a structural motif, cleverly, that mimics the normal cellular host ligand. When pathogenic bacteria evolve mechanisms that supplant a normal host function as a means to take advantage of their biology, it is termed **molecular mimicry**. When invasin binds, it oligomerizes. The accumulation of invasin facilitates the clustering of integrins, which send a downstream signal into the host cell. A cell signaling linker enzyme that recognizes the clustered integrins, termed focal adhesion kinase, likely conveys the information to downstream proteins through phosphorylation. The exact mechanistic steps are still unclear, but the recruitment of a GTPase, the actin polymerization complex arp2/3, and addi-

tional host kinases results in the extension of actin filaments (*i.e.*, the cup lips) outward and around the bacteria. Listeria also usurps this cellular machinery to promote entry, albeit with different players. The elegant studies of **internalins**, InlA and InlB, serve as excellent examples here. Like invasin, they stimulate a zipper entry but do so by engaging different host receptors. InlA binds to the junctional protein E-cadherin. This is notable because E-cadherin's cytosolic tail recruits alpha and beta catenin, which physically links E-cadherin and listeria to the cytoskeleton. Although the exact mechanism by which actin polymerization occurs is unknown, small GTPases and arp2/3 are involved, just as we observed for yersinia. InlB induces the same activation of GTPases (the GTPase Rac is an example) and energizes the arp2/3 complex but not through E-cadherin. Instead, InlB ligates the tyrosine kinase Met, which induces its dimerization and activation. In both cases, and similar to invasin, the two internal ends of yersinia bind their host receptors at the same location as the natural host ligand. By interjecting into already established pathways, these bacteria brilliantly manipulate the host to do its bidding. They signal: "take me in".

One can only marvel at how one simple manipulation by a single outer membrane protein of a key host receptor can do so much for a pathogenic bacterium. But such simplicity is not evolution's only route to induce cell entry. At the other end of the successful invasion spectrum is sophistication, the Aston-Martin of biological engineering. Here we speak of the type III secretion system (T3SS), which we learn more about

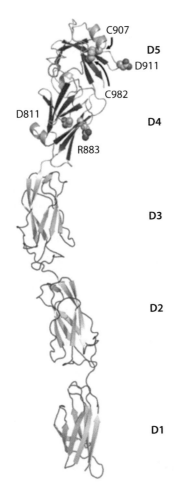

in the next chapter but touch upon briefly here to introduce another concept. Instead of one protein mediating entry into the host cell, more than two dozen are involved. T3SS, as it's abbreviated, is an injection system that delivers bacterial proteins in the host cytosol with the ability to exert mind control. The results are similar to what happens with invasins/internalins, just with more complexity. It begins with the assembly of the type III needle. Once formed, the tip of the needle docks onto the host cell. These proteins form a translocon that pass bacterial effectors through the plasma membrane of the host and into the cytoplasm, appropriately called injection. There may be specific regions on the host cell membrane where this occurs. For example, salmonella uses a type III secretion system as an inducer of cell entry. Its system engages host receptors located in cholesterol-rich regions

of the membrane, also known as **lipid rafts**. These specialized host membrane micro-domains harbor much functional diversity, thus targeting them is a way to efficiently place the bacterial effectors where signaling molecules cluster.

After the injection of effectors through the needle, their enzymatic activity immediately begins to de-stabilize the host cytoskeleton. This targeted deconstruction has one main objective: to use the individual G-actin monomers to re-create a new structural narrative. While one set of effectors deconstruct, another set begins assembly, only this time the purpose is to polymerize F-actin filaments. So extensive are these filaments that the plasma membrane forms structures visible with a light microscope. If not for their insidious control by bacteria, one might even find them beautiful. The larger segments of these structures look like giant tidal waves about to overtake the bacterial cell. These are called **lamellopodia**. Smaller tentacle-like protrusions are also present. These are termed **filopodia**. Both structures surround the bacterium, which leads to the final stage of invasion - engulfment. Here, the action of injected bacterial effectors now reverse the process and completely de-polymerizes the actin filaments. With no underlying support to maintain the structure, the invagination now enters the host-cell cytoplasm. The bacteria are in! The overall process is termed the **trigger** mechanism to reflect that injected effectors build an actin-filament extension that moves beyond the length of the bacterial cell and eventually encloses it in a vacuole upon fusion of the two extensions. A schematic diagram of the steps in the zipper and trigger mechanisms of cell entry are shown in ◪ Figs. 8.3 and 8.4. A representative real-life example of invasion is shown in ◪ Fig. 8.5 and some examples of cell protrusions that promote the process shown in ◪ Fig. 8.6.

8.4 Host Killing and Bacterial Survival Strategies

"Getting in" is only half the struggle. Staying inside and surviving, and subsequently getting back out, is the other half. "Out" in this case means exiting from both the compartment the bacterium used to enter the cell as well as the entire cell itself. These two processes may be mutually exclusive. The process of getting out is eventually addressed below. In between getting in and out are any number of dozen different ways bacteria manipulate host cell physiology to survive. In ▶ Chap. 4 (innate immunity), we learned that the host cell has a designated pathway to kill its bacterial invader. The uptake of bacteria in most cases is through an invagination of the plasma membrane. Other than the membrane containing toll- or nod-like receptors that sound the alarm, the resulting vacuole the pathogen finds itself in is rather inert and poses no inherent threat to the pathogen. Instead, the vacuole must mature into a killing machine. Only the most skilled intracellular pathogens can avert this fate.

From the host's standpoint, it wants to mature the vacuole from what is termed an early endosome (the fusion of the invaginated membrane carrying the bacterium with vesicles

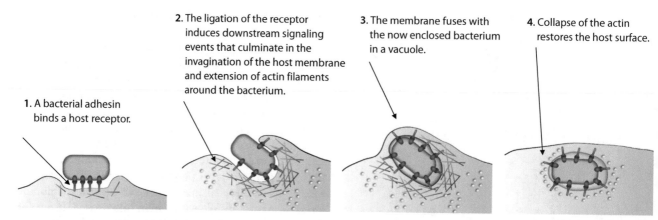

1. A bacterial adhesin binds a host receptor.

2. The ligation of the receptor induces downstream signaling events that culminate in the invagination of the host membrane and extension of actin filaments around the bacterium.

3. The membrane fuses with the now enclosed bacterium in a vacuole.

4. Collapse of the actin restores the host surface.

Fig. 8.3 The zipper mechanism of entry by invading bacteria. If not directly phagocytosed, bacteria can induce their entry into host cells. One such mechanism is referred to as the zipper effect due to the entry process resembling the peeling of a zipper from a surface. Shown above is the mechanism thought to occur for various species of yersina and listeria. The process begins with the ligation of a host receptor by a bacterial adhesin. The binding of the adhesion induces actin filament formation that somehow promotes the invagination of the membrane or formation of a pocket that the invading bacterium slips into. Once in, the membrane around the bacterium closes on itself and the resulting vacuole now contains the engulfed pathogen

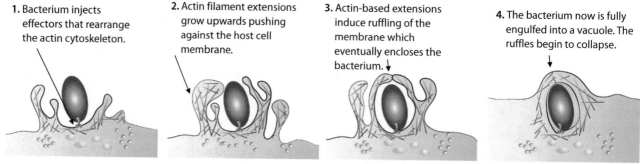

1. Bacterium injects effectors that rearrange the actin cytoskeleton.

2. Actin filament extensions grow upwards pushing against the host cell membrane.

3. Actin-based extensions induce ruffling of the membrane which eventually encloses the bacterium. ↓

4. The bacterium now is fully engulfed into a vacuole. The ruffles begin to collapse. ↓

Fig. 8.4 The trigger mechanism of entry by invading bacteria. If not directly phagocytosed, bacteria can also induce their entry into host cells through a mechanism referred to as the trigger effect. After binding to the host surface, the bacterium uses the type-III secretion system to inject bacterial effector proteins into the host cell cytoplasm. These proteins rearrange the actin cytoskeleton to induce the formation of long F-actin filaments that push against and extend the host plasma membrane well over the plane of the invading bacterium. The filaments will eventually collapse, perhaps induced by other injected effectors themselves, resulting in the complete engulfment of the pathogen. This is the preferred mechanism of entry for salmonella and shigella species

derived from the endocytic pathway) to a late endosome capable of combining with the host **lysosome**. The resulting body, the phago-lysosome, is a killing vacuole. At all costs, the intracellular pathogen will attempt to avoid this maturation process. Scientists have studied the stages in the formation of these structures, usually "marked" with specific host proteins in the membrane of the vesicles, which has led to knowledge of how specific pathogens arrest maturation before phago-lysosome formation, often considered the penultimate step in bacterial death.

The phago-lysosome, as a microbial death bag, leaves no stone unturned. The shear diversity of different harmful substances that attack the enclosed bacterium is a testament to the strong evolutionary push for bacteria to avoid the maturation of this vacuole. One of the earliest changes is the recruitment of the so-called **V-ATPase proton pump** to the late endosome-phagosome membrane. The V-ATPase cleaves free ATP to generate energy to transport hydrogen ions (H$^+$) from the host cytoplasm into the lumen of the phagosome. These ions concentrate to the point of eventually lowering the pH to about 5, which is acidic enough to kill most bacteria. Thus, one of the more prominent defenses of intracellular bacteria against killing is to prevent the acidification of the compartment. In some cases, acidification promotes virulence because it enhances the translocation of certain bacterial toxins across the lumen into the cytoplasm.

At a somewhat later stage, the phagosome also increases its level of either **reactive oxygen species** (ROS) or **reactive nitrogen species** (RNS). The NAPDH oxidase system, located on the phagosome membrane, uses NADPH and oxygen to make superoxide (O$_2^-$), which is converted in the presence of hydrogen ions made by the V-ATPase to hydrogen peroxide (H$_2$O$_2$) and eventually hydroxide ion (HO$^.$). These ROS wreak havoc on the bacterium; they destroy certain amino acids, lipids in the membrane, and can break DNA. The enzyme **inducible nitric oxide synthetase** (iNOS), located in the host cytoplasm, generates nitric oxide (NO) which diffuses into the phagosome and becomes NO$_2^.$, a highly reactive RNS that also reacts with the bacterium. Intracellular bacteria have a counter for these oxidative

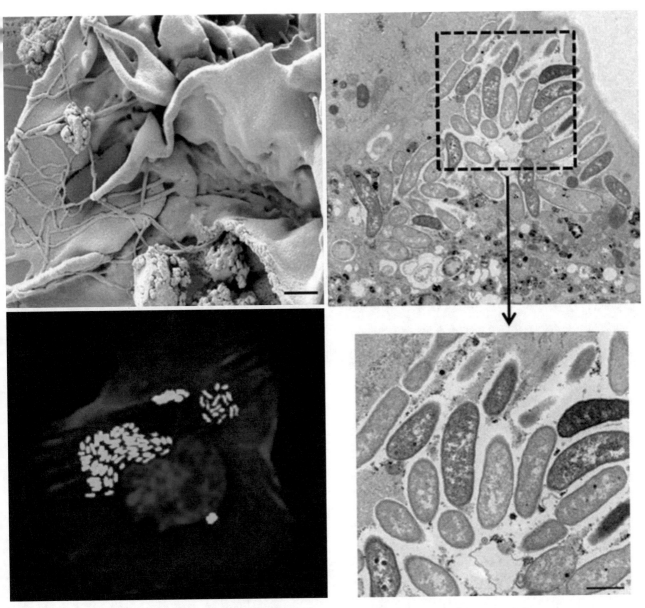

Fig. 8.5 Bacterial invasion and replication. The top left image shows a transmission electron micrograph of *Vibrio parahaemolyticus* (color coded purple) being wrapped in a host membrane-ruffle like structure. The bottom left image demonstrates many *V. parahaemolyticus* (expressing green fluorescent protein) inside a HeLa cell. Note that the cytoskeleton is stained red with rhodamine-phalloidin and the nucleus blue (Hoechst stain). The right panel is an electron micrograph that shows *V. parahaemolyticus* has seemingly escaped from any membranous structure and is free in the cytoplasm (boxed area). (Adapted from Orth et al (see *suggested readings*) under a creative commons license. (▶ https://creativecommons.org/licenses/by-nc-sa/3.0))

species as well. This includes making the enzyme **catalase**, which destroys the reactive radicals before they encounter critical bacterial molecules. Pathogenic bacteria also prevent the function or formation of the two enzyme complexes (NADPH oxidase and iNOS) that make these radicals.

We will examine the topic of bacterial nutrient acquisition in ▶ Chap. 11. Suffice it to say at this point that another strategy to limit intracellular bacteria is to starve them. This is more easily achieved in the phagosome then in the host cytoplasm. Specifically, the host secretes **lactoferrin** into the lumen to chelate iron, a metal most desired (and often absolutely needed) for microbial growth. Iron and other metals, including the metal manganese (which is a co-factor for bac-

terial enzymes that break down free radicals), are also exported out of the phagosome by the action of **natural resistance-associated macrophage protein 1** (NRAMP1). Bacteria can resist these changes by upregulating high-affinity metal transporters on their surface or secreting small molecules that chelate iron, termed siderophores.

Finally, lysosome fusion brings other obstacles to bacterial survival, including a small armamentarium of host enzymes that target key surface bacterial structures. The most substantial is lysozyme, which degrades bacterial cell walls. **Antimicrobial peptides** (AMPs) such as defensins will integrate into bacterial membranes, leading to their disruption and eventual collapse. There are **lipases** that also cleave

8

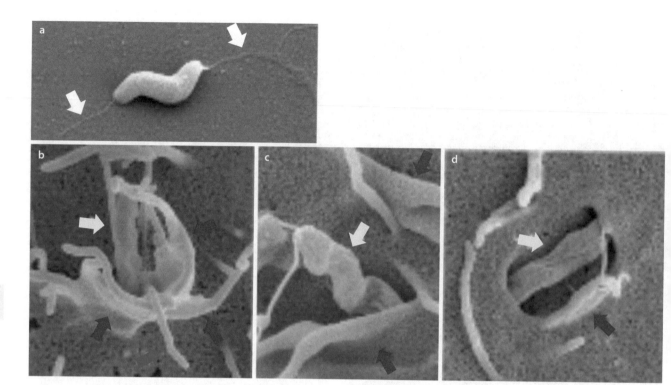

◻ Fig. 8.6 Membrane ruffling and filopodia during bacterial invasion. High resolution field emission scanning electron microscopy of *Campylobacter jejuni* infection of host cells. **a** Shown are *C. jejuni*, with prominent flagellar structures (white arrows) adhering to the surface of host cells. **b, c** A single *C. jejuni* cell (yellow arrows) being partially engulfed by a ruffled membrane (red arrows) and filopodia (blue arrows). **d** Here, the membrane ruffles have seemingly collapsed on the bacterial cell while an additional ruffle (red arrow) is still extended. (Adapted from Backert et al (see *suggested readings*) under a creative commons license. (▶ https://creativecommons.org/licenses/by/4.0/))

the phospholipids in bacterial membranes and **proteases** that cleave bacterial proteins and peptides. **Hydrolases** may degrade important bacterial sugars, especially those that constitute a portion of the cell wall. The pathogenic intracel- lular bacterium responds in turn by making its own proteases to degrade AMPs or host enzymes. Bacteria also rearrange their cell wall or membrane to be less susceptible to host enzymes or AMPs that target them.

Out of the Box

In June of 1976, 2000 veterans of the American Legion cel- ebrated the bicentennial of the birth of the United States of America in the Belleuve-Stratford Hotel in downtown Philadelphia. Over the following days to weeks, some of the veterans present at the meeting began to develop strange symp- toms; malaise, vomiting, coughing, and fever. More time passed, more Legion members showed symptoms. The number grew to nearly 200 (10% of the attendees) and sadly some of them died, apparently diagnosed of heart attack or heart failure. A physician that treated some of them noticed they had in common the fact that they attended the convention. The American Legion also reported an abnormal number of deaths amongst its members. The health department was notified; something very terrifying was occurring.

In total, 29 American Legion members died within the first week following the convention.

The U.S. Centers for Disease Control mounted an investiga- tion. A break-through came when samples from the patients yielded the growth of a strange new bacterium – more than 6 months after the conference. It was named *Legionella pneumophila* to designate its first appearance among the veterans at the conference and its characteristic respiratory symptoms which resemble the flu. We now know legionella to be part of a larger genus that contains more than 50 species that primarily inhabit waterways and ponds. Notable among them is their association (and infection) of amoeba. In fact, *L. pneumoph- ila* infects the alveolar macrophages of the human lung, can lyse these cells, and then infect new macrophages, no doubt an evolutionary carry-over from the amoeba-infecting property of the genus. It turns out, *L. pneumophila* had somehow made its way into the cooling tower of the hotel's air conditioning system. As the warm air passed by the tower to get cold, it picked up the bacterium and distributed it to those in the conference room.

Since then, there have been at least a dozen more large scale outbreaks of legionella, as it is now commonly called. Even a retrospective analysis has concluded that some past outbreaks were caused by this organism. What is remarkable about this story is that the bacterium was unclassified as a human pathogen even in an era of what one can say was and still is very advanced medicine and knowledge of Microbiology. Just 10 years earlier, Neil Armstrong walked on the moon. It makes one wonder. What other bacteria, viruses, parasites, or patho- genic fungi lurk amongst us, hidden, waiting for their time? And what diseases do we already know about that are attributed to something else but have an underlying infectious origin? The microbe hunter must be vigilant, and ready!

8.5 Bacterial Manipulation of Intracellular Host Physiology

When a pathogenic bacterium enters the host via a vacuole, we term the inclusion a **Pathogen Containing Vacuole** or **PCV**. Depending on the pathogen that has entered, it is not uncommon to name the PCV after the pathogen. If salmonella is entering, the inclusion would be called a salmonella containing vacuole (SCV), and so on. The singular purpose of the bacterium engulfed in such a compartment is to avoid being killed by the normal cellular process that directs the maturation of this vacuole into an acid filled bag of hydrolytic enzymes, as stated above, the phago-lysosomes. This structure is meant to dissolve the entrapped pathogen and is the main mechanism by which intracellular bacteria are eliminated. Bacteria employ many different mechanisms by which they avoid this fate, often turning the PCV into their own little cytoplasmic submarine. Invasion represents a challenge to modern medicine because the prophylactic or therapeutic must somehow also work inside host cells and inside vacuoles of host cells. Let's take a closer look at how pathogens manipulate normal clearance mechanisms to maintain their survival in the host.

8.5.1 Railroads

Host cells contain directional pathways by which they move vesicles, including those containing engulfed antigens, around the cell. Normally, these vesicles contain precious cellular cargo that is meant to be transported from the external environment to inside the cell or from inside the cell to be released into the surrounding tissues. Think of them as a railroad system, going two ways, each cargo container housing a unique payload to deliver important molecules to the host. The tracks themselves are called **microtubules**, which are small cellular filaments with directionality. The vesicle is linked to the microtubule tracks by a complex of proteins that includes a fascinating family of motor proteins called kinesins, of which there are more than a dozen different types that have been described. Kinesins link the hydrolysis of high energy phosphate bonds of ATP with mechanical movement, or "walking." Two kinesin proteins forming a dimer, each having long coiled-coiled regions, intertwine to create "legs" that translate the energy released from ATP cleavage to leg over leg walking of the kinesin down the microtubule shaft, taking the vesicular cargo along. Like a stowaway secretly boarding a train for a free cross-country ride, enclosed bacteria can use this railroad system to their advantage. Unlike a passenger whose destination is fixed in one direction, bacteria actually have the ability to re-route the cargo to a location that suites them. Such is the case with salmonella. Once internalized, salmonella not only directs vesicles to come its way but also lays down an entire new set of railroad tracks to direct the entire transport cargo around the

cell. A salmonella effector secreted by the type-III secretion system, termed **salmonella-induced filament A**, functions to recruit the motor protein kinesin and its accessory factors to the SCV. This complex directs the SCV to the microtubule tracks and the motor system propels the vesicle to a perinuclear region of the cell. The exact reason for this localization is unknown; maybe it's a gathering locale of several vesicle structures, some housing salmonella, which fuse into a larger structure with extended vesicles termed the **endosomal tubules** or ETs, also known as salmonella-induced filaments (SIFS) because they are constructed by the activity of secreted salmonella effectors. The ETs are essentially a long railroad system of cargo on microtubules that extends near to the plasma membrane and is likely salmonella's escape route once it decides to exit the cell.

8.5.2 Chemical Control

Laying your own railroad is one thing, but making a lipid-sugar conjugate that resembles host bioactive membrane molecules is another. This is exactly what M. tuberculosis and related mycobacterial species appear to do. Called phosphatidylinositols, these lipids are found in the mycobacterial cell wall. One in particular, termed **mannose-capped lipoarabinomannan** (ManLAM), is shed by mycobacterium during intracellular infection of host cells, and has at least three distinct effects on the host that promote the safe persistence of mycobacterium in an intracellular vacuole. The first is it inhibits the production of two proinflammatory molecules, interleukin 12 and interferon gamma. IL12 stimulates natural killer and T-cell activity, directing them towards infected host cells. Interferon gamma promotes the maturation of the phagolysosome. By suppressing these molecules, both the mycobacterial vacuole and the entire host cell that is infected remain a safe domain for the bacteria. Second, ManLAM activates cellular pathways that enhance cell survival while suppressing those that lead to host cell apoptosis. This too ensures the host cell is kept alive, thereby maintaining the reservoir mycobacteria needs to survive. Finally, ManLAM can also alter host signaling pathways that keep the mycobacterial vacuole in an immature, and thus hospitable, place. One of the more potent signals of phagolysosome maturation is the release of cytosolic calcium from the ER. This secondary messenger activates the well-studied calcium binding protein Cam-dependent protein kinase II which is recruited to the phagosome membrane upon cytosolic increase in calcium. ManLAM brunts the release of calcium, shuttling CAM-II kinase away from the phagosome. This in turn prevents recruitment of early endosomal antigen 1 (EEA1), which tethers early endosomes to late endosomes, a necessary step in vesicular maturation. With the tether, the endosomes are locked in a harmless state, which is of course perfect for mycobacteria (Fig. 8.7).

8

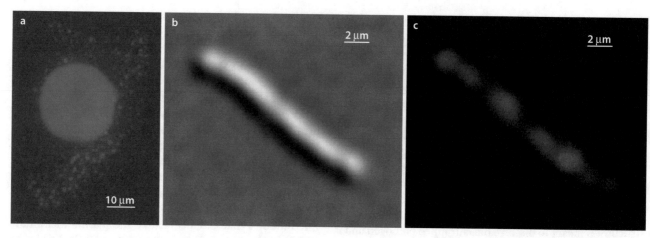

Fig. 8.7 Bacterial manipulation of intracellular host cell physiology. In this experiment, host macrophages were labeled with fluorescent fatty acids (red) and then washed to remove excess unincorporated lipids **a**. The nucleus is shown in blue. The macrophage cells were then infected with *M. tuberculosis*, which enters the macrophage cytoplasm, and then extracted and analyzed for the presence of fluorescent fatty acids originally incorporated into the host macrophages. The red fluorescence in panel **c** is indicative of Mtb (panel **b**) having acquired the fatty acids from the infected macrophage. (Adapted from Kolattukudy et al (see *suggested readings*) under a creative commons license. (▶ https://creativecommons.org/licenses/by/4.0/))

8.5.3 Treasure to Trash

Another major way in which bacteria modulate intracellular signaling processes is through the manipulation of key signals. One such signal are the post-translational modifications that are placed on host proteins. A good example is the manipulation of the **ubiquitylation/ubiquitin** pathway. Ubiquitination is the host's way of targeting proteins for disposal. Ubiquitin can also direct the localization of proteins or can modify their activity or their interaction with other proteins. The process of ubiquitination occurs by three well-characterized steps. Each step has an enzyme dedicated to its execution. The first step is termed activation. The name given to the enzyme in this pathway is ubiquitin-activating enzyme (E1). The E1 uses ATP to catalyze the transfer of ubiquitin to itself. In the next step, conjugation, the ubiquitin is transferred to an E2 enzyme. The final step is carried out by a ligase, termed E3. E3 bridges E2-ubiquitin to an acceptor protein or target, which is to be ubiquitinated. The E3 catalyzes this reaction, thereby facilitating the transfer of ubiquitin to the substrate.

One of the fascinating traits of *Legionella pneumophilus* is that it encodes for a half dozen or so effectors that resemble host E3 ligases. One function of these ligases is to ubiquitinate host proteins, a signal that will get rid of them, which allows for bacterial control of their levels. Remarkably, this ubiquitination step does not require E1 or E2 enzymes, thus bypassing the host requirements for this, giving legionella an advantage to jumpstart the pathway. Instead, legionella activates the ubiquitin via another modification, that of ADP-ribosylation, which generates a highly reactive chemical moiety that is used to link ubiquitin to host proteins that legionella wants to control, including RAB proteins and proteins involved in ER vesicle function such as RTN4.

8.5.4 Redecorating

In addition to manipulating endocytic cycling, forming their own interstate to travel on, puppeteering the RAB complex, altering host signals and checkpoints, intracellular bacteria such as legionella must also shape the composition of the vacuolar membrane. Two masters at this are mycobacterium and legionella. The lipids of a phagosome do more than just create an enclosed container that separates the pathogen from the cytosol. They are also biologically active signaling molecules that stimulate and recruit proteins involved in vesicular formation. Again, we turn to legionella, which uses a two-step shell trick to make a key host signaling lipid that redirects ER-derived vesicles. Legionella encodes what is called the **dot/ICM system**, which secretes a number of effectors including SidF. SidF is an enzyme that contains phosphoinositide phosphatase activity. Phosphotydial inositol 4 phosphate is a highly influential signaling lipid that is a marker for Golgi vesicles. The Golgi system receives vesicle derived from the ER, a normal cellular trafficking pathway for export of important molecules. SIDF, being a phosphatase, cleaves a key phosphate from two prominent phosphotydial inositols that are substrates for another host phosphatase that is deceptively recruited to the LCV by a second legionella effector, LpnE. This host phosphatase generates phosphotidal inositol 4 phosphate (PtdIns4P) from these precursors right at the LCV surface. The buildup of PtdIns4P on the LCV confers a Golgi-like appearance and likely acts as one of the signals to redirect ER-derived vesicles away from the true Golgi and towards the growing LCV. This type of vesicle laundering not only provides key building materials for the LCV, it does so without the host knowing too much about it, a mastery of cell manipulation.

8.6 Bacterial Exit Strategies

To this point, we have discussed the reasons bacteria invade their hosts, some mechanisms of invasion, the host's response to invasion, and some examples of how bacteria manipulate host physiology to survive. Our last foray into the biology of intracellular bacteria survival is their exit. Once the intracellular invader has co-opted host cellular endocytic function for its own sinister purpose, it may need to get out, especially if its primary purpose was to exhaust nutrients and reproduce. There are several ways pathogenic bacteria exit the pathogen-containing vacuole.

8.6.1 Fire and Ice

The first is **lysis exit**. Like we saw with the invasins, the exiting process can be simple and mediated by a single factor. Such is the case with another important listerial protein, that of listerial lysin O or LLO. While still encased in the vacuole, listeria secretes this protein into the vacuole compartment. Remarkably though, the protein is not active. As the vacuole acidifies (an event normally meant to destroy the enclosed bacterium), LLO becomes active, reaching optimal functionality around pH 5.5. It then inserts into the vacuole membrane as a beta barrel multimer creating a pore which destabilizes the membrane. Listeria can then simply move through the dissolving membrane. An elegant control feature is built into this system because LLO will turn back to being inactive once the contents of the vacuole spill into the cell cytoplasm where the pH is neutral. This ensures that the same membrane destroying activity does not behold the plasma membrane, a process that might sound the alarms and draw the immune system to the dying cell. A quiet exit of this type means listeria can move about the cytoplasm while the host cell is still intact. When ready, it will then spread laterally to the adjacent cell, propelled by an actin-rich tail, in another secret move that is meant to avoid alarming the host (◘ Fig. 8.8).

Direct lysis of the vacuole is one way to exit. Other ways play on the theme we encountered during vacuole/phagosome manipulation. This includes the induction of known cell-death pathways to fulfill a pathogen-directed objective. When a host cell dies, there is the possibility of inflammation. Any signal from an exploding host cell that tells the host to concentrate all fire power on this dying entity may result in the attack and death of the bacterium, an obviously undesirable outcome from the pathogen's standpoint. To prevent such an inflammatory response, the bacterium may induce **apoptosis** via the cytochrome C/caspase pathway. Apoptosis is the mechanism by which eukaryotic cells initiate their own death, silent and cold, and without alarm or harm to nearby neighbors. It is often termed programmed cell death. A hallmark of cancer are cells that have lost this ability and thus continuously divide, unchecked, until they spread throughout the body. Apoptosis is the method of choice to exit its host cell for the cause of tularemia, a highly fatal disease initiated by the pathogen *Franciscella tularensis*. The reservoir for this bacterium is usually small mammals like rabbits, but people can become infected if they encounter a carcass. The organism has also been weaponized owing to its high rate of mortality. In some cases, there is evidence that the exiting bacterium is enclosed in a membrane compartment following apoptosis, termed the **apoptotic body**. Decorated with a lipid signal on its surface that is recognized by phagocytes, here we see how apoptosis leads to silent entry into a new host cell, all undetected by the host immune system (◘ Fig. 8.9).

There is also a form of programmed cell death that does result in the induction of inflammation – the process of **pyroptosis** which we first encountered in our discussion of the host response to invasion. In this unique cell death response, intracellular NOD-like proteins recognize bacterial PAMPS after they emerge from the vacuole. Take Listeria, which uses a flagella during its escape and infection of a neighboring cell. A common component of the flagella is the protein flagellin, which makes up the filament of the flagellar

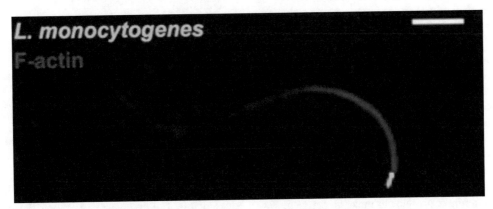

◘ **Fig. 8.8** Bacterial propulsion inside host cells. A prime example of the manipulation of host cell physiology for the benefit of an intracellular bacterium is that of *L. monocytogenes*. Shown above is a listerial cell (green) moving through a hepatocyte via the polymerization of F-actin (the so called "comet tail") that is induced by secreted listeria effector proteins. This image was taken 8 hours post infection. The tail is particularly long because the hepatocytes lack a key innate immune factor involved in adapting to infection with intracellular bacteria. (Adapted from Woodward et al (see *suggested readings*) under a creative commons license. (▶ https://creativecommons.org/licenses/by/4.0/))

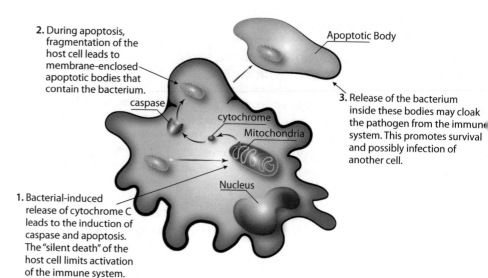

Fig. 8.9 Apoptosis as a bacterial exit strategy. Apoptosis is a form of programmed cell death that generally results in little to no activation of the immune system. Pathogenic intracellular bacteria may induce apoptosis as a means to escape the host cell in a quiet manner without further inflammation

2. During apoptosis, fragmentation of the host cell leads to membrane-enclosed apoptotic bodies that contain the bacterium.

3. Release of the bacterium inside these bodies may cloak the pathogen from the immune system. This promotes survival and possibly infection of another cell.

1. Bacterial-induced release of cytochrome C leads to the induction of caspase and apoptosis. The "silent death" of the host cell limits activation of the immune system.

8

whip. NOD-like receptor 4 recognizes flagellin and activates caspase-1, which culminates in the production of two fever-inducing cytokines, IL-18 and IL-1B (hence the play on "fire" or "pyro"). *F. tularensis* may undergo autolysis resulting in the release of DNA, which can stimulate interferon-inducible protein AIM2, a PAMP that also stimulates pyroptosis. Salmonella, like francisella, which prefers to replicate in macrophages, stimulates pyroptosis as well. It is tempting to speculate that these bacteria *want* to draw macrophages to the dying cell via this inflammation so that a fresh new phagocytic cell can be infected, thereby repeating the process anew – spread by fire!

8.6.2 Morphological Observations of Exit

Exiting cells without lysis seems to be a common, and very successful, theme, and other types have been described. These include **protrusion**, **extrusion** or **budding**, and **exocytosis**. There are shared themes among the four of these mechanisms, discussed here as separate entities. Regarding the above mechanism of exit for *L. monocytogenes*, this can be described as protrusion, the process by which the infecting bacterium "protrudes" out of one cell and directly into another (**Fig. 8.10**). After exiting the vacuole by the action of LLO, listeria secretes another protein termed ActA (actin assembly inducing protein A). This protein is responsible for the characteristic "comet-tail" often observed with listeria as it moves within the host cell cytoplasm. ActA promotes actin nucleation next to listeria by pretending to be the host protein WASP, which recruits the actin nucleator Arp2/3 close to the listeria in the cell. As the actin filament grows, it pushes listeria towards the cell membrane. At the membrane, listeria controls the rho family of proteins to make an active filopodia. When the filopodia extends out and touches a neighboring cell, the listeria can enter the new cell through these tentacles.

This differs from the process of extrusion, in which vesicles are pinched off from the infected cell, best exemplified by

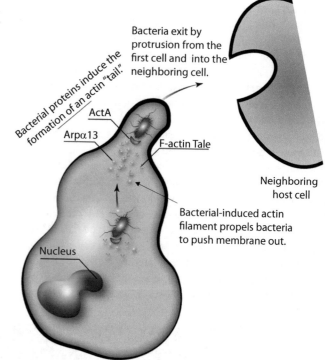

Bacteria exit by protrusion from the first cell and into the neighboring cell.

Bacterial proteins induce the formation of an actin "tail."

ActA

Arpα13

F-actin Tale

Neighboring host cell

Bacterial-induced actin filament propels bacteria to push membrane out.

Nucleus

Fig. 8.10 Protrusion as a bacterial exit strategy. Bacterial protrusion is an exit strategy mastered by *L. monocytogenes*. By budding through the host cell plasma membrane without its rupture, the bacterial cell can enter the neighboring cell, often at cell junctions, without detection by the immune system. The original cell membrane then dissolves leaving the bacterium engulfed with the membrane of the newly infected cell

chlamydia species (**Fig. 8.11**). Here, bacterial effectors released into the cytoplasm rearrange the cytoskeleton to construct a contractile ring around a vesicle that has juxtaposed itself next to the membrane. After squeezing into the plasma membrane, the vesicle containing the chlamydia is released extracellularly. A similar process occurs in what may be called budding exit, as exemplified by *Orientia tsutsuga-*

Extrusion

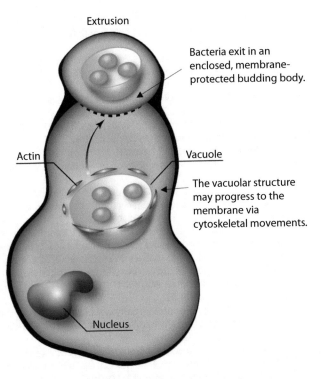

Bacteria exit in an enclosed, membrane-protected budding body.

Actin

Vacuole

The vacuolar structure may progress to the membrane via cytoskeletal movements.

Nucleus

◻ **Fig. 8.11** Extrusion as a bacterial exit strategy. During extrusion, the exiting bacterium is enclosed in a membranous structure derived from the host cell. Being cloaked with host membrane avoids detection by the immune system and can facilitate the movement of infective inclusion bodies to other parts of the same or different hosts

mushi, which can be found associated with lipid rafts at the plasma membrane that pinch from the host cell with often a single encased bacterium. The molecular factors involved in budding are unknown.

Finally, bacteria like *Porphyromonas gingivalis*, which causes cavities and gum disease, employs the process of exocytosis to leave the host cell. Exocytosis is the normal cellular process by which endocytic vesicles carrying cellular cargo fuse with the plasma membrane to release their cargo. *P. gingivalis* simply hitches a ride on this normal exit pathway. Like protrusion and extrusion, exocytosis is non-destructive to the cell, which is most likely the major reason for the evolution of such exit strategies. These are discrete processes that do not alert the immune system. Such vesicles are likely seen as "host" and may even circulate in the blood, being deposited at other locations in the body which facilitates bacterial dissemination. In addition, they may include parts of the host cell cytoplasm full of snacks and goodies that provide the nutrition these deviate invaders need until they arrive at their next location in the body.

Whether the objective is for long-term hiding and persistence or a means to access nutrients to make more of themselves, some pathogenic bacteria have evolved to enter the lion's den of the host itself. These bacteria bid the host to take them in and then cleverly subvert host vesicle fusion pathways and antibacterial strategies to avoid detection and death. There is a clear dearth of therapeutic activity and medicines against such bacteria and their strategies, largely

because the challenges of accessing these pathogens are greatly different than extracellularly localized bacteria. Since many of the world's bacterial infections involve intracellular dwelling bacteria, the microbe hunter should be aware of their survival tactics in hopes of generating new approaches that undermine their insidious intent.

Summary of Key Concepts

1. Natural selection has favored the adaptation of some bacterial species to survive (even thrive) inside eukaryotic hosts. Advantages for the bacteria include being hidden from the immune system, increased access to nutrients, and Trojan horse-like dissemination deep inside the unsuspecting host. Some bacteria are obligate (required) in this regard while others are facultative (can live both inside and outside of host cells).

2. The process by which bacteria enter eukaryotic cells is termed invasion. Morphologically and molecularly, distinct mechanisms of bacterial-induced entry have been observed and studied.

3. Inside their hosts, bacteria usurp normal host signaling processes to rearrange host biology to meet their needs. This includes structural (remodeling of actin cytoskeleton), physiological (redirecting metabolism and cell signaling), and immunological (inhibiting phagosome pathways) alterations.

4. The control of these bacterial processes is executed by a diverse group of secreted protein effectors with structural or enzymatic activity that sometimes replace endogenous host functions or manipulate them altogether via novel mechanisms.

5. Bacteria can exit the host through controlled and discreet mechanisms that avoid immune detection.

❓ Expand Your Knowledge

1. You wish to design a new vaccine strategy that leads to the killing of host alveolar cells infected with *M. tuberculosis*, one of the most common worldwide bacterial infections. Using what you learned in ▶ Chap. 5 on Adaptive Immunity, and your new knowledge of mycobacterial intracellular biology here, formulate a T-cell based approach that will clear infected host cells but spare uninfected ones.

2. Read about Rab-based vesicular trafficking of eukaryotic cells from a recent scientific review on the topic. Explain how three steps in this pathway can be manipulated by bacterial pathogens.

3. Download three recent review articles on the biology and invasion of salmonella, listeria, and mycobacterium. Compare and contrast the ways these pathogens enter, manipulate, and persist in host cells.

Suggested Reading

Boehm M et al (2011) Major host factors involved in epithelial cell invasion of Campylobacter jejuni: role of fibronectin, integrin beta1, FAK, Tiam-1, and DOCK180 in activating Rho GTPase Rac1. Front Cell Infect Microbiol 1:17. https://doi.org/10.3389/fcimb.2011.00017

Cossart P, Sansonetti PJ (2004) Bacterial invasion: the paradigms of enteroinvasive pathogens. Science 304:242–248. https://doi.org/10.1126/science.1090124

Daniel J, Maamar H, Deb C, Sirakova TD, Kolattukudy PE (2011) Mycobacterium tuberculosis uses host triacylglycerol to accumulate lipid droplets and acquires a dormancy-like phenotype in lipid-loaded macrophages. PLoS Pathog 7:e1002093. https://doi.org/10.1371/journal.ppat.1002093

Davis BK, Wen H, Ting JP (2011) The inflammasome NLRs in immunity, inflammation, and associated diseases. Annu Rev Immunol 29:707–735. https://doi.org/10.1146/annurev-immunol-031210-101405

de Souza Santos M, Orth K (2014) Intracellular Vibrio parahaemolyticus escapes the vacuole and establishes a replicative niche in the cytosol of epithelial cells. MBio 5:e01506–e01514. https://doi.org/10.1128/mBio.01506-14

Fields KA, Hackstadt T (2002) The chlamydial inclusion: escape from the endocytic pathway. Annu Rev Cell Dev Biol 18:221–245. https://doi.org/10.1146/annurev.cellbio.18.012502.105845

Hybiske K, Stephens R (2015) Cellular Exit Strategies of Intracellular Bacteria. Microbiol Spectr 3. https://doi.org/10.1128/microbiolspec.VMBF-0002-2014

Knuff K, Finlay BB (2017) What the SIF Is Happening-The Role of Intracellular. Front Cell Infect Microbiol 7:335. https://doi.org/10.3389/fcimb.2017.00335

Kumar Y, Valdivia RH (2009) Leading a sheltered life: intracellular pathogens and maintenance of vacuolar compartments. Cell Host Microbe 5:593–601. https://doi.org/10.1016/j.chom.2009.05.014

Mambu J et al (2017) An Updated View on the Rck Invasin of. Front Cell Infect Microbiol 7:500. https://doi.org/10.3389/fcimb.2017.00500

Leone P, Méresse S (2011) Kinesin regulation by Salmonella. Virulence 2:63–66

McFarland AP et al (2018) RECON-Dependent Inflammation in Hepatocytes Enhances Listeria monocytogenes Cell-to-Cell Spread. MBio 9. https://doi.org/10.1128/mBio.00526-18

Mikula KM, Kolodziejczyk R, Goldman A (2012) Yersinia infection tools characterization of structure and function of adhesins. Front Cell Infect Microbiol 2:169. https://doi.org/10.3389/fcimb.2012.00169

Qiu J, Luo ZQ (2017) Legionella and Coxiella effectors: strength in diversity and activity. Nat Rev Microbiol 15:591–605. https://doi.org/10.1038/nrmicro.2017.67

Ribet D, Cossart P (2015) How bacterial pathogens colonize their hosts and invade deeper tissues. Microbes Infect 17:173–183. https://doi.org/10.1016/j.micinf.2015.01.004

Vergne I, Chua J, Singh SB, Deretic V (2004) Cell biology of mycobacterium tuberculosis phagosome. Annu Rev Cell Dev Biol 20:367–394. https://doi.org/10.1146/annurev.cellbio.20.010403.114015

Weiss G, Schaible UE (2015) Macrophage defense mechanisms against intracellular bacteria. Immunol Rev 264:182–203. https://doi.org/10.1111/imr.12266

Bacterial Secretion Systems

© Springer Nature Switzerland AG 2019
A. W. Maresso, *Bacterial Virulence*, https://doi.org/10.1007/978-3-030-20464-8_9

Learning Goals

In this chapter, we discuss the structure, mechanism of action, and function of bacterial secretion systems as they relate to the delivery of polypeptides into the host environment. These systems encompass those that deliver proteins into the extracellular milieu where they can diffuse to nearby cells or tissues as well as those that are directly delivered into eukaryotic or other prokaryotic cells. Since many of these secreted proteins are effectors or toxins, the relationship between their delivery and pathogenesis is explored using specific examples of their action for certain pathogens. The learner will be well versed in the basic biology of bacterial secretion, especially relevant concepts as they relate to the negative effects on host physiology.

9.1 Introduction

A bacterium is puny. The average *E. coli* cell is volumetrically about 2000 times smaller than the average epithelial cell and 5000 times smaller than a typical macrophage. This is about the difference between a large human and a small mouse. For a bacterium, physical distance is a matter of life or death. If it must engage the host to survive, it will need to overcome the fact that its ability to gain access to critical areas of the host cell are limited by distance. A macrophage extending out lamellopodia or filopodia, large tentacle-like structures, can stop a bacterium from coming anywhere near its surface, much like an adult, arms extended to a child's head, can prevent being hit by swinging fists.

Pathogenic bacteria solve this problem by "action from afar", namely, the secretion of protein-based toxins or effectors that can diffuse to far greater distances than the bacterium can readily travel. These molecules extend the territory over which a pathogen can assert its influence. A rogue nation state with limited air or navy power but which possesses long-range missiles is a threat regardless of its size. Similarly, a bacterial protein toxins helps close the distance gap because its enzymatic properties can negatively affect a host cell that is a great distance from the bacterium.

Toxins also allow the bacterium to exert fine motor control over what it wishes to target. A long-range missile system capable of targeting a nation's capital of government or its military center can produce a lethal blow in one quick strike. A bacterial toxin or effector secreted into the blood may ignore the thousands or millions of harmless epithelial cells until it finds a mobile, lethal macrophage. Taking down a macrophage from a distance, which may have eventually phagocytosed the bacterium, short-circuits the host attack before it even begins. So, in addition to "action from afar", bacterial toxins also allow for specific targeting of host tissues, cell types, or important processes. This surgical approach balances the equation a bit; size and distance matters less with such sophisticated molecular weapons systems.

9.1.1 Challenges and Types

Before we explore the extraordinary properties of the long-range action of bacterial missile technology, we must first consider the problems associated with their launch, or as it is referred to by the microbe hunters that study it, their secretion. The first is **topology**. The transport of such complex proteins must transverse the bacterial cytoplasm, across sometimes two membranes and a cell wall, and then in some cases, also cross either the host plasma membrane or the membranes and cell walls of other bacteria. The second is **protection**. The bacterial proteins may be sensitive to osmolarity, pH, additional chemistry, and their maturation (in terms of their folding) may not be complete until they exit the cell. As such, they must be protected in their transit from the harsh external environment, with different ions, ligands, and proteases, that may catastrophically harm them before they are ready. The third condition is **temporal control**. A launch system allows one to control the exact moment of the release of the payload, as well as the order of release. Temporal and hierarchical control of a dozen or so bacterial proteins, each with its own target and activity, is a powerful way to sleigh a giant. The solutions to these problems come in the form of the **bacterial secretion system**.

Secretion systems are ubiquitous to all bacterial genera, but not all bacteria contain secretion systems whose function is to cripple mammalian host defenses or offensives. Some span both the inner and outer membranes, while others only span a single membrane and rely on an auxiliary process to complete secretion. Common to most of them are some type of cytoplasmic docking complex that recognizes the substrate to be secreted, a membrane-spanning channel or pore that allows for transit of the substrate across a bilayer, and a mechanism to release the substrate either into the periplasm or the extracellular environment. The simplest of them contain a few proteins; the grandest contain upwards of twenty. All are elegant in form and function.

There are seven secretion systems (types 1–7), numbered for the most part in the order they were discovered. There are other secretion systems not numbered, but not less important, including the very common Sec YEG translocon. Because of their transit from cytoplasm to the cell surface, the curli and chaperone-usher pathway may also be considered secretion systems in and of themselves. Their description was considered in ▶ Chap. 7. The first recognition that bacteria may move a substrate through a defined structure from one location to another occurred with the discovery of conjugation, circa the mid-1940s. Pili were recognized in the 1950s. By then, it was becoming clear that bacteria made all types of different surface structures. A 25 year period of intense investigation beginning in the early 1980s would result in the elucidation of six types of secretion systems. Their functional and structural characterization, including some of the most elegant high resolution electron microscopy visuals, shortly followed. Today, much of what remains uncharacterized include the exact mechanism by which substrates are transported, and ways the microbe hunter can exploit this knowldge for therapeutic gain. All of these systems are applicable o Gram-negative, double-membraned bacteria. As such, every system except the type 5 and pili systems transport substrates across both the inner and outer membrane.

9.2 The Sec Translocon

We start with a description of the **Sec translocon** because its function transcends most of bacterial secretory biology (□ Fig. 9.1). It also aids in the secretion of substrates associated with the main secretion systems involved in killing bacteria or the host cell. The translocon is also fundamental to the health of the bacterial cell. Many inner and outer membrane proteins – porins, transporters, adhesins, etc. – make their way to their membranous locations via secretion through this system. The components of this system are referred to as Sec proteins. The process begins with the newly transcribed nascent pre-protein emerging from the ribosome. Four separate structural and functional components then work together to ensure secretion. From the ribosome, the pre-protein is picked up by SecB whose primary job is to keep the still unfolded pre-protein stable and pass it to SecA, the translocon ATPase. An N-terminal signal on the pre-protein is largely responsible for directing the substrate to the Sec pathway since SecA recognizes both the pre-protein bound SecB as well as the free N-terminus of the pre-protein (□ Fig. 9.2 shows the structure of SecB). SecA is directly associated with the inner membrane system that will move the

protein into the periplasmic space. This grouping is called the SecYEG translocon, a three protein complex that makes up the channel. The association of SecA with the translocon leads to its opening, which can then receive a substrate. SecY forms the channel walls and is absolutely needed for secretion. SecE probably stabilizes the translocon while SecG, although dispensable, does seem to provide some level of control having the ability to accelerate protein translocation. There is debate, and this is for just about every secretion system discussed herein, as to how the substrate is transported into the periplasmic space. One model calls for an alternating on/off cycle of a SecA monomer that drives conformational changes in the translocon that push the substrate through the channel. Another model suggests SecA acts as a type of ratchet, powered by ATP, each power stroke feeding a defined length of amino acids into the bore. Regardless of the exact mechanism, in addition to hundreds maybe thousands of different surface proteins transported in this manner, the type 2 and 5 secretion systems, as well as the secretion pathways that generate pili, all need the Sec translocon to transport proteins across the inner membrane.

9.3 The Twin-Arginine Translocation System

What is not handled by the Sec secretion system may be secreted by another, similar system termed the **twin-arginine translocation system** (Tat for short – □ Fig. 9.3). The system is named because the N-terminal secretion signal contains

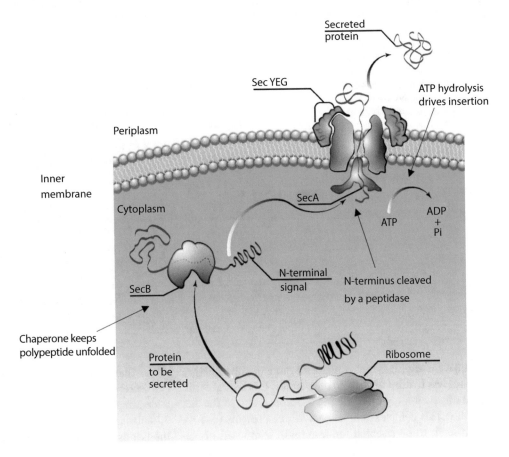

□ **Fig. 9.1** The Sec translocon. A significant fraction of extracellular bacterial proteins are secreted by the Sec translocon. Newly synthesized polypeptides are recognized by the chaperone SecB which then delivers the unfolded substrate to the SecA which uses the energy from ATP hydrolysis to insert the polypeptide into the YEG translocator complex. Following passage through the YEG complex the secreted protein folds in the periplasm. Not shown: the N-terminus, which helps direct the polypeptide to the membrane, is cleaved by a membrane-localized peptidase

9

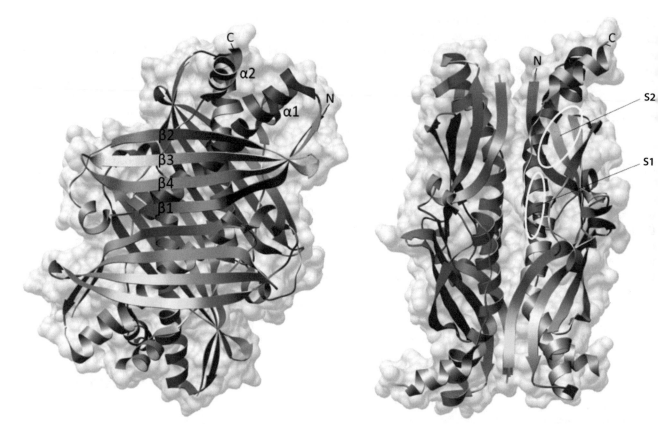

◘ Fig. 9.2. The Sec chaperone. The sec translocon consists of at least three separate functional entities that are critical for proper protein secretion. One of these is the behavior of the chaperone, which keeps the to-be-secreted protein unfolded and protected as it guides it to the membrane ATPase. Shown here is the ribbon structure of the SecB chaperone, as a tetramer, from *E. coli* overlayed with a molecular surface representation (light grey). The regions thought to interact with the substrate are circled (S1 and S2). (Adapted from Genevaux et al (see *suggested readings*) under a creative commons license. (► https://creativecommons.org/licenses/by/4.0/))

◘ Fig. 9.3 The twin arginine secretion system. A dual arginine signal located at the N-terminus of the polypeptide is recognized by the TatBC complex, which then recruits multiple TatA proteins to form a pore. The passenger domain of the polypeptide, partially or fully folded, then inserts into the TatA pore and is translocated after removal of the N-terminus

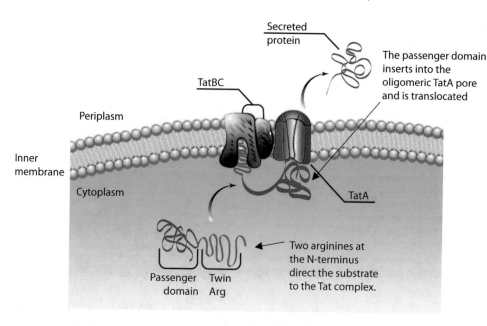

two adjacent arginines that confer a bit more positive charge, and thus less hydrophobicity, to the peptide. It is thought this signal directs it away from the Sec translocon and to the Tat complex. This complex is small, only three proteins (two of which seem to be essential for secretion), composed of Tat

ABC. The Tat system is not as universally distributed as the Sec secretion system and does not handle the secretion of as wide range of substrates as its Sec colleague (in *E. coli*, about 30 substrates are predicted compared to the hundreds or thousands for Sec). The major defining difference between

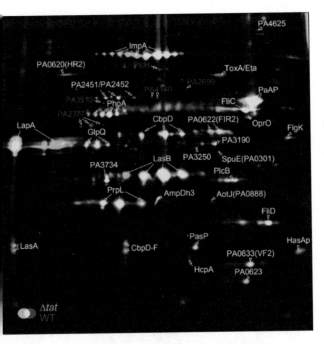

Fig. 9.4 Twin arginine secretion substrates. In this study, the authors aimed to identify new secreted substrates of the *P. aeruginosa* dual arginine secretion system. Shown is an overlay of a two-dimensional gel of the "exoproteome" (the secreted proteins) from a wild-type (red) strain and a strain lacking a functional dual arginine secretion system (green). Dots that are red represent proteins that are less abundant in the mutant strain, which would be potential substrates of dual arginine secretion. (Adapted from Ize et al (see *suggested readings*) under a creative commons license. (▶ https://creativecommons.org/licenses/by/4.0/))

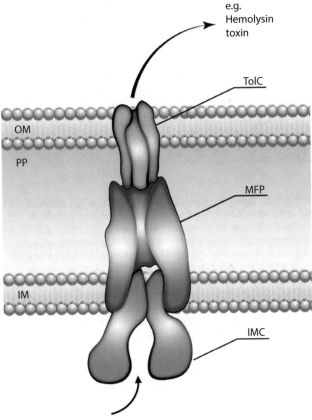

Fig. 9.5 The type 1 secretion system. The bacterial protein to be secreted is first engaged by the IMC which uses the energy from the hydrolysis of ATP to propel the polypeptide to the periplasmic MFP protein. Moving through the MFP channel, the substrate is next received across the outer membrane by the membrane-spanning tolC protein

Sec and Tat secretion is their capability; whereas the Sec translocon only accepts unfolded protein substrates, the Tat system can transport a fully-folded polypeptide. This is quite an amazing and logistical accomplishment. Not only must the diameter of the system be wider (perhaps 70 angstroms[1] compared to 10–20 angstroms for Sec), but it also must recognize different shapes of the folded protein. Scientists believe the Tat evolved to handle the secretion of substrates that absolutely need to be folded first in the cytoplasm. This includes proteins that may be sensitive to the periplasmic environment (and thus can't fold there) or those that need to protect functionality of the folded protein that would be lost extracellularly. A good example of the latter is **allostericism**, the idea that a co-factor (such as a metal) is associated with the protein and necessary for its full activity. The metal can only be added during folding. By protecting the co-factor during folding in the cytoplasm (metal co-factors are inserted after translation from the ribosome, for example), the bound metal, being blanketed by the surrounding folded protein, is safe from competition with other, different metals, that may poison it.

Some common pathogens that use the tat system include *E. coli*, *P. aeruginosa*, and *M. tuberculosis* (□ Fig. 9.4 demonstrates the discovery of some of these substrates for *P. aeruginosa*). Energy for transport comes from the protein motive force and is costly. The N-terminal double arginine peptide is bound by TatC in the inner membrane. The C-terminal passenger domain of the substrate, fully folded, is then recognized by TatA which, upon substrate coupling to TatC, assembles into an oligomer that forms a secretion-competent translocon. The passenger domain inserts through the TatC complex and into the periplasm. As is true for the sec system, a periplasmic signal peptidase then cuts the signal peptide, leading to the release of the substrate into the periplasm.

9.4 The Type I Secretion System

The first numbered secretion system to discuss is the **type I secretion system**, or T1SS (□ Fig. 9.5). The T1SS is responsible for two main functions that contribute to the pathogenesis of bacteria that use them. The first is the secretion of potent cytotoxins, which are discussed further in ▶ Chap. 10. The T1SS is present in many Gram-negative bacteria but are most studied in *E. coli*. Some strains of *E. coli* that cause urinary tract infections use a T1SS to secrete the cytotoxin hemolysin. As its name implies, hemolysin lysis red blood cells (□ Fig. 9.6), but various homologs in other pathogenic bacteria can also target other host cells including immune and epithelial cells. It is believed the system assembles after the production of hemolysin and recognizes the toxin

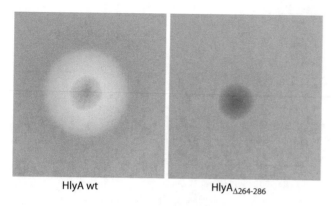

HlyA wt   HlyA$_{\Delta 264-286}$

◘ Fig. 9.6 Type 1 secreted hemolysin toxin. The type 1 secretion system is notable for being the mechanism by which a prominent bacterial toxin termed hemolysin is pumped into the host extracellular environment. Shown here are *E. coli* spotted on a bacteriologic plate that has red blood cells. The *E. coli* in the left panel secrete wild-type hemolysin (HlyA). Notice the zone of lysis of the red blood cells around the bacteria. The panel on the right side is the same experiment except the toxin contains a deletion in residues 264-286 and thus lacks red blood cell lysing activity. (Adapted from Ludwig et al (see *suggested readings*) under a creative commons license. (▶ https://creativecommons.org/licenses/by/4.0/))

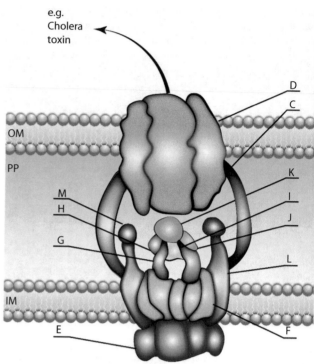

◘ Fig. 9.7 The type 2 secretion system. The bacterial protein to be secreted is loaded into the periplasmic GspJHKI component after transversing the inner membrane (likely through the sec translocon). The secreted substrate may be pushed by the periplasmic complex into the membrane-spanning GspD secretin complex, a multimer that forms a pore which spans the outer membrane. One of the more substantial toxins that induces profuse watery diarrhea, cholera toxin, is secreted by this system, but there are others including lipases and proteases. *E. coli* is used as the model organism here with only the final letter of the name provided for clarity

through a C-terminal signal. The T1SS system also exports non-proteinacious small molecules, the most notable being antibiotics. By exporting antibiotics, the bacterial cell may be spared death by the antibiotic, thus making treatment of the infection more difficult. The homologs of the T1SS that export antibiotics are a large family of protein exporters that are present in cells in all kingdoms of life.

The T1SS structurally consists of three proteins that, as a unit, span the bacterial surface. The first protein is the inner membrane part known as the IMC, or **inner membrane compartment**. The IMC is part of a large family of diverse exporters termed ATP-binding cassette transporters or ABC transporters for short. They contain a cytoplasmic domain that binds the high energy molecule ATP and the substrate, and a transmembrane β-barrell domain that crosses the inner membrane and contacts the periplasm. This protein couples the release of chemical energy from the cleavage of ATP to the mechanical energy needed to move the substrate across the membrane. The second component is the periplasmic adaptor protein, also known as the **membrane fusion protein** (MFP). The MFP can form a channel and it is presumed the substrate passes through the channel after export via the IMC ABC transporter. The final component, **TolC**, receives the substrate from the MFP and transports it across the outer membrane. The various components of the T1SS may mix and match with others to provide specificity as to which substrate to be secreted.

9.5   The Type II Secretion System

The **type II secretion system** (T2SS – ◘ Fig. 9.7), also known by its *E. coli* common name the general secretory pathway (Gsp), is one of the most ubiquitously distributed of all the systems and is thus present in a wide-range of pathogenic

bacteria. It is best studied in *E. coli* where each individual component of the system is referred to by the preface Gsp and a corresponding letter. The most nefarious of toxins are secreted by the T2SS, including cholera toxin, which, for the most part, is responsible for the massive fluid loss and diarrhea observed when one ingests cholera's causative agent *V. cholerae*. It has also been described in other human pathogens such as klebsiella, which can cause intestinal, bloodstream, and lung infections. Structurally, the T2SS is composed of four distinct locational components, a total of ~ 12 proteins in all. There is a **cytoplasmic ATPase** (GspE) coupled to the **inner membrane platform** consisting of GspM, F, L and C. GspC may be the key linker protein here, binding to the outer membrane complex of GspD (sometimes termed the secretin complex – ◘ Fig. 9.8) thereby making a continuous conduit by which the periplasmic components can operate (GspJ, H, K, and I). This periplasmic spanning region of four proteins resemble proteins belonging to the type 4 pilus. These assemble into a pilin-like shaft system inside the GspC-D shell. The exact mechanism by which a secreted substrate is released from the bacterial cell to the outside via this system is still unknown. However, some data and conjecture suggest that substrates are first transported into the periplasm by another secretion system and then

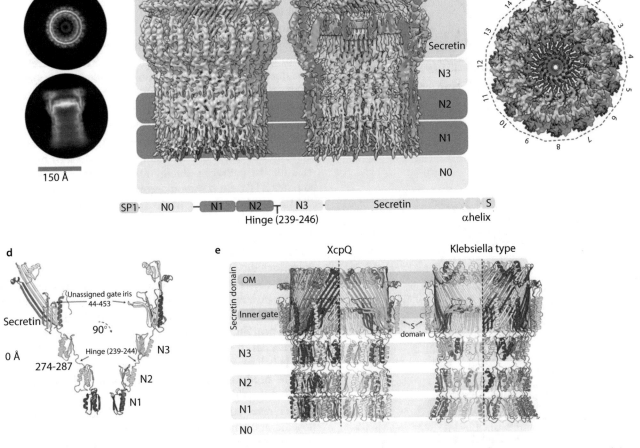

Fig. 9.8 Type 2 secretion system outer membrane secretin structure. In *P. aeruginosa*, the GspD homolog is a protein named XcpQ. Shown here is an elegant cryo-electron microscopic structure of XcpQ (the secretin complex) as a multimer forming a central channel through which type 2 substrates can pass through the outer membrane. **a** Top and side views of electron microscopic images of purified XcpQ complexes. **b** The complex of XcpQ from the side showing the multimeric structure (left) and a sagittal slice of the multimer (right). **c** A top-down view showing the symmetry of the multimer (15 fold). **d** A protomer of the complex showing domain organization (color coded). **e** A comparison of XcpQ with its secretin homolog from klebsiella. (Adapted from Lithgow et al (see *suggested readings*) under a creative commons license. (► https://creativecommons.org/licenses/by/4.0/))

inserted into the GspC-D complex. Transport through the periplasm and outer membrane may occur by the ATP-driven formation of a short pilus comprised of GspJ/H/K/I and its homologues in other bacteria. As the pilus is built, like a piston in an engine, it pushes the loaded substrate through the C-D shaft and outer membrane. Interestingly, somehow the pilus stops growing after the release of the substrate so, in this sense, it is not a true pilus structure. Alternating cycles of this process may lead to the release of additional substrates.

9.6 The Type 3 Secretion System

The level of complexity, elegance, and some would even say dangerousness increases when we consider the next system, the **type 3 secretion system** (■ Fig. 9.9). The T3SS typifies the immense imagination of evolution. What better then to evolve something that looks exactly like a needle to inject toxic bacterial proteins into host cells? The "injectisome" as it is sometimes called, is exactly that – a molecular syringe by which pathogenic bacteria such as salmonella, yersinia, shigella, and others, directly and continuously, pump more than a dozen types of bacterial proteins, sometimes termed **effectors** (see ► Chap. 10) into host epithelial and immune cells. Strains that lack the T3SS or one of its many critical components are often avirulent, a finding that demonstrates the importance of such a system to the development of disease. The substrates that move through this needle complex are guided across two bacterial membranes, the periplasm, are protected from the extracellular environment and, amazingly, transferred directly into the host cell since the needle tip permeates the host plasma membrane. More than 20 proteins make up the structure, in some cells a dozen or more effectors run through it, and perhaps a dozen additional chaperone proteins in the bacterial cytoplasm guide their cognate substrates to the syringe base, also called the **sorting platform**. The secretion process begins with a **chaperone** bound to its paired effector/toxin substrate, keeping it unfolded. In fact, all substrates are transported through the system in such a state because the diameter of the needle is

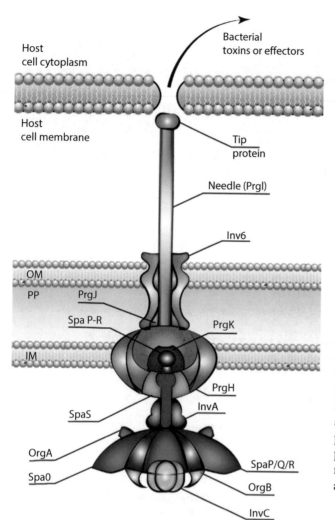

Fig. 9.9 The type 3 secretion system. The type 3 secretion system resembles a syringe and needle structure that pierces the host plasma membrane to deliver bacterial toxins or effectors that alter host cell physiology. Secreted substrates are received from chaperones by the sorting platform located at the base of the inner membrane. Movement through the periplasm and outer membrane may be guided by the Prg proteins with the needle protein PrgI directing the substrate to the host cell. Salmonella is used as the model organism here

quite small, perhaps ten nanometers. Effectors refold upon entry into the host cytoplasm, a seemingly miraculous event considering *it's in another cell.*

The first hundred or so amino acids of the T3SS constitute a **secretion signal** and guide the substrate to the sorting platform. There is much specificity here; the order of secretion is not stochastic. The precise delivery of different effectors into the host cell, each with different activities, is critical for the bacterium's ultimate goal of manipulating its host. Without this hierarchal secretion, as it is called, middle or late secreted effectors may short-circuit the process, or not work at all, creating an imbalance in host manipulation that may not bode well for the pathogen. Energy for this process comes from another ATPase, a common occurrence in secretion, here the dominant player being **InvC**. The **inner membrane base** forms two rings stacked on each other by homologs of the proteins PrgH and PrgK. They sit in the inner membrane, stabilizing the rings. About a half dozen other proteins line the rings, including **InvA**, which may have a role in controlling the signal for secretion. Two outer membrane rings, again stacked close to each other, are made of a single protein, **InvG**, which also connects to the inner rings spanning the periplasm. A **needle protein**, termed **PrgI** can extend up to 70 nanometers from the base to the outer rings; this is essentially the channel. PrgI is helical, which explains the narrow channel it forms, and the need for the substrates to be kept unfolded as they pass through the bore. The needle tip protein pierces the host plasma membrane, has affinity for host lipids, can be immunogenic, and is necessary for injection. A visual and structural analysis of the T3SS is demonstrated in Fig. 9.10.

9.7 The Type 4 Secretion System

Not all secretion systems work to transmit protein toxins as their primary substrate; some influence a bacterial cell's virulence in far more sinister ways. This is the characteristic of the **type 4 secretion system** (Fig. 9.11), also known as the **conjugative pilus**, whose one of several functions includes the

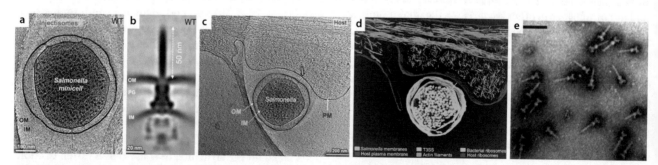

Fig. 9.10 Visualization of the type 3 secretion system. The enteric pathogen salmonella has served as an excellent model organism to visualize and study the type 3 secretion system. **a** A cryo-electron image of a single *S. typhimurium* cell with three type 3 secretion systems visible (blue arrows labeled "injectisomes"). **b** A magnified central section of one type 3 complex showing clear plate and needle structures. **c** A cryo-EM image of a salmonella cell with a single type 3 needle complex (blue arrow) engaging the plasma membrane of a host

cell (HeLa). **d** A 3-D rendering of the image in panel C with added color and labeling of cell structures. PM plasma membrane, OM outer membrane, IM inner membrane, PG peptidoglycan. **e** Purified type 3 secretion "syringes" from salmonella showing the elegance inherent in this bacterial structure. (Adapted from Liu (panels **a–d**) and Wagner et al (panel **e**) (see *suggested readings*) under a creative commons license. (▶ https://creativecommons.org/licenses/by/4.0/ and https://creativecommons.org/licenses/by-nc-sa/3.0))

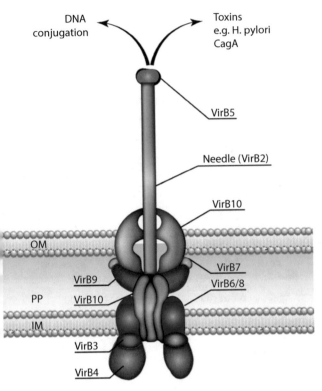

DNA
conjugation

Toxins
e.g. H. pylori
CagA

VirB5

Needle (VirB2)

VirB10

OM

VirB7
VirB6/8

VirB9

PP   VirB10

IM

VirB3

VirB4

☐ **Fig. 9.11** The type 4 secretion system. The type 4 secretion system includes an inner membrane complex that recognizes the substrate and propels it into the central channel (VirB10) with energy from cleavage of ATP. The substrate is delivered long distance through the needle complex (VirB2). *Agrobacterium* tumefaciens, a plant pathogen, is used as the model organism to illustrate the structure

transmission of DNA from one bacterium (donor) to another (recipient). The bacterial equivalent of sex, conjugation is one mechanism that facilitates the exchange of genetic information among consenting bacterial partners. As such, genes that encode antibiotic destroying enzymes, toxins, and potentially secretion systems themselves can be transmitted, thereby conferring instant virulence potential to the recipient. The conjugation system is widespread; most bacteria, even Gram-positive species, are capable of it. Proteins can be transmitted as well, including pertussis toxin, the major virulence factor of the causative agent of the respiratory disease pertussis. Even pathogens that prefer to enter host cells, such as the bacterium *Legionella pneumophila* (see ▸ Chap. 8), uses this system to secrete its Dot/Icm effectors. The T4SS is very complex, rivaling that of the T3SS, with as much as 12 proteins participating in its structure and function. At least two cytoplasmic ATPases are associated with translocation, so-named **VirB** with a numeral (*e.g.* VirB4 and B11), and, much like the pilin-like T2SS, which it is related to, the T4SS is powered by ATP binding and hydrolysis. The inner membrane component consists of at least five VirB proteins, the outer membrane having another three or four, and a "glue" protein that holds both components together, termed VirB10. A cytoplasmic protein, VirB11, is thought to facilitate substrate secretion via a two-step process that first involves pilus-like assembly and then loading of the main substrate, DNA, into the channel.

9.8   The Type 5 Secretion System

Of the seven types of secretion systems, the **type 5 secretion system,** may just be the weirdest. Similar to the curli, chaperone pili, and twin arginine systems, which essentially direct their own secretion through the outer membrane, the T5SS has an inherent ability to move across the outer membrane in a pore structure that forms in the transported substrate. The literature sometimes refers to this system as the "autotransporter" system, largely named because of the observation that the substrate could transport itself. More recent data though indicates that although such a function is encoded in the substrate polypeptide, a complex of at least four additional outer membrane lipoproteins is also involved. Each substrate has two functional domains, an N terminal **passenger domain** and a C terminal **transporter domain**. The substrate is first secreted across the inner membrane by the Sec secretion system as an unfolded polypeptide. A dedicated periplasmic chaperone recognizes the substrate, keeping it unfolded, and delivers it to the outer membrane and a complex, the **Bam lipoprotein assembly** (four outer membrane proteins). How this assembly helps the substrate insert into the membrane is unknown, but the transporter domain forms a β-barrel pore through which the passenger domain will be inserted and threaded. On the extracellular side, the passenger domain folds into its native conformation. Although discovered in the 1980s and considered relatively obscure for a long time, the recent sequencing of many bacterial genomes has revealed that the type 5 secretion system may be the most numerous of them all. Many bacterial proteins that modify host cell actin, proteases, as well as adhesins that recognize host receptors, are secreted via this system. They are prominent in the pathogenesis of heliobacter, escherichia, bordetella, and shigella species. Thus, the T5SS is important in the pathogenesis of bacterial infections.

9.9   The Type 6 Secretion System

The **type 6 secretion system** (☐ Fig. 9.12), the most recently discovered (circa 2006), rivals the T3SS in its complexity and size. The T6SS is found mostly in the proteobacteria, in particular pathogenic pseudomonas, and, interestingly, is primarily used to kill off competing bacteria. This may, on its surface, not seem like a mechanism that would lead to increased virulence, but pathogenesis is more than just the sum of a bacterium's virulence factors. Pathogenesis is also outcompeting beneficial commensal bacteria for a critical host niche. Pseudomonas species, being a normal inhabitant of the human microbiome, indeed encounters such a scenario. This is best seen in the lung of cystic fibrosis patients where, over many years, *P. aeruginosa* slowly becomes the dominant species. This outcome can be deadly. The T6SS delivers protein toxins to recipient bacteria that do not contain an antitoxin protective mechanism. Transfer of these toxins can kill the recipient, thus clearing a competitor. A remarkable facet of this system is that it may be an evolutionary Frankenstein-

◻ Fig. 9.12 The type 6 secretion system. The bacterial type 6 secretion system delivers antibacterial toxins into competing prokaryotes. The current model is that the VrgG spike protein and Hcp spike tube assemble into a "spring-cocked" configuration awaiting the loading of the secretion substrate into a complex formed by TssJ/M/L/K. Once loaded, extension of the spike through the complex pushes the substrate, and needle, into the membrane of the recipient cell

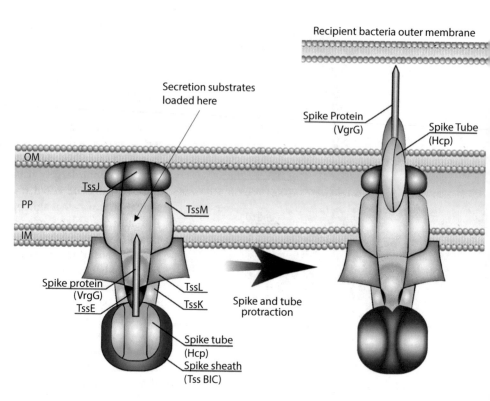

9

like monster. Somehow, the T6SS formed as a hybrid of T4SS components and the contractile injections system common to tailed phages (viruses that infect bacteria).

The inner membrane component, which consists of two proteins, including one lipoprotein, resembles that of the T4SS. Unlike any secretion system discussed thus far, the T6SS seems to grow its needle from the cytoplasm; thus, the inner membrane complex is not the most proximal component. Instead, the two phage-like proteins, **VgrG** and **TssE**, come together in a complex that resembles the baseplate of tailed phages. Three VgrG molecules form a "spike" that serve as a point of nucleation for what is called the tail tube. This is similar to the tube by which phage, upon binding to their bacterial hosts, inject their nucleic acid into the target bacterium. The tube is made of the protein **hemoly-** sin co-regulated protein (Hcp) which self-assembles into a ring structure with an internal diameter approaching 50 angstroms. How this tube transmits proteins, or even assembles, is still under investigation, but the mechanism likely resembles a similar property observed when phage contract their tails to push nucleic acid into the bacterial cytosol. Somewhat like a pin-prick device used to draw a drop of blood to measure glucose levels, once the baseplate and its tube are assembled, rapid contraction leads to propelling of the needle forward through both donor and recipient membranes. If the substrates to be transported are loaded into the needle, the injection mechanism would push these effectors into the recipient cell. It is not known how the bacterial cell knows when to assemble and disassemble the sheath.

Out of the Box

Microbial Surgeons

The author can't help but ponder the elegance and machine-like qualities of say a type 3 and 6 secretion system. Electron microscopy images clearly show these systems are highly organized and efficient. Bacterial cells are more than just blobs and chemistry.

Such structures, which are so near to a syringe and needle in form, makes one wonder if these bacterial tools can be used or engineered for other functions. If a bacterial cell is capable of making these instruments so to speak, and they can execute a designed function, is it fair to say that we can change these instruments to do something else? Maybe bacteria can be made that pump a killer protein into cancer cells, or deliver a hormone to a tissue; and it begs the question as to how far we can go with such biotechnology. Miniature spy robots or robots that enter tiny crevices of a collapsed building are being used already. It is not too much of a leap to envision cellular versions of these that can be commanded to go to a diseased tissue and use their "tools" to correct the problem. If one thinks of biology as a combination of chemistry and mechanics, where all proteins and other molecules have precise fits and forms, it would seem that only a lack of knowledge into the nature of these fits and forms prevents us from making microbial tools that can do precise work and tasks at our bidding. If bacteria can manipulate a host to such a degree just to survive, imagine what is possible if we expand that concept to all eukaryotic biology.

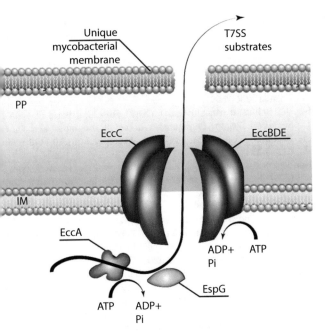

Fig. 9.13 The type 7 secretion system. Secreted substrates are directed by the chaperone protein EspG to the Ecc complex. Energy from the hydrolysis of ATP may assist in moving the substrates through the complex. *M. tuberculosis* is used as the model organism in this depiction

9.10 The Type 7 Secretion System

The final secretion system, that of the **type 7 secretion system** (□ Fig. 9.13), was also uncovered in the past 20 years, and as such we know little about its actual secretion mechanism. Although gene clusters can be found in Gram-positive bacteria such as *S. aureus*, most of what we know of the T7SS comes to us from mycobacterial species, primarily *M. tuberculosis*, the cause of tuberculosis. In this species, a mutant lacking these genes is actually the basis of an attenuated and licensed vaccine for tuberculosis, thereby highlighting its importance in disease and virulence. The core system, (termed **Ecc**), consists of a double barrel structure of three Ecc proteins and associated cytoplasmically-oriented ATPase (EccC). Substrates are recognized by a chaperone (EspG) and another cytoplasmic ATPase (EccA) that likely direct the protein to the Ecc inner membrane complex (EccBDE), which somehow moves the substrate into the periplasm. Unique to mycobacteria, the outer membrane is composed of a waxy lipid, mycolic acid. This "mycomembrane" may present additional secretion obstacles but how Ecc-secreted substrates transverse it is currently a mystery.

Secretion systems should rightfully occupy a seat at the table of discussion of important virulence factors for bacterial diseases. Be it the secretion of so-called exotoxins, the intracellular injection of effectors that muck up host physiology, or the elimination of beneficial host microbes, they should be considered suspect number one for the microbe hunter. There are many unanswered questions about their mechanism, and possibly still undiscovered systems working in relevant human pathogens. The important point is that

their substrates often negatively affect host health, and as such, either their substrates or the machinery itself, lend themselves to promising vaccine or small molecule targets.

Summary of Key Concepts
1. Bacteria can affect the host "from afar" through the secretion into the environment of proteins such as toxins and effectors.
2. These proteins are secreted through highly organized secretion systems that vary in structure and function.
3. Some of these systems secrete polypeptides directly into the extracellular environment, others use a needle-like apparatus to puncture targets cells. Bacterial proteins can then transit through this conduit into the recipient cell.
4. Secretion systems often are encoded in an operon, are important for bacterial virulence, and have specialized components that carry out key functions.
5. These specialized components may include a membrane localization complex that structurally anchors the system to the cellular surface, chaperones that aid in the folding of substrates before, during, or after secretion, a translocon that acts as the actual translocation unit through which the substrate transverses the membrane (s), and extracellular components that engage recipient cells.
6. The toxins and effectors these secretion systems transit contribute to the diseases bacteria cause.

? Expand Your Knowledge
1. Purchase a poster board. On this board, sketch out the structure of each secretion system discussed in this unit. Label any parts that are known then include a column or section that lists their known or proposed function. Write a summary of how a substrate moves through each system and list a representative example of a species that houses such a system. Discuss how each system may help that species be pathogenic or survive in the host. Finally, list key features that are not let worked out in the study of these systems.
2. You work for VaccMake, a startup of Biomedical Company whose purpose is to make a vaccine for every lung pathogen of humans. As division leader, you are charged with the construction of a vaccine for *P. aeruginosa* infections, a common cause of serious lung infections in people, especially those with cystic fibrosis or chronic pulmonary obstructive disease. You decide to target the secretion systems of this pathogen and first propose to determine

which ones are absolutely necessary for virulence in a murine model of pneumonia. You create a strain lacking the T1, T2, T3, T5, and T6 secretion systems and are astonished to find that the mean time to death and lethal dose 50 are only marginally reduced compared to the wild-type strain. You notice that in in vitro models of lung epithelial cells the mutant strain is still highly toxic but that it requires contact with the host cell for this activity. A proteomic analysis of host cells after contact with Pa indicates many of the host map kinase proteins have lost about 5 kDa from their N-terminus. What could be happening?

3. Using your knowledge of the secretion systems discussed in this Chapter and that of your reading of ▶ Chapters 4 and 5 (Innate and Acquired Immunity), and using at most a 5-gene cluster, design the perfect secretion/injection system for a bacterium to cripple the host immune system. Then, use your knowledge of the host immune system to come up with a way it may stop this system.

Suggested Reading

Ball G et al (2016) Contribution of the Twin Arginine Translocation system to the exoproteome of Pseudomonas aeruginosa. Sci Rep 6(27):675. https://doi.org/10.1038/srep27675

Benz R, Maier E, Bauer S, Ludwig A (2014) The deletion of several amino acid stretches of Escherichia coli alpha-hemolysin (HlyA) suggest that the channel-forming domain contains beta-strands. PLoS One 9:e112248. https://doi.org/10.1371/journal.pone.0112248

Delepelaire P (2004) Type I secretion in gram-negative bacteria. Biochim Biophys Acta 1694:149–161. https://doi.org/10.1016/j.bbamcr.2004.05.001

Hay ID, Belousoff MJ, Lithgow T (2017) Structural Basis of Type 2 Secretion System Engagement between the Inner and Outer Bacterial Membranes. MBio 8. https://doi.org/10.1128/mBio.01344-17

Henderson IR, Navarro-Garcia F, Desvaux M, Fernandez RC, Ala'Aldeen D (2004) Type V protein secretion pathway: the autotransporter story. Microbiol Mol Biol Rev 68:692–744. https://doi.org/10.1128/MMBR.68.4.692-744.2004

Houben EN, Korotkov KV, Bitter W (2014) Take five - Type VII secretion systems of Mycobacteria. Biochim Biophys Acta 1843:1707–1716. https://doi.org/10.1016/j.bbamcr.2013.11.003

Monjarás Feria JV, Lefebre MD, Stierhof YD, Galán JE, Wagner S (2015) Role of autocleavage in the function of a type III secretion specificity switch protein in Salmonella enterica serovar Typhimurium. MBio 6:e01459–e01415. https://doi.org/10.1128/mBio.01459-15

Palmer T, Berks BC (2012) The twin-arginine translocation (Tat) protein export pathway. Nat Rev Microbiol 10:483–496. https://doi.org/10.1038/nrmicro2814

Park D et al (2018) Visualization of the type III secretion mediated. Elife 7. https://doi.org/10.7554/eLife.39514

Sala A, Bordes P, Genevaux P (2014) Multitasking SecB chaperones in bacteria. Front Microbiol 5:666. https://doi.org/10.3389/fmicb.2014.00666

Tsirigotaki A, De Geyter J, Šoštaric N, Economou A, Karamanou S (2017) Protein export through the bacterial Sec pathway. Nat Rev Microbiol 15:21–36. https://doi.org/10.1038/nrmicro.2016.161

Bacterial Protein Toxins and Effectors

© Springer Nature Switzerland AG 2019
A. W. Maresso, *Bacterial Virulence*, https://doi.org/10.1007/978-3-030-20464-8_10

Learning Goals

In this chapter, we discuss the function and mechanism of action of secreted or delivered bacterial protein toxins and effectors. The multitude of their effects on host cell physiology, architecture, signaling, and survival is framed in the context of the advantage their activity has on the success of the bacterium during infection. Concepts that lead the learner to consider how targeted intervention disables the disease-causing ability of the pathogenic bacteria are stressed, as is how the bacterium regulates such proteins to be maximally effective. The learner will be well versed in the basic biology of bacterial protein toxin/effector concepts and the important role these microbial agents of warfare play in the subversion of their eukaryotic hosts.

10.1   Introduction

It would be an injustice to the microbe hunter to talk about the deviate ways of pathogenic bacteria and not state that much of their study and modes of making ill health are most directly aligned with their ability to make toxins. Even in the earliest days of Microbiological research, even after peering under the microscope and observing a patient's blood or tissues teaming with squirming bacteria, the main investigators of the day suspected they produced "poisons." The earliest reports were from Koch and Friedrich Loeffler (late 1800s), both examples that also highlight the history of this topic in its fullest grandeur. Koch used the term "toxicosis" to describe the ill effects of cholera, but his experimentation on the topic lead him emptyhanded; direct injection of vibrio culture filtrates did not induce disease in animals. Loeffler was more successful in experimentally suggesting a toxin may exist. Working with the etiological agent of diphtheria, which he discovered and which we have encountered several times in this volume, he demonstrated how, despite there not being any *C. diptheriae* in distant organs, these tissues were substantially compromised. How could this be unless "a poison … has circulated in the blood?" Koch would eventually be validated, but it took a century. Dutta and De would show in the 1950s that *V. cholerae* supernatants could in fact induce fluid accumulation in a modified ileal loop experiment; 20 more years would pass before scientists would purify the toxin, appropriately named cholera toxin, and conclusively show the activity was from a protein made by the organism. It took ten more years (early 1980s) for the gene to be cloned by John Mekalanos at Harvard and another 10 years before its widespread distribution in many other types of bacteria were noted. Regarding the diptherial poison, Loeffler's vindication came sooner, a mere 4 years later when Yersin and Roux, at the Pasteur institute (~ 1888), detected poisonous activity in the filtrates from this bacterium. It can be said this was the first demonstration of a diffusible and soluble bacterial compound producing a disease. However, it would take John Collier, to demonstrate that diphtheria toxin is in fact an enzyme, as just about all bacterial toxins are, and that they behaved by catalyzing a very specific reaction that, once complete, was detrimental to the host.

To date, nearly 400 bacterial toxins have been either cloned, purified, or identified by sequence analysis of bacterial genomic repositories. There are probably double that number of what we describe here as **bacterial effectors**, proteins with enzymatic activity that are not necessarily acutely toxic to a host cell but modify the host cell physiology in a way that benefits the pathogen. Not all of these are unique; here, we make an attempt to classify them on their activity, and from this type of framing, we can observe clear concepts that every microbe hunter should consider when squaring off against their invisible invaders.

We start first with a simple idea. Bacterial toxins, and the damage they do, are nature's version of what the military calls a surgical strike. From a biochemical perspective, they are enzymes, first and foremost. Generally, this means they target a narrow range of host cell substrates, which in turn usually means they influence a specific cellular function. Because they are delivered by one of the elegant launch machines discussed in ▶ Chap. 9 and guided by a global positioning system that consists of a receptor that may be selectively expressed by the host, it also means they also execute this function in a specific cell type or tissue. Such toxins are a large part why some bacterial pathogens are so good at the game of disease. This is evidenced by the fact that diphtheria, pertussis, and tetanus, once a terrible scourge of human children, have been relegated to sporadic cases by vaccination programs that induce immunity against these proteins.

The medical success of vaccinating with inactivated toxins as a way to protect ourselves against deadly bacterial infections should seemingly compel the microbe hunter to study them. So, in the spirit of this idea we begin, namely, by working first from the fundamental premise that if we understand their delivery, specificity, structure, and function, interventions can be devised that neutralize their disease-causing activity. We need to think like the pathogen. If for your survival you had to target critical host processes, what would you take out? When thinking in this manner and viewing the field of toxin biology from the clouds rather than the ground, one begins to realize that despite the discovery of hundreds of different bacterial proteins that manipulate the host, most of their activity can be grouped into simple-to-digest themes. Patterns emerge. Whether the pathogen is simply trying to secure food or silently disable an endocytic pathway that would normally lead to its digestion, toxins really represent very economical and efficient ways to survive. In some ways the word "toxin" confuses our understanding of the topic. The elegant and often subtle ways these proteins work to manipulate the host is far more interesting than there sometimes "toxic" effect. Like little mechanical robots preprogramed to follow logic gates, they bid their master's wishes with near flawless execution. In most cases, their intended goal is to do less, not more, harm. Less is more when it comes to activation of the immune system and potentially just finding a convenient little host niche to set up shop. A summary of some of the main cellular actions of bacterial protein toxins is shown in ◻ Fig. 10.1.

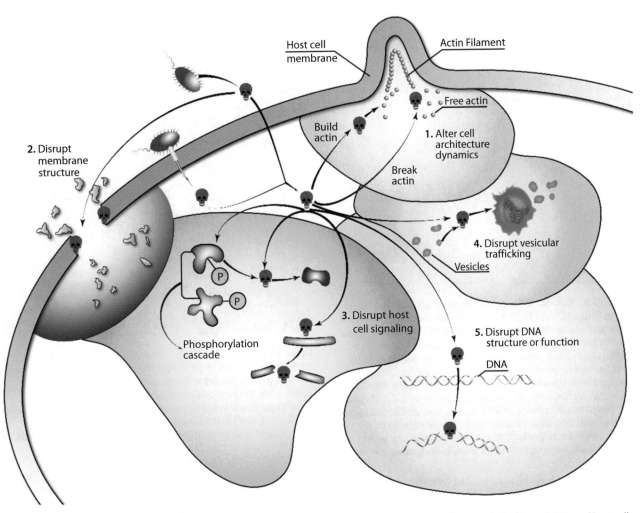

Fig. 10.1 Subversion of host balance with bacterial protein toxins and effectors. One of the fundamental hallmarks of a successful bacterial infection is the pathogen's ability to subvert, control, or down-right cripple host cell function via secreted or delivered bacterial protein toxins or effectors. Although their molecular mechanisms of action are diverse and numerous, some core functional consequences of their activity are evident. These include the modulation of host cell architecture, disruption of the plasma or intracellular membranes, manipulation or attenuation of host cell signaling, control of phagosomal or endocytic vesisular trafficking, and the direct targeting of protein synthesis (not shown) or DNA integrity

10.2 Toxins that (de)Engineer Cell Infrastructure

10.2.1 Non-covalent Tunability

Returning to the question "what host process would you target?", maybe the most obvious answer is anything that has to do with the immune system. We will return to that shortly. But you might be surprised to learn that many secreted bacterial proteins whose function is to manipulate host physiology actually are directed to cell infrastructure. No matter what is happening inside the eighty story office skyscraper of a cell – catabolism, anabolism, all the organization of all the reactions of biochemistry – none of it matters if the entire building collapses. The complex chemistry needed to make life stands, literally, on the foundation of that structural unit. Without it, even the most basic of functions become impossible. Cell structure is a way to compartmentalize stochasticity, to separate quanta of chaos into distinct units so they are more manageable to organize; and, what gives all human cells their structure is the rebar lattice of actin strings and microtubule tracks that stretch from nucleus to membrane, binding processes and even cells together at their junctions. This cell architecture is controlled by a large family of eukaryotic proteins termed small **monomeric GTPases**. So many of the bacterial pathogens we have encountered in this volume in one way or another expend energy manipulating these G-proteins, as they are called. The intense investigation that deduced G-proteins were the target of bacterial proteins from the 1990s until the present is one of the great stories in the history of molecular microbiology.

The small monomeric GTPases have hundreds of members but their functions can be conceptualized into a few key areas of activity. Their name arises from their ability to fluctuate between binding a small guanine nucleotide, either guanosine triphosphate (GTP) or guanosine diphosphate (GDP). They are often called the Ras superfamily because of early focus on the GTPase Ras and their structural and functional

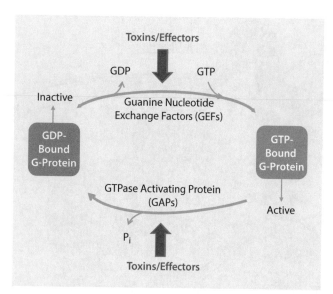

Fig. 10.2 Pathogenic bacteria target small monomeric GTPases such as RHO, RAC and CDC42 to modulate cell-host actin cytoskeleton. Although there are many examples of how toxins and other effectors can alter host cell physiology, perhaps none are more thoroughly studied or serve as a prime teaching example than the ways pathogenic bacteria target monomeric G-proteins. GTPase-activating proteins (GAPs) stimulate the hydrolysis of GTP bound to the GTPase. This inactivates the protein. Guanine Exchange Factors (GEFs) remove GDP, promoting the binding of GTP. This activates the GTPase. Bacterial toxins or effectors, either covalently or non-covalently, modify monomeric GTPases in ways that resemble GAPs or GEFs, among other mechanisms, thereby controlling these key host signaling pathways

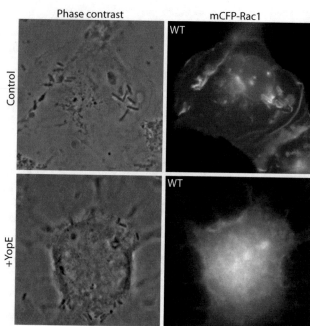

Fig. 10.3 GTPase targeting bacterial effector in action. In this study, the small monomeric GTPase Rac1 has been fused to cyan fluorescent protein (CFP) and expressed inside COS1 host cells. The fusion of Rac to CFP allows for its visualization by fluorescence microscopy. Notice in the fluorescence panel (top) in this image that CFP-Rac1 localizes to the plama membrane of the cell, particularly concentrated in what looks like membrane ruffles. The cell also looks flat in the phase contrast image on the left of the panel. However, when the COS1 cells expressing CFP-Rac1 are infected with *Y. pseudotuberculosis* expressing the bacterial effector YopE, which mimics and contains GTPase activating protein (GAP) activity and targets Rac1, the fluorescence of CFP-Rac1 shifts to the cell cytoplasm, a sign that the GAP activity of YopE has converted Rac1 to the GDP bound state, thereby making it inactive (lower flourescence panel). The left panel shows the phase contrast; noticeable cell rounding is evident, a sign the actin network has been targeted via inactivation of G-proteins. (Adapted from Isberg et al. (see *suggested readings*) under a creative commons license. (▶ https://creativecommons.org/licenses/by/4.0/))

relatedness, but have now expanded to include the subfamilies of Rho, Rac, Rab, and Cdc42. We have already encountered several of these proteins in our discussions of intracellular pathogenic bacteria, particularly the Rab family, which regulates vesicular trafficking. GTPases are often described as molecular switches. The guanine nucleotide in which they bind represents an allosteric regulator of their function. In the GTP bound state, they are "ON." In the GDP bound state, they are "OFF." By simply regulating whether they are bound by GTP or GDP, these binary states can be controlled (◘ Fig. 10.2). Since each small G-protein and its related family members are each involved in distinct but specific cellular functions, this binary control strategy can be applied to a plethora of different cellular processes within the context of a central theme by simply modulating the bound state of guanine phosphate. For example, if a pathogen wants to hone in on vesicular traffic, target the Rab proteins; for actin polymerization, one targets the Rho proteins.

The "ase" part of the GTPase comes from the fact that the G-protein can convert GTP to GDP by cutting off the terminal phosphate of the bound guanine nucleotide. Whereas the small G-proteins do have this intrinsic ability, a protein cofactor can influence this activity many orders forward. These accessory factors are **GTPase activating proteins (GAPs)**. They cleave bound GTP to GDP on the small G-protein – an inactivation event! Small G-proteins prefer to conduct their business at the membrane, a perfect place to regulate dynamic changes in cell shape. The inactivation of a small G-protein

will often release it from this location, along with the help of other factors that keep the protein in the inactive state. Conversely, **guanine exchange factors (GEFs)** promote the release of GDP, which, by virtue of its higher concentration in the cytosol, allows GTP to now occupy this space. This is an activation signal! The inactivation and activation of small G-proteins coordinates the dynamic cytoskeletal changes often associated with host cell migration, phagocytosis, filopod extension, vesicular budding, and so forth (◘ Fig. 10.3).

The G-protein regulatory apparatus is certainly an elegant way to control cell macromolecular function. The limitation, though, is that a binary system also leaves the host vulnerable to exploitation by crafty bacteria. If one could manipulate the guanine bound state of small G-proteins, one might imagine you could gain access to a cell's structural control center. Pathogenic bacteria have cleverly solved this problem. One way they do this is though **functional** or **molecular mimicry**. They "mimic" the host proteins normal function or structure, and, in doing so, take control of that function for themselves

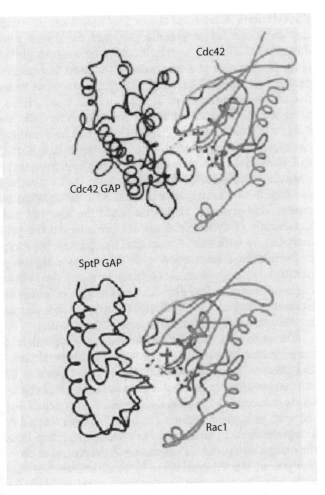

Cdc42

Cdc42 GAP

SptP GAP

Rac1

◼ **Fig. 10.4** Structural molecular mimicry by a bacterial effector. One mechanism pathogenic bacteria use to usurp host cell function is through structural mimicry. An example of this the salmonella protein SptP. This protein contains two distinct activities, one being phosphatase activity and the other a GTPase activating (GAP) activity. The crystal structure of the GAP domain of SptP resembles very closely the structure of the host GAP (shown here as Cdc42 GAP), especially in the local area of the protein that stimulates the cleavage of GTP to GDP (highlighted yellow here) on its substrate Rac1. (Adapted from Galan et al (see *suggested readings*) with permission from Springer-Nature)

(◼ Fig. 10.4). For example, GAPs stimulate the nucleophilic attack of the terminal phosphate of GTP by coordinating a well-placed water molecule. At the molecular level, this is achieved with the perfect placement of a water-loving positively charged arginine residue in the site near the water and bound nucleotide. Bacteria have evolved toxins that mimic this exact activity. Take exoenzyme S (ExoS), a type-III secreted toxin made by *Pseudomonas aeruginosa*. ExoS is a potent inducer of host cell rounding. It targets the small G-proteins Rho, Rac, and Cdc42, converting them to the GDP bound state. With no activation of actin assembly via active G-proteins, the cytoskeleton collapses, a representative example of functional mimicry. This feature is shared by other pathogens, including *Yersinia pseudotuberculosis* and its GAP protein yersinia outer membrane protein T (YopT). Thinking like these pathogens, it also becomes evident that breaking the cytoskeleton could disable phagocytosis or cell

migration, two anti-immune responses. In some cases, the bacterial protein mimics the structure (overall structure or the region concerned with catalysis) of the host protein.

Certainly, these host-modifying activities can disable host defenses, particularly phagocytic ones that require GTPase function. But what if the pathogen *wants* to be absorbed by the host cell, as is the case with numerous intracellular replicating pathogens. In this context, activation of skeletal changes that promote engulfment and then the release of effectors to promote its collapse, might just be what the invader desires. Such a narrative is consistent with the functional mimicry of GEF activity, which stimulates the activation of small G- proteins and is the modus operandi of escherichia, shigella and salmonella species. Perhaps the best studied example of this is the salmonella outer membrane protein SopE. This effector, also delivered by the type-III secretion system, acts as a GEF (GDP for GTP) for Rac proteins by inserting a non-polar region of amino acids into the area where magnesium coordinates the GDP, thereby destabilizing it. Once released, the higher concentration of GTP favors its association, thereby activating the Rac protein.

10.2.2 The Covalent Hammer

The manipulation of host proteins by bacterial effectors/toxins with GAP and GEF activity are prime examples of the type of non-covalent temporal control bacteria can exert over host processes. Because the action is non-covalent, there is no permanent modification affixed to the host target. Thus, it can be readily reversed. Masterful is this strategy because it gives the bacterial pathogen control, turning the action on or off readily. For example, if the injection of Yops into the host cell leads to membrane ruffling and an extension of an engulfing lamellopod (alterations that may facilitate bacterial entry), once in, the bacterium can reverse the process by simply removing the effector or releasing another one that performs the opposite modification. Reversal of the process leads to collapse of the actin extension and invagination of anything trapped in it.

There are bacterial toxins that covalently modify host proteins as well. These modifications, from a practical standpoint, are irreversible. The intent with these toxins seems to be the absolute and relentless subversion of host function in a single direction. Perhaps they evolved to counter the host's ability to reverse the process, or this type of chemical addition was the single best strategy to get a favorable outcome. Whereas a non-covalent modification certainly allows the bacterium to tune the temporal control of the process, it also exposes the action to being reversed by the corresponding host enzyme. This tit for tat competition may be a vulnerability to the bacterium when it absolutely needs the process to be unidirectional. Hence, the covalent (long-lasting) modification of host proteins as a solution. There is no shortage of examples to draw upon, but here we discuss the most prevalent and their outcomes to highlight the concept.

10

Evolution has produced a wide swath of different modifications that bacteria place on host proteins. Some of them occur by the addition of a chemical, some by the taking away of one. Others result in a subtle structural change with dramatic changes in function. One common covalent modification is the glycosylation of host proteins, *i.e.* the addition of some type of freely available sugar substrate to a protein's amino acids. It would take a lot of energy and ingenuity to make a new substrate not normally present in the cell for this purpose. When an abundant metabolite or substrate that is often in molar excess over the enzymes that convert it to products can be used, it is economical to evolve the use of this substrate as a chemical messenger. In this regard, the use of sugars makes sense. They are very abundant because of their importance in central metabolism, and in general there are many different structural types. The main type of sugar modification of a host protein by a bacterial toxin is probably **glucosylation**. During glucosylation, a glucose moiety is attached to the host protein, usually to the amino acid side chain of threonine. A good example of this are the clostridial toxins **TcdA** and **TcdB** (associated with colitis, a painful inflammatory condition of the large intestine). These toxins glucosylate Rho at threonine residues near to where GTP binds. The modification leads to the activation of the Rho protein. The permanent glucosylation of Rho prevents its interaction with the activating GEF while changing the structure so that an active conformation is not readily available. The result is collapse of the signaling pathway Rho controls.

Sugars are not the only thing bacteria put on host proteins. They also attach nucleotides. As you might imagine, being the building blocks of DNA, nucleotides are quite abundant in host cells. They also comprise energy-releasing molecules such as ATP and signaling molecules like GTP. It comes as no surprise then that the precursors to these molecules might be used as covalent modifiers. Such is the case with adenine, and the specific **adenylation** (attachment of adenine monophosphate, also called AMPylation) of host proteins by pathogenic bacteria. Perhaps the best example of this is the modulation of Rab proteins by *Legionella pneumophila*. As we discussed in the chapters on intracellular bacteria and secretion systems, *L. pneumophila* secretes effectors like SidM that target Rab-dependent control of vesicular trafficking. SidM adenylates Rab1B at the amino acid tyrosine (theonine can also be a target of adenylation), leading to its activation. Interestingly, and perhaps the most elegant example of the bacterial puppeteering of host processes, *L. pneumophila* also can de-adenylate Rab1 with another of its effectors. The de-adenylated Rab1 is then a target by a third effector that inactivates its function. This mosaic of successive chess moves gives legionella almost complete control of Rab-dependent vesicular fusion.

The creativity of bacterial toxins becomes even more evident with an entire class of toxins known as the ADP-ribosylators. These toxins have evolved to attach both a sugar (ribose) and adenine (in the form of ADP), which are linked as one molecule, to host substrates (termed **ADP-**

ribosylation). There is no shortage of toxins and effectors that carry out this enzymatic step, and the diversity of downstream effects these modifications have on cell physiology is extensive and astounding. The most historically prominent of human bacterial pathogens, as well as those that are major causes of nosocomial and community infections use ADP-ribose as a host modifier. This includes *Bordetella pertussis* toxin (Ptx), several toxins from various clostridial species, diarrhea-causing bacteria like *E. coli* and *V. cholerae*, and skin and soft tissue infections from staphylococcus. At least three toxins from the lung pathogen *Pseudomonas aeruginosa* also use ADP-ribosylation to modify host proteins. Without a doubt the Rho and Ras superfamily of cytoskeletal control proteins are the primary targets, with ADP-ribosylation being an effective way to inhibit their interaction with downstream signaling partners. But heterotrimeric G- proteins, which themselves are important signaling proteins that function primarily as a trimeric complex to amplify signals from the host plasma membrane, are targets of ADP-ribosylation as well.

The above examples all share the common mechanism of the addition of a chemical to a host protein. Bacterial toxins and effectors can also covalently modify host proteins by subtraction. Here, something is removed from the host protein to induce a new function that benefits the bacterium. For example, pathogenic bacteria can inject effectors that act as phosphatases and thereby remove a phosphate group from their target host protein. Phosphate, and the process of phosphorylation, is a universal signal by which information travels in cells. Toxins or effectors that remove this signal kill the message; downstream proteins do not then receive the signal and stay inactive. Yersinia produces Yops that act as phosphatases and behave in this manner. Other modifications that are subtractive include proteolysis, including the removal of signals that localize host proteins to specific locations in the eukaryotic cell. Again, Rho proteins are the unfortunate recipients of such an activity, and yersinia again acts as master of this technique. YopT is a yersinia effector that cleaves the isoprenyl (fatty) moiety that localizes Rho to the membrane, where it is active. Removal of the lipid group makes it less likely to be able to associate with hydrophobic membranes and therefore blunts its activity via delocalization.

Finally, even the most subtle of changes induced by toxins or effectors can matter. Take **cytotoxic necrotizing factor 1** (CNF1), which is common in the many different pathotypes of *E. coli* that cause a wide range of clinical infections. CNF1 removes an amide group (consisting of only 11 atoms!) from the amino acid glutamine. This converts glutamine to the amino acid glutamic acid. It would seem like a harmless perturbation except for the fact that the modification occurs in the most critical region of Rho needed to stimulate the GAP (inactivation) activity. By blocking the ability to be inactivated, the Rho remains permanently active. This is referred to as **constitutively active**. Activated Rho constitutively activates its downstream effectors, pumping up cytoskeletal activity. Here we see the elegance of molecular pathogenesis at an atomic scale.

Out of the Box

Reductionism and Holism

For nearly 130 years, microbe hunters have discovered, classified, and characterized bacterial protein toxins. With each decade, our understanding of their poisonous effects on our cells increases. And with each decade, our biases of how bacteria hurt their hosts has also evolved. The paradigm of bacterial induced disease has shifted from the mere presence of the microorganism as cause of disease (Koch's postulates in the late 1800s) to the products of the microorganism's activity, more specifically virulence factors, as the culprits (Falkow's molecular postulates of the present). In the last 10 years, however, a portion of the field of Microbiology that explores the relationship between our body and its multitude of bacterial inhabitants (the human microbiome) has shifted back to a consideration of the cellular basis of the association with disease. What was a trend towards a reductionist approach to science, breaking about the individual parts to arrive at mechanistic function (*the how*) is now more concerned with the outcome (*the why*). It will be quite exciting for the young microbe hunter to also explore if the many associations of more chronic human diseases with the composition of the microbiome can also be distilled to a few key molecular determinants in contrast to a holistic mindset where all parts are uniformly integrated and important.

10.3 Membrane-Dissolving Toxins

When the tides of molecular warfare have rushed close to the most privileged of areas, the host cell plasma membrane may be all that stands between a bacterial victory or defeat. By virtue of its importance in cell osmotic balance, amongst other things, the membrane represents the ace of diamonds as a target for bacteria. There are no shortage of bacterial toxins that disrupt this organelle, which brings us to the **pore-forming toxins**, or PFTs (◘ Fig. 10.5). As their name implies, they poke small holes in the membrane; the holes then leak important ions like potassium or bundles of energy like ATP. The membrane may also depolarize, a catastrophic occurrence. The pore-forming toxins are an extensive family of surface acting bacterial toxins present mostly in Gram-positive bacteria but also found in Gram-negatives. Professional human pathogens such as staphylococcus and streptococcus secrete numerous different versions common in structure and function but varying in target cell specificity via the membrane receptor they bind. As a family, they can be further divided by their secondary structure into alpha and beta PFTs, a topic we will address shortly.

PFT activity can be divided into three stages. Stage 1 involves the secretion of the inactive pore-forming toxin and its *association* with its receptor on the surface of the host's plasma membrane. As more and more of the monomers bind the surface, the local concentration of the monomers increases and facilitates stage 2, *oligomerization*. This stage facilitates the formation of the pre-pore intermediate which, when maximized in oligomerization, will then form the active pore which activates stage 3, *insertion* into the plasma membrane.

The binding of a single unit of toxin, sometimes termed a protomer, to a receptor on the plasma membrane initiates an escalating cascade of association of additional units that stimulates self-oligomerization. The broad diversity of the PFTs has led to an equally diverse list of host receptors. These include protein, lipid, and carbohydrates. The receptor drives the specificity of PFTs for a particular cell or location on the cell membrane. For example, the targeting of immune cells by one type of PFT, the cholesterol-dependent cytolysin (see below), occurs because they bind to the chemokine receptors present on macrophages and T-cells. Neutralizing the most elite of highly trained killers from the host immune system, such specificity prevents the diffusion of toxin to superfluous bystander cells that may limit the local concentration increases needed for oligomerization. The second receptor, that of lipids, consist of specialized fatty acids found only in eukaryotic membranes, such as cholesterol or sphingomyelin. These are enriched in lipid rafts, subareas of the host membrane that also contribute to the concentration of the toxin protomers. Finally, numerous sugars are also receptors, including the GPI tails used to localize host proteins to the cell surface. Some PFTs contain specialized regions in their folded polypeptide that bind these carbohydrates.

Of the two main families, alpha and beta PFTs, the beta version have the most notoriety for the topic of pathogenesis. They include hemolysin, cholesterol-dependent cytolysin, and aerolysin families. The hemolysins acquired their name due to the observation that they lyse red blood cells. This is a notable property of PFTs at high concentrations. At the ribbon diagram level of molecular structure, and when inserted into the membrane, hemolysins resemble a bushy maple tree viewed from the side and a ninja star when viewed top down. They are potent membrane lysing toxins that also demonstrate specificity for immune cells. The pathogenesis of *Staphylococcus aureus* is well connected to PFTs like hemolysin; about a half dozen related toxins including the immune cell targeting leukocidins are copiously produced by these bacteria. One the one hand we see the leukocidins destroying the first responders of the innate immune system before they even arrive to confront a staphylococcal cell; on the other hand we observe hemolysins lysing red blood cells releasing a treasure chest of iron cargo for "staph" to consume.

Not too distant second on the scale of notoriety of the beta PLTs are the cholesterol-dependent cytolysins (CDCs), which, as their name implies, require cholesterol for their activity. Prominent in Gram-positive bacteria such as streptococcus, staphylococcus, and listeria, the CDCs use a cholesterol rich area in the plasma membrane to accumulate fifty or more protomers, which by virtue of their abundant numbers then assemble into pores with some of the largest diameters known amongst this family of toxins. The large pore

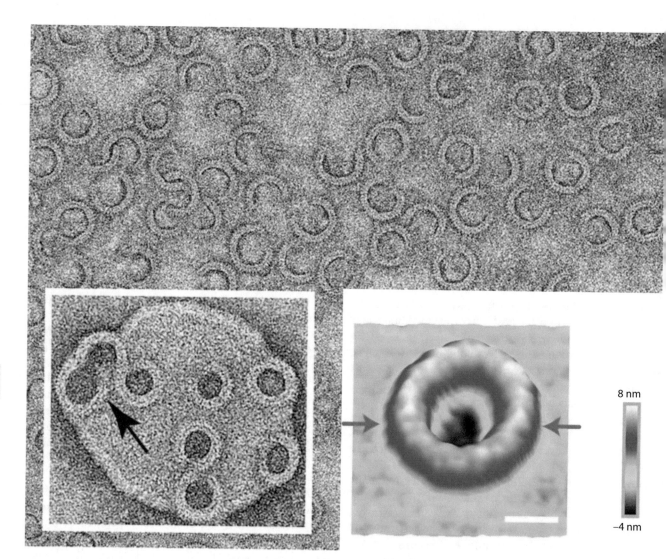

☐ **Fig. 10.5**   Pore formation by a cholesterol dependent cytolysin. Bacterial toxins can form elegant nanostructures. Shown here is a cholesterol-dependent cytolysin (suilysin) from the bacterial pathogen *Streptococcus suis*. The gray rings are oligomeric structures of monomers of suilysin that have come together to form a pore-like structure on a lipid membrane (as viewed by electron microscopy). The colored image represents atomic force microscopy of suilysin with the ring clearly highlighted against the green lipid background. Notice the dark hole in the middle, suggestive of a pore. (Adapted from Hoogenboom et al. (see *suggested readings*) under a creative commons license. (▶ https://creativecommons.org/licenses/by/4.0/))

diameter probably accounts for the potent activity of CDCs. Finally, the aerolysin family, prominent amongst *Clostridial perfringens* (the cause of gangrene), form a mushroom-like structure on the plasma membrane after oligomerization. Aerolysins are notable because post-translational cleavage of their C terminus is required to initiate oligomerization.

The alpha PFTs are comprised mostly of the cytolysins and colicins. These PLTs are commonly found in Gram-negative bacteria such as shigella, salmonella, and escherichia. Like the CDCs above, cholesterol is a common receptor for the cytolysin family, possessing a hydrophobic region in their overall structure. Termed the beta-tongue, it associates with cholesterol via non-polar interactions. A side view of their inserted pore into the membrane resembles a large weeping-willow tree; top down, they look like a vibrant sunflower. Being prominent among pathogenic enterics, these toxins might be important in the stimulation of fluid loss via the pores they create, a leakage of ions from the cell would be followed by water. Secreted by such enterics and with strong affinity for outer membrane receptors of Gram-negative bacteria, colicins are thought to kill competing bacteria in the GI microenvironment. In this manner, they may eliminate beneficial microbes and open a niche for pathogenic enterics to bloom.

10.4   Disruption of Osmotic Balance and Cell Signaling

The 1994 Nobel Prize in Medicine was awarded to Alfred Gilman for "for the discovery of G-proteins and the role of these proteins in signal transduction in cells." It was known at the time that certain hormones could bind to cells and stimulate the production of "signals", sometimes called secondary messengers like cyclic AMP. These signals would direct the cell down a certain physiological path and culminate in some altered biological function. What was not known was how the stimulation by the hormone was transmitted to changes in secondary messenger concentration. Gillman uncovered a series of proteins that linked the hormone-bound receptor on the cell surface with the activation of the enzymes that produced secondary messengers; these proteins were termed **heterotrimeric G-protein** (because they formed a complex of several proteins that also bound GTP, an allosteric regulator of the proteins) **coupled receptors** (because they also were linked to the receptor carrying the ligand, in this case a hormone). Subsequent work confirmed G-proteins are actually a composite of a complex of proteins that each perform a different role in the transmission of the signal, including regulatory ones. The prize was well deserved. The human genome alone encodes for greater than 1000 different types of G-proteins (about 5% of the entire proteome), and their diversity is testament to the myriad of different functions in human physiology they control, from cardiovascular maintenance to brain activity. Their primary purpose is to relay, and in large part control, soluble signals that originate from outside of the cell to actionable items that change things inside the cell. These proteins are fundamental to all life.

It must come as no surprise then that bacteria set their toxin eyes on heterotrimeric G-proteins. To understand this, we have to learn a bit about how G-proteins function. The G-protein trimer consists of alpha, beta, and gamma subunits that come together and are associated with a receptor in the GDP bound state. Upon engagement of the receptor externally with a ligand, conformational changes are transmitted to the G-protein which, with the help of a GEF, may exchange its GDP for GTP. The alpha subunit, which binds the GTP, is then active and thus leaves the complex to activate its downstream effector. This action is what leads to transmission of the signal from the cell exterior to the cell interior. Bacterial toxins essentially short-circuit the G-protein's connection to downstream signaling partners. They do so in two main ways. The first way is to directly modify the G-protein. This is expertly achieved by a toxin secreted by *Bordetella pertussis*, the cause of whooping cough, known as **Pertussis Toxin** (PT). PT is an ADP-ribosyltransferase, transferring the ADP-ribose after entry into the cell to the G-alpha subunit of the trimeric complex. G-proteins are amplifiers of signals in some cases but suppressive of them in others. This facilitates more control over the amplitude of the signal. The G-alpha subunit that PT modifies is actually an inhibitor of the cAMP-generating enzyme adenylate cyclase. ADP-ribosylation locks this protein into an inactive state, which actually means it activates adenylate cyclase by not inhibiting it! The result is a jump in the levels of cAMP.

What bacterial-favoring function would this have? It is known from animal studies that pertussis toxin seems to slow down the immune special ops during bordetella infections. This bacterium causes a terrible infection of the lungs that leads to difficulty breathing; in the worst cases, the characteristic "whoop." The toxin can enter into lung macro-phages. The toxin also enters lung epithelial cells. Elevated cAMP in these cells likely dampens the release of chemokines that draw in neutrophils, which of course promotes bordetella survival in the lung microenvironment. ADP-ribosylation is a direct modification of the heterotrimeric G-protein. But bacterial toxins can often bypass the G-protein conduit altogether by encoding the necessary activity in the toxin itself. Such is the case with edema toxin, one of the three components of anthrax toxin, a potent tripartite killing machine encoded by the cause of anthrax, *Bacillus anthracis*. Edema toxin enters the host cells, but, instead of modifying the heterotrimeric G protein complex, the toxin bypasses the complex by acting as an adenylate cyclase, thereby directly controlling the levels of cAMP in the host cell. We learn more about the amazing properties of anthrax toxin when we discuss toxin trafficking and movement below.

We see from pertussis and edema toxins that the direct manipulation of heterotrimeric G-proteins alters the levels of important secondary signaling messengers. The downstream result, at least for these toxins, is likely a suppression of immune cell recruitment. Targeting of the heterotrimeric G-proteins may not always be to cripple innate immune responses. Manipulation of these key proteins also allows the bacteria *to disseminate into the environment*. In these cases, the purpose of the toxin is to manipulate the G-protein that is involved in the control of fluid balance. The most-wanted in this example is **cholera toxin**. Cholera is one of a few bacterial infections where the cause of death is the catastrophic loss of water. The patient simply dries to death. The cause of cholera, *V. cholerae*, is an enteric pathogen that infects the intestinal tissue of mammals after ingestion of contaminated water. As much as 1–2 liters of water per hour, in the form of profuse diarrhea ("rice water"), can be ejected, a rate that may exceed the ability of one to rehydrate. A testament to their amazing activity, this level of diarrhea is caused by a single toxin - cholera toxin. After secretion, cholera toxin enters mammalian cells through its binding component and ADP-ribosylates the heterotrimeric G subunit alpha S (or "stimulatory"). The active form of this protein increases the activity of adenylate cyclase when in the GTP form. But, the ADP-ribose moiety blocks its GTPase function. It remains always "on" and thus so does adenylate cyclase. The over active cyclase activity dials up the concentration of cAMP, which stimulates protein kinase A to phosphorylate an important chloride channel importer known as the cystic fibrosis transmembrane conductance regulator (CFTR). You may recall that CFTR is also the protein that is mutated in cystic fibrosis patients, a mutation that confers hypersensitivity to *Pseudomonas aeruginosa* infection. The opening of CFTR channels moves chloride ions out of the cell, and with them (for osmotic balance), water. This water represents the fluid lost in diarrhea. With the water goes any cholera bacillus that reproduced in the intestine. By ejecting their progeny back into the environment, a new cycle can begin once an unsuspecting host drinks the contaminated water.

10.5 Targeting the Protein Factory

Cholera toxin represents perhaps the clearest example of the notion that the toxin's main evolutionary role is to promote the dissemination of cholera progeny into the water so a new infectious cycle can begin. Massive water loss is a means to get there. Unfortunately, the host sometimes succumbs to dehydration, hence the pathogenesis, which may be considered a consequence of another bacterial objective. But some bacterial toxins leave little doubt as to their purpose. Of all the host cell activities essential for function, the translation of mRNA into protein may be the most important. Proteins are the engines of biology. Their enzymatic activity yields the small molecules that fuel metabolism. Their structural roles hold the cell together and compartmentalize function. It should not be a surprise then that bacteria have evolved toxins to cripple the host's protein production machinery.

During translation, message of RNA is made, read, and converted into a mature protein. Among the many vital mechanistic steps that ensure it happens efficiently, there are two structural components essential for the process. They are the formation of the synthesis platform and the extension of the growing polypeptide chain from this platform. The platform consists of the two ribosomal subunits (the 40S and 60S units), each themselves composed of smaller proteins and ribonucleic acid. One may think of the ribosome as the factory where polypeptide production occurs. In the early 1900s, Kiyoshi Shiga, a young Japanese bacteriologist and protégé of the great German Microbiologist and Chemist Paul Ehrlich (and an ardent student of the methods of Koch), was sent to investigate "sekiri" or "red diarrhea" during an outbreak of dysentery. This disease was, and still is in parts of the globe, responsible for the deaths of many people. Characterized by bloody diarrhea, intense pain and sometimes organ failure, its mortality rate can approach 20% if left untreated. Shiga used Koch's postulates, popular at the time because of the master's publications about 20 years earlier, to cultivate what is now known as the cause of shigellosis, the "bacillus dysenterie", later renamed Shigella after its diligent scientist. Shiga would also go on to describe toxic activity associated with the bacterium. They were later purified and named **Shiga toxin** (of which there are two!). Recall that our description of this work opened with the 2011 outbreak of an enteroaggregative *E. coli* strain that acquired Shiga toxin; a potent combination of intestinal stickiness and cell cytotoxicity that bred a deadly outbreak and testifies to the seriousness of the damage bacterial toxins can induce. Shiga toxin goes straight for the jugular. The toxin binds to the 60s ribosomal subunit and removes a single purine nucleotide (adenine) from the RNA/protein complex. Thus, the toxin is an RNA glycosidase. The adenine is a landing pad for the host protein elongation factor 2 (EF2). Without the adenine, EF2's contribution to extending the chain is eliminated, an action that halts protein synthesis on all ribosomes it modifies. Thus, Shiga toxin is a translation targeting toxin that shuts down host cell protein production.

Shiga toxin is not the only bacterial toxin that targets protein synthesis. Two other toxins closely related to each other also modify the translation machinery, but do so with a mechanism different than that of Shiga. The most well studied of these is **diptheria toxin**, produced by the *Corynebacterium diphtheria*, the "Spanish Strangulator" known for its infection of the throat and closing of the trachea from inflammation. One of the more potent toxins known, with a barely visible amount to the naked eye needed to subdue an adult human, diphtheria toxin traffics into the cell and ADP-ribosylates (remember this is an adenine and sugar moiety covalently attached to the target) elongation factor 2 on a modified histidine amino acid. This amino acid is important for the interaction of EF2 with the translation machinery. By placing a bulky ADP-ribose at this site, EF2 is sterically hindered and cannot maintain its association with the machinery. As a result, elongation of the growing polypeptide, a principal function of EF2, ceases and protein production again terminates. The toxin's importance in disease is further highlighted by early studies in the 1900s that showed anti-toxin could treat the disease and that the current vaccine which contains the toxin is highly effective at protecting recipients. *Pseudomonas aeruginosa* Exotoxin A is also an ADP-ribosylating toxin that targets elongation factor 2 and is very similar to diphtheria toxin. The presence of ToxA, as it is sometimes called, correlates with worse outcomes from pseudomonas infection in humans and is necessary for cornea and lung infections in experimental animals.

Shiga, diphtheria, and ToxA are all examples of what are termed **A-B toxins**. The "A" refers to the active domain of the toxin – essentially the part that contains the enzymatic activity. The "B" domain refers to the binding portion of the toxin – essentially the region that binds to and mediates entry of the toxin into the host cell. Thus, exotoxin A contains its ADP-ribosyltransferase activity in the A domain and its host cell binding portion in the B domain. Some toxins have more than one B domain. A-B toxins are **exotoxins**; that is, they are secreted into the surrounding environment by the bacterium and then mediate their own entry into the host cell. This contrasts with the toxins discussed in the following sections which are delivered into host cells not by virtue of having a B domain but by their delivery through one of the secretion systems we encountered in ▶ Chap. 9. With Shiga toxin and ToxA we observe two activities, one targeting RNA (Shiga) and the other targeting the ribosome translation complex, that both result in the same outcome, the inhibition of protein synthesis. This highlights different molecular strategies that benefit the bacterium but with the same functional outcome.

10.6 Bacterial Dicers

The next focus takes us back to activities which subtract from host factors, only in a bigger more malicious way. This leads us to the **bacterial protease**. Some will say that a protease is not a toxin, but there are very clear examples of where the protease function is highly effective at inducing disease. In fact, the most effective protein toxin on the planet, and pound for pound one of the most potent substances period, is a protease. It is botulinum toxin secreted by *Clostridium botulinum*. Just a few nanograms, equivalent to about 50,000 times less than a single grain of table salt, is enough to kill an adult human being. The toxin is likely secreted by the bacterium as it contaminates foodstuffs. Upon ingestion, the toxin traffics to and inside neurons where it cleaves a key neuronal protein, a SNARE, that is needed to deliver vesicles containing the neurotransmitter acetylcholine to the synapse. Without the signal for nerve transmission, paralysis ensues. The patient may lose complete control of muscle function. If this happens in the lungs, breathing can stop. The contraction of muscles in the face and forehead is one cause of wrinkles; botulinum toxin, or botox, became an international sensation when it was realized that paralyzing these muscles takes away wrinkles. There may not be a bigger contrast in medicine between the disease-causing ability in one context and the use for cosmetic upgrades in another context as that seen with botulinum toxin.

Botulin toxin aligns the ledger for this section in an educational way. This is because the toxin contains many of the structural features present in bacterial proteases that are linked to pathogenesis. Included in this description is the need for a metal cofactor for protease activity, most often the metal zinc. The metal atom is located in the active site of the protein, the part that grabs the polypeptide substrate, and helps aid the cleavage of the peptide backbone by stabilizing a nucleophilic, or "attacking" water molecule. If the metal is removed, the protease is almost completely defunct of its cleaving ability. This may be one of the reasons why the metal chelator EDTA is so effective as a food preservative. In addition to taking away key metals bacteria absolutely need for growth, it also prevents the breakdown and spoiling of the food induced by bacterial proteases. A second structural component common to proteases is that the metal atom is stabilized by two histidine residues spaced a few amino acids apart (often HXXXH). This is referred to as **coordination**, where amino acids coordinate a metal in the active site as part of the necessary catalytic machinery. Finally, a third structural component is a coordinating glutamic acid residue, which although not positioned linearly close to the histidines, is found in close 3-dimensional proximity in the folded protein. The family of metalloproteases in bacteria is extensive, with many subfamilies and lineages classified by their arrangement of the histidines and glutamic acid. The take home point is that bacterial proteases are metal-dependent, structurally-conserved and very potent purveyors of host destruction. We highlight there many different actions below.

10.6.1 Breaking Barriers

The human body is a highly ordered system of cells, tissues, and organs connected together by a fibrous substance called extracellular matrix, or ECM. A major component of ECM is collagen. Without collagen, humans might look like an amorphous blob. Collagen is the hidden network that helps us have form. ECM is also an effective barrier between cells. It is no surprise then that an entire family of proteases with metals as active site co-factors can degrade ECM components, especially collagen. Here we observe the first function of a bacterial protease, as general artillery launched from afar to weaken the structure of enemy strongholds. Blasting holes in the brick and mortar of cell and tissue networks creates an opportunity for pathogens to infiltrate these breaches. Proteases that break down collagen (collagenases) and other ECM components enhance pathogenesis by facilitating deep penetration of the human host. In addition to what holds host cells to the substratum as a target, the stuff between host cells is also acted upon by bacterial proteases. *P. aeruginosa* elastase is a good example. This protease targets zonula occludens 1, the major crosslinking protein that links tight junction fibrils to the actin cytoskeleton. Destruction of this protein decouples cell and junction structure, paving a narrow but accessible path to breaching the epithelial barrier. This path may be travelled by the pathogen, seeking refuge from the immune system or greener pastures with more nutrients, or the path may be taken by another bacterial toxin whose main mechanism of action functions more systemically. Nevertheless, breaking barriers is a major pathogenic mechanism brought on by secreted bacterial proteases.

10.6.2 Liberation of Nutrients

Proteases are also the knives of bacterial dinner parties. They are important for the acquisition of essential nutrients that aid in the growth and replication of pathogenic bacteria in an environment where nutrients are tightly controlled. The digestion of a single 100 kilodalton host protein can release hundreds of distinct peptides and about a thousand individual amino acids, usually all twenty varieties as well. Small peptides and amino acids are transported into the bacterial cell and used as building blocks for the construction of new proteins or for energy. Proteases may also facilitate the release of metal cofactors from host metalloproteins, examples being iron, zinc, calcium and magnesium. A classic example of this is the InhA1 protease secreted by *Bacillus anthracis*. InhA1 recognizes a multitude of host proteins but one important feature is the recognition of mammalian hemoglobin. Cleavage of hemoglobin by InhA1 is a twofer: it releases the bound iron in the center of the globin fold while also liberating branched amino acids, in particular valine. Vibrio species, often the causative agents of enteric infections, require proteases for the release of iron from iron binding proteins such as transferrin; the released iron is then captured at the bacterial cell surface. In this case, we see how proteases allow bacteria to overcome nutrient immunity, the topic of the next chapter.

10.6.3   Jamming Signals and Transmissions

A strength of multicellularity is communication. One part of the organism can provide important biological signals to another part. That part in turn can respond accordingly, and so forth. During bacterial invasion, communication is critical in defeating the invader. The cells at the wall need to communicate with the immune cells that provide reinforcements and the immune cells in turn must communicate with those at the barrier to mount an appropriate response. Individual cells must transmit signals from the outside in and the inside back out. In all cases, the signals come in the form of small chemical messengers. These messengers can be inorganic atoms such as calcium, small molecules such as dinucleotides (e.g. cyclic AMP) or more complex molecules such as an entire polypeptide or larger protein (e.g. chemokines). Bacterial toxins often claim as a central purpose the activity to decapitate these signals by either preventing them from being made or degrading them all together. Our final example of toxin activity in the chapter investigates a case study of how anthrax toxin, made by *B. anthracis*, jams host communications to dampen innate immunity, and serves as an excellent model for many of the concepts put forth in this chapter (◘ Fig. 10.6).

B. anthracis encodes the toxin on a plasmid it carries. Without the toxin, the organism is thought to be much less virulent and it is believed that the addition of the toxin and a capsule (incidentally encoded on another plasmid it carries), are the two main reasons why *B. anthracis* is so much more virulent then it's still serious but less harmful cousin *B. cereus*. The toxin, in an inactivated form, is also the basis for the licensed U.S. vaccine, thereby highlighting its importance. The toxin consists not of one polypeptide, but three, each part playing a distinct and important role in the overall activity of the complex. The first component is arguably the most critical – protective antigen or PA. So named because immunization with this component can confer protection in challenge models of infection, PA can be considered the "B" portion of the toxin. When secreted by bacilli, it binds to a host receptor on a variety of cell types and is cleaved by a host protease. Cleavage opens the protein up to oligomerization, the final product being a heptameric ring of monomers on the surface of the host cell. The ring acts as a docking platform for the other two factors, which can be considered "A" domains. These are lethal and edema factor, so named because of original studies in the 1950s that associated them with tissue necrosis and swelling. Here we see the targeting or specificity of the toxin, acting from afar.

◘ **Fig. 10.6** Multi-modality capability of bacterial protein toxins. Anthrax toxin, secreted by the bacterium *B. anthracis*, serves here as a good example of the varied abilities bacterial toxins possess. Secreted as a tri-partite toxin, the protective antigen 83 kDa fragment binds to its cellular receptor (depicted here as TEM8 and/or CMG2). Cleavage by the host furin protease yields the PA 63 fragment which oligomerizes, itself serving as a receptor for either lethal factor (LF) or edema factor (EF). After the complex is internalized, the low pH of the endosome induces the formation of a PA 63 pore that now facilitates the transfer of EF and LF to the cytoplasm where they modify their host targets. (Adapted from Sausa et al. (see *suggested readings*) under a creative commons license. (▶ https://creativecommons.org/licenses/by/4.0/))

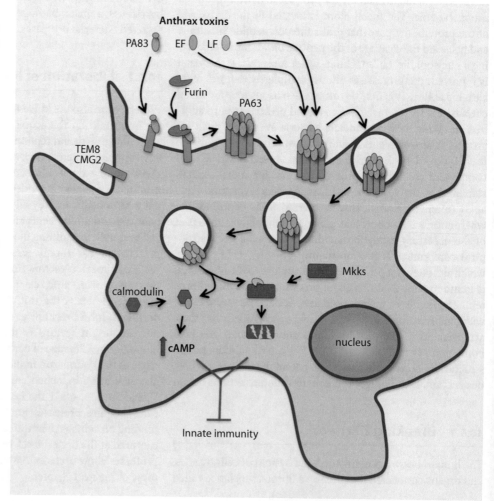

After the lethal and edema factor are secreted, they dock onto the PA complex, upwards of three at a time. Docking induces the endocytic engulfment of the complex which progresses to an internal endosome whose luminal pH is rapidly lowered. The lower pH triggers a conformational change in the PA complex which now inserts into the endosomal membrane and becomes a pore. The toxins, either lethal factor or edema factor or both, bound to the luminal side of the pore, now translocate into the host cell cytoplasm. There, edema factor turns on its adenylate cyclase enzymatic activity and generates high levels of cAMP. As a secondary chemical messenger, cAMP has many cellular functions but the one that may matter most in this context is cAMP-regulated opening of ion channels. The toxin essentially scrambles intra and extracellular osmotic balance leading to an exit of ions out of the cell and water with it (tissue edema). The exact mechanism by which this promotes the survival of bacilli is not entirely understood, but systemic multi-organ failure is correlated with edema toxin activity in animals. From the standpoint of *B. anthracis'* objective of wanting its host to die (so it can sporulate in the deceased carcass), such a systemic meltdown makes evolutionary sense.

The other toxin, lethal factor, also jams cell signaling pathways, but by a different mechanism. After its release from the endosome into the cell cytoplasm, lethal factor, a zinc-dependent protease, cleaves members of the mitogen-activated protein kinase (or MAP kinase) family. MAP kinases are regarded as some of the more important signal transducers in eukaryotic biology, a phosphate transferred to protein substrates of the kinases being the transmitted chemical message. Cleavage of the terminus of the MAP kinases by lethal factor inactivates their kinase activity thereby rendering their phosphate transduction capability obsolete. This cripples cell signaling and leads to a death signal that results in apoptosis. It is clear that apoptosis of macrophages, T- or B-cells or other host cells critical for barrier and organ function would substantially impact the host's ability to operate while infected, an obvious advantage for the growing bacilli.

With anthrax toxin we see it all when it comes to the concepts in toxin biology. The secreted toxin can bind to specific host receptors via its "B" domain. The B domain serves as a platform for the active "A" domains and mediates their entry into the cell. With the toxins now delivered into the cytoplasm, two different enzymatic activities cripple two distinct cell signaling processes, all resulting in the destruction of host function and better survival of the bacterium.

10.7 Code-Disrupting Toxins

Left out of the discussion to this point has been a toxin that acts upon host cell DNA. Leaving no beach shell unobserved, bacteria have made them as well. In fact, they are some of the more intriguing and recently discovered toxins of the group. Collectively referred to as **cytolethal distending toxins (CDTs)**, they are so-named because of their ability to increase the size and volume of the cell's they effect. The mechanism

behind this observation seems to be the arrest of the host cells before they enter into mitosis, the cell-dividing stage where one cell becomes two daughter cells. The host cells move to the point of wanting to divide but don't, and for good reason. CDTs are DNAses. They enter the host cell through classic A/B toxin mechanisms and the "A" portion can cleave host DNA in half – a double-strand break. Too many double strand breaks in DNA is catastrophic and, rather than perpetuate these errors to daughter cells which by nature can be harmful to the host in other ways (think cancer or loss of cell functionality), the cell arrests itself and eventually undergoes programmed cell death. These toxins are commonly found in proteobacteria that inhabit the human gastrointestinal tract, such as *E. coli* or shigella, and as such may be associated with colitis and inflammation in these tissues.

10.8 Regulation of Toxin Production and Activity

There are three main ways in which bacteria exert control over toxin or effector activity. These are: (i) regulated gene expression, (ii) spatial or locational control, and (iii) temporal control. Regulated gene expression involves transcriptional control, either positive or negative, of the gene that encodes the toxin. For example, the above-mentioned diphtheria toxin was difficult to purify because sometimes it was not expressed in culture of growing *C. diptheriae*. By chance, it was found that the toxin is produced in accordance with the concentration of extracellular iron in the media. Molecular studies confirmed that indeed a small repressor protein, which is sensitive to iron levels, controls diphtheria toxin production. Other toxins are also controlled by iron levels, usually turned on by low iron, a sort of universal signal that the bacterium is in a host[1]. Other central regulators of toxin production are common; staphylococcal toxin production is controlled by two perhaps three cytoplasmic regulatory proteins and pathogenic bacilli that produce anthrax toxin is controlled by a cytoplasmic protein termed AtxA. Two component regulatory systems, which we encountered in ▸ Chap. 6, control some of the toxins made by the causative agent of gangrene (*C. perfringens*). By evolving proteins that integrate information from the host microenvironment and translate that information into the production of toxins or effectors, it allows the bacteria to produce these actionable proteins when needed, which also conserves energy and resources for later.

Bacteria also control toxins and effectors by keeping them in distinct locations. We saw with anthrax toxin above that its entry into the host cell cytoplasm is controlled by at least three events (activation of its receptor on the host cell surface, engulfment in host vesicles, and exit in a pH-dependent manner from the vesicle). Considering that more than one anthrax toxin is delivered via this manner, one can view such a strategy as keeping the activity clandestine until it can be executed upon with a wave of cytosolically-delivered toxins. Finally, bacteria also order the entry of their toxins or effectors into host cells to maximize building upon the activities occurring in a precise sequential order on some host process. This is best exemplified by the type III secreted (see ▶ Chap. 9) toxins of yersinia species. A dozen or so effectors can be delivered by this system. Their order of delivery is important for their total manipulation of host actin dynamics and cell signaling, with one effector's activity preceding and enhancing the downstream activity of others. Thus, both spatial and temporal control allows for bacteria to introduce more sophistication into their already complicated and precise molecular enzymatic activity.

Summary of Key Concepts
1. Bacterial protein toxins are secreted or injected polypeptides that target host cells, tissues, organs, and the immune system.
2. Most often, they are enzymes that catalyze distinct biochemical reactions, usually acting on host proteins or lipids as substrates.
3. The products of these reactions are favorable to the bacterium and detrimental to the host. Although many molecular outcomes are possible, bacterial toxins often target host cell membranes, cell architecture, cell signaling, or cell protein production.
4. Bacterial protein toxins can covalently modify their substrates or non-covalently modify them. Both activities can destroy, accentuate, or rearrange host function.
5. Toxins are prominent targets for therapeutic development. Several commonly used vaccines are composed of important bacterial toxins.

❓ Expand Your Knowledge
1. As we have touched upon throughout the volume, *P. aeruginosa* is a Gram-negative bacterium that can infect the lungs, blood, bladder, and damaged skin of humans. The pathogen produces three different cytotoxins that each execute one of the activities highlighted in this chapter. Exoenzyme S inactivates GTPases and disrupts actin dynamics. Exoenzyme U is a lipase that cleaves host cell membranes. Exotoxin A or ToxA shuts down protein synthesis. Describe how each of these activities would specifically disable the innate or adaptive immune response to Pa in the mammalian lung. Devise a vaccine strategy that neutralizes each of these functions with a single but multivalent polypeptide that is both safe and effective for people.
2. Group A streptococcus (GAS), known by its scientific name as *Streptococcus pyogenes*, is the cause of strep throat, a highly contagious infection that results in swelling and pain in the throat. Normally, the infection can be treated with antibiotics and will resolve within a week's time without severe complications. As a public health epidemiologist in New York, you are called to investigate a strep outbreak at a New York middle school that is associated with severe hemolysis and kidney failure resulting in the hospitalization of many children. After culturing the bacterium, you find that culture media supernatants can lyse red and white blood cells and kills guinea pigs when injected intravenously. What is the likely mechanism of pathogenesis of this bizarre strain?
3. Go to Genbank. Search for anthrax toxin. In one of the sequenced genomes of *B. anthracis*, identify the gene number and locus tag for anthrax lethal factor. Copy and paste the coding region plus 500 bases of its upstream regulatory sequence in a word processing program. Now, use the ExPASy bioinformatics resource portal to translate the sequence, identify functional and/or enzymatic domains, and propose a methodology by which you can clone and express the toxin in a heterologous protein expression system (bacteria, yeast, etc). Then, devise a multi-step purification strategy to isolate the toxin and study its enzymatic activity against its known MAP kinase substrates.

Notes
1 = This protein is called DtxR, diphtheria toxin regulator. We learn in the next chapter about the concept of nutritional immunity, namely, that the host keeps the extracellular concentration of iron very low by sequestering iron in heme and transferrin/ferritin/lactoferrin. A low iron signal is often one that lets bacteria know they are "in host" and that its time for battle.

Suggested Reading

Aktories K (2011) Bacterial protein toxins that modify host regulatory GTPases. Nat Rev Microbiol 9:487–498. https://doi.org/10.1038/nrmicro2592

Alouf J, Ladant D, Popoff M (2006) The Comprehensive Sourcebook of Bacterial Protein Toxins. 4th Edition. May 2015. Elsevier, 1200 pages

Carbonetti NH (2010) Pertussis toxin and adenylate cyclase toxin: key virulence factors of Bordetella pertussis and cell biology tools. Future Microbiol 5:455–469. https://doi.org/10.2217/fmb.09.133

Dal Peraro M, van der Goot FG (2016) Pore-forming toxins: ancient, but never really out of fashion. Nat Rev Microbiol 14:77–92. https://doi.org/10.1038/nrmicro.2015.3

do Vale A, Cabanes D, Sousa S (2016) Bacterial toxins as pathogen weapons against phagocytes. Front Microbiol 7:42. https://doi.org/10.3389/fmicb.2016.00042

Duarte AS, Correia A, Esteves AC (2016) Bacterial collagenases - a review. Crit Rev Microbiol 42:106–126. https://doi.org/10.3109/1040841X.2014.904270

Gill DM (1982) Bacterial toxins: a table of lethal amounts. Microbiol Rev 46:86–94

Gordon VM, Leppla SH (1994) Proteolytic activation of bacterial toxins: role of bacterial and host cell proteases. Infect Immun 62:333–340

Greaney AJ, Leppla SH, Moayeri M (2015) Bacterial exotoxins and the inflammasome. Front Immunol 6:570. https://doi.org/10.3389/fimmu.2015.00570

Ingmer H, Brøndsted L (2009) Proteases in bacterial pathogenesis. Res Microbiol 160:704–710. https://doi.org/10.1016/j.resmic.2009.08.017

Krueger KM, Barbieri JT (1995) The family of bacterial ADP-ribosylating exotoxins. Clin Microbiol Rev 8:34–47

Leung C et al (2014) Stepwise visualization of membrane pore formation by suilysin, a bacterial cholesterol-dependent cytolysin. elife 3:e04247. https://doi.org/10.7554/eLife.04247

Miyoshi S, Shinoda S (2000) Microbial metalloproteases and pathogenesis. Microbes Infect 2:91–98

Schiavo G, van der Goot FG (2001) The bacterial toxin toolkit. Nat Rev Mol Cell Biol 2:530–537. https://doi.org/10.1038/35080089

Stebbins E, Galan J (2001) Structural mimicry in bacterial virulence. Nature 412:701–706. https://doi.org/10.1038/35089000

Williams JM, Tsai B (2016) Intracellular trafficking of bacterial toxins. Curr Opin Cell Biol 41:51–56. https://doi.org/10.1016/j.ceb.2016.03.019

Wong KW, Isberg RR (2005) Yersinia pseudotuberculosis spatially controls activation and misregulation of host cell Rac1. PLoS Pathog 1:e16. https://doi.org/10.1371/journal.ppat.0010016

Zhang YZ, Ran LY, Li CY, Chen XL (2015) Diversity, structures, and collagen-degrading mechanisms of bacterial collagenolytic proteases. Appl Environ Microbiol 81:6098–6107. https://doi.org/10.1128/AEM.00883-15

The Acquisition and Consumption of Host Nutrients

© Springer Nature Switzerland AG 2019
A. W. Maresso, Bacterial Virulence, https://doi.org/10.1007/978-3-030-20464-8_11

Learning Goals

In this chapter, we discuss the basic concept that pathogenic bacteria must have a source of energy and other nutrients to power their growth, replication, and virulence during host infection. Since the host itself harbors nearly everything to fulfill these basic needs, bacteria have evolved clever ways to acquire these essential nutrients from its host. The host, in turn, sequesters essential nutrients that bacteria need, a sort of nutritional immunity that limits bacterial success. The varied mechanisms bacteria use to acquire, transport, and use host nutrients are discussed in terms of the constant give-and-take between pathogen and host and the unique adaptations pathogenic bacteria can undergo to undermine this balance. The learner will be well versed in this interplay as it pertains to the determination of an outcome of infection.

11.1 Introduction

All life requires energy to power its ordered existence. Without energy, the basic cellular reactions needed for metabolism, build cells or tissues, and reproduce – all organized processes - cannot occur. In our own species, energy is acquired in two main ways. First, the very air you breathe brings with it oxygen which is used during respiration to make ATP. In essence, every inhalation is a tiny burst of fuel designed to keep your cells running even when your entire body may be resting or fasting. Second, you eat. The sugars, fats, and proteins from each meal are pushed through half a dozen different energy generating pathways used by your cells, all of which directly or indirectly yield more ATP. If the air you breathe is a continuous supply of small units of energy for near perpetual metabolic activity, a meal represents a top-off of the gas tank, meant to sustain you at peak performance over the next few hours. What is not used in that time can be stored. Meals also bring essential elements or other nutrients that your body may not be able to synthesize but nonetheless requires. They nourish your cells with stored chemical energy, are used as building blocks, or are co-factors for complex reactions all to ensure your cells can perform at an optimal level.

11.1.1 Bacterial Hunger

Bacteria must also eat. Unlike us, they are more often at the mercy of their environment to deliver what they may need in the present. Because of this, the breadth of the biosynthetic reactions that bacteria are able to perform is abundant. They also possess a rather extensive array of versatile transporters that can import many chemically distinct nutrients. Indeed, many bacteria can use or make metabolites that humans cannot, and as a kingdom[1] of organisms, they cover just about every reaction known in the natural world. Humans have recognized this very fact and employ bacteria in numerous agricultural or industrial settings to harness these useful reactions. The wide metabolic capacity of bacteria also comes at a great price to human health for it also means that patho-

genic bacteria are less constrained by the nutritional environment of the host. Indeed, the most capable of pathogenic bacteria are not only able to make what they need, they also have absolute mastery of the use of what *we make*. When it comes to symbionts or pathobionts that live in and on us, bacteria are so good at making useful metabolites that we even depend on some of them for nutrients, including amino acids and vitamins. They also catabolize complex molecules like sugars and lipids. As we learn in ▶ Chap. 13, many of the biosynthetic reactions performed by the gut microbiome effect human health and metabolism.

The process by which a molecule is broken down to biochemically useful metabolites or energy is termed **catabolism**. The process by which these metabolites and energy are used to make other molecules, especially ones that may not be found in the environment, is termed **anabolism**. Cellular life if really just the product of the two reactions moving in different directions. Cells use what the environment gives to make different molecules that can in turn be used to make more cells. Bacteria live and die by this simple premise and as such can shift their metabolic focus to changing needs. In the absence of energy, human beings can tap into stored reserves or move to a different environment to get more energy. Most bacteria are limited by a narrow geographical range, which, in the literal sense, may be a single rock on the ground. If the intestinal tract or blood or skin is their world, they must be crafty at using what is available in these places. And, even if the nutrient is available, bacteria are at the mercy of the concentration of this nutrient. In most cases, the concentration of the nutrient outside the bacterial cell is much lower than inside. In other words, bacteria must transport the solute against a concentration gradient. This requires energy. It is no surprise then that many of the bacterial transporters discussed here will sacrifice an ATP to import a nutrient or use stored energy that exists across their membranes. Some atoms like metals are the stuff of stars. They cannot be made and are, in soluble forms, quite scarce. So bacteria must also solve this problem. Bacteria dedicate entire gene operons to the acquisition of such rare nutrients.

Like us, bacteria dine on sugars, lipids, proteins, peptides, oligonucleotides, xenobiotics, vitamins, minerals, and other inorganic compounds and elements, the **bacterial nutriverse** (◘ Fig. 11.1). Sugars like glucose are fed into the glycolytic and pentose phosphate pathway. Lipids are broken down by β-oxidation and their products fed into the tricarboxylic cycle. Proteins are digested by proteases into peptides and peptides into single, di, or tri-peptides by peptidases; the products are imported and also fed into the TCA cycle. All of these processes result in the production of useful energy. Oligonucleotides can be divided into individual bases, much of which is recycled for use during DNA synthesis or fed into other pathways to generate energy. Xenobiotics are compounds not readily observed in the immediate bacterial environment or host and often are the result of human production or ingestion. Caffeine for example is a blood xenobiotic, so are some synthetic antibiotics. Bacteria can often use xenobiotics as a source of carbon for the biosynthesis of other metabolites,

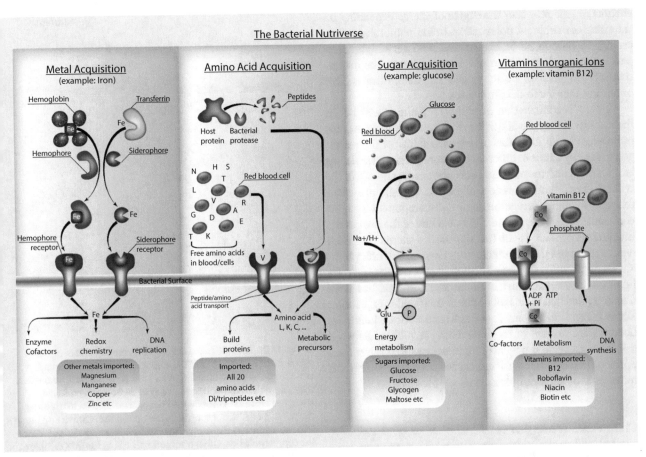

□ Fig. 11.1 The bacterial nutriverse. Pathogenic bacteria acquire many of the essential nutrients needed to power their metabolism, growth, and replication from the hosts they infect. As such, bacteria have evolved sophisticated mechanisms to pry, bind, relay, transport, and breakdown these nutrients, including pathways that target metals, amino acids, sugars, and vitamins, amongst others. The host also attempts to sequester these molecules, a growth limiting strategy

a process termed **bioremediation**. Bioremediation is being harnessed by the industrial sector to clean made-made pollutants in the environment. After all, bacteria are some of the most voracious scavengers on Planet Earth. Vitamins are transported into pathogenic bacteria as well, which become chemical co-factors to broaden the biological output of metabolism. Minerals and other inorganics like metals serve as co-factors, often tightly affixed to bacterial protein enzymes whose biochemical capacity is enhanced when the metal partakes in the reaction. All of these compounds can be considered nutrients and all of them are important in the growth of bacteria during infection.

11.2 The Porins

To understand nutrient acquisition, we start at the bacterial surface, and its interaction with the host. The membranes (outer and inner for Gram-negatives and the single membrane for Gram-positives) are effective barriers against the import of hydrophilic (water loving) compounds (oil and water do not mix). In addition, the charged LPS (Gram-negative) and teichoic acid (Gram-positive) are effective barriers against hydrophobic compounds. This means that bacterial cells must contain specific systems to move these substances across these barriers. A common conduit that nutrients encounter at the bacterial surface of the Gram-negative bacterium is the **porin**. Discovered in the mid-1970s, the porin does exactly what its name implies; it forms a pore in the outer membrane that allows for the diffusion of nutrients. Nutrients in this case include simple molecules like glucose to more complex and large ones such as certain vitamins. Some porins are very selective, the selectivity based on the charge and size of nutrient and the chemical properties of the porin channel. Other porins are more promiscuous. The porin is arranged as a transmembrane β-barrel, essentially a tube opened at both ends with each end protruding from the membrane. The inside of the channel is often lined with charged residues. This makes it more conducive to the passage of hydrophilic substrates through the pore. The outside lining of the barrel contains lipophilic residues which allows for the interaction with non-polar lipids of the membrane. In the case of selective porins with higher levels of specificity in what they allow through, the extracellular opening may contain an **eyelet**. This flap may swing between open and closed conformations and thus serve as a gatekeeper. In addition, transport may also be regulated or blocked by the voltage of the membrane, termed "**gated**." The ionic or charged environment of the channel or gate may alter the degree of charge depending on the extent of membrane polarization. In the membrane, porins arrange as monomers or trimers and with very high abundance; thousands can be present in a single cell. The magnitude of this level of porin production demonstrates how important they are to cell physiology.

The main contribution of porins to pathogenesis lies in their ability to rapidly allow the diffusion of important biomolecules. In addition, they endear the ability of the pathogen to rapidly adjust to different host conditions. Osmolarity, temperature, and the nutrient concentration in and out of the cell all effect the expression of porins. Signals are often relayed via phosphorylation, and two-component systems contribute to sensing the nutritional status of the host at the membrane. Similar to all the transport systems discussed here, a pathogen that is nutritionally satisfied will often initiate its replication during times of plenty. Porins also are involved in the transport of some antibiotics. It has been demonstrated that the loss of porins or their under-expression allows bacteria to become resistant to antibiotics. Mutational hotspots are present in the intervening sequences between β-folds; such regions may acquire mutations that select for a porin variant that allows for enhanced adaptation to a certain nutritional or antibiotic state.

11.3   ABC Transporters

Once a solute gets through a porin, it enters the periplasm. It may diffuse through the periplasm or be bound and carried by specific **periplasmic-binding proteins**. From the periplasm, the nutrient makes its way to the inner membrane. The inner membrane provides much of the selectivity in allowing the nutrient to pass. This is the location of many different types of transporters that facilitate entry. The most visible and well-studied of these may be the ABC transporters, which are conserved in all forms of life. **ATP-Binding and Cassette transporters** (ABC) couple the energy released from the hydrolysis of ATP on the cytoplasmic side of the transporter with the thermodynamically unfavorable movement of the nutrient across the membrane into the cytoplasm (◘ Fig. 11.2). Most ABC transporters are characterized by two structurally and functionally distinct regions. The first is the **transmembrane domain** (TMD) which spans the membrane with a channel opening in the periplasm that can receive the nutrient. The second region is the **nucleotide binding domain** (NBD) which contains so-called Walker A boxes that bind nucleotides. The NBD is located on the cytoplasmic side of the transporter linked to the TMD. This facilitates the interaction with sources of chemical energy made in the bacterial cytoplasm. The mechanism by which ABC transporters move nutrients into the cell is a tale of two states. In the ATP-free form, the NBD is positioned in a more open conformation which pulls the TMD in a more closed form. When nucleotide binds to the NBD, the NBD is pulled together since multiple interactions in the NBD cleft collapse to surround the nucleotide. This pulls the TMD domains

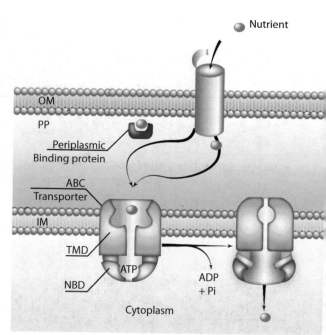

◘ **Fig. 11.2**   The ABC transporter. A fundamental unit of bacterial nutrient acquisition is the ABC transporter. Typically, nutrients first cross the outer membrane through porins (in Gram-positive bacteria, they may diffuse through the cell wall or be bound by cell wall anchored proteins). Once they diffuse or are delivered to the inner membrane, an ABC transporter will recognize the nutrient and pump it into the cytoplasm via energy released from the hydrolysis of ATP on the cytoplasmic side. Other transporters, such as the MFS complex and its related systems, propel nutrients or solutes in by coupling the process to the proton motive force. ABC transporters can also expel metabolites into the periplasm by reversing this process

inward thus opening the periplasmic region to receive a nutrient. Once bound, and after the ATP is hydrolysed releasing ADP and a phosphate, the conformation returns back to the original state thereby squeezing the nutrient through the channel. Because these systems import amino acids, vitamins, metals, sugars and other useful substances, their role in bacterial growth during infection is essential. To date, most reports on the importance of ABC transporters during infection have involved those that transport iron or other metals (◘ Fig. 11.3). We will visit this topic shortly.

11.4   Major Facilitator, Multidrug, and Small Drug Resistance

11.4.1   The MF Superfamily

Whereas the ABC transporter superfamily encompass the largest group of nutrient transporters, a close second are the **Major Facilitator Superfamily** also known as the MFS transporters. The MFS superfamily serves a similar function as the ABC transporters but does so through a different mechanism. Instead of using the energy from the cleavage of a phosphate bond, MFS proteins power translocation by exploiting stored energy inherent in chemical and ion gradients. The cumulative effect of this gradient, sometimes

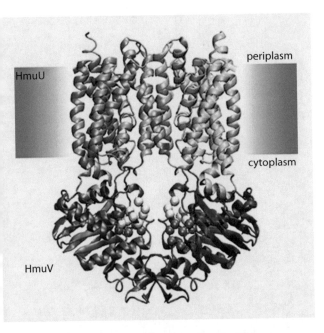

periplasm

HmuU

cytoplasm

HmuV

☐ **Fig. 11.3** Ribbon structure of an ABC transporter. Three-dimensional ribbon structure of the HmuUV heme transporter showing transmembrane domains (purple and green) spanning the inner membrane and nucleotide binding domains (blue and red) in the cytoplasm. The site of ATP binding is shown with the yellow and orange balls. (Adapted from Flechsig et al. (see *suggested readings*) under a creative commons license. (▶ https://creativecommons.org/licenses/by/4.0/))

referred to as the electrochemical gradient, leads to a disbalance of both ions and chemicals across a biological membrane. Because these ions and chemicals will tend to want to equilibrate on both sides of the membrane, small bits of energy liberated from the process of doing so can be applied to the transport of other more complex compounds. Thus, electrochemical gradients represent a kind of stored and inherent potential energy that is converted to kinetic energy when a compound moves from one side of the membrane to another. As such, three types of MFS transporters are recognized. **MFS uniporters** move in one type of solute. **MFS symporters** and **antiporters** transport two types. Symporters couple the transport of a smaller ion with another substrate in the same direction whereas antiporters do this but in different directions. In the latter two cases, the movement of the main substrate piggybacks on the natural transfer of a small ion from high to low environments. It's a clever harnessing of a natural phenomenon; since ions will move in that direction anyway, cells have evolved to generate channels that bring in a useful nutrient along for the ride.

The MFS transporters constituent about 1/4th of all bacterial transporters. Collectively, just about every nutrient is imported or exported using these systems. Individual transporters are often highly specific. This differs from porins and the ABC transporters. They share a common structure; 12 transmembrane extensions governed by an alpha-helix topology. The connection between each helix is often exposed to the cytoplasm or the periplasm. This gives an alternating feature to the structure that dips in and out of water-loving

areas. Unlike porins and ABC complexes, the pore is less obvious but is formed between the two halves, or domains (N and C terminus) of the protein. These domains are linked by a cytoplasmic hydrophilic loop of about fifty amino acids which is probably flexible enough to convey conformational changes between the two regions during transport. A rocker-switch mechanism of movement is proposed whereby the two domains rock between each other to move solutes from one to the other end. By bringing a solute along its concentration gradient, the activation energy needed to induce the rocker motion is lowered thus favoring its spontaneous conversion without the need for ATP.

11.4.2 Drug Influx/Efflux Transporters

Like MFS transporters, two additional classes of transporters, the MATE (**multidrug and toxic compound exclusion**) and SMR (**small multi-drug resistance**) families also couple the electrochemical gradient to the transport of small compounds. MATE transporters resemble MFS transporters in size with 12 TM helices while SMRs are much smaller (4 TMs). MATEs and SMRs are important in the pathogenesis of bacterial infections because they can be used to export fluoroquinolone and macrolide antibiotics. Common carrier ions for MFS, MATEs, or SMR transporters are protons, sodium, or phosphate. **Sodium solute symporters** (SSSs) are a family of transporters that function similarly to MFS transporters. These transporters couple the import of a sodium ion with sugars but peptides, vitamins, and nucleosides can be co-ligands. The concept is similar to MFS transporters; the nutrient of interest is "symported" with the sodium ion using large differences in the sodium concentration across the membrane as stored energy to facilitate transport. It is believed the sodium binds to the receptor first, then the nutrient binds, with conformational changes occurring at each new binding event that drives emptying onto the cytoplasmic side.

11.5 A Third Arm of Immunity: Starvation

There are three major nutrients of central importance for a bacterial infection. These include amino acids such as peptides, a source of readily useable energy such as a sugar like glucose, and a source of metals, most often iron. This is not to say other transported nutrients are not important for pathogenesis. They are. But much of what we understand concerning the relationship between nutrient uptake and infection comes from these three key sources of food. Although differing in many ways when it comes to their infective lifestyle, just about all bacterial pathogens must in some way tap into such sources. The challenge for the microbe hunter interested in exploiting this knowledge, however, is not in revealing so much in how bacteria utilize these nutrients, but in how they get them. For the most part, with perhaps the exception of free glucose or larger

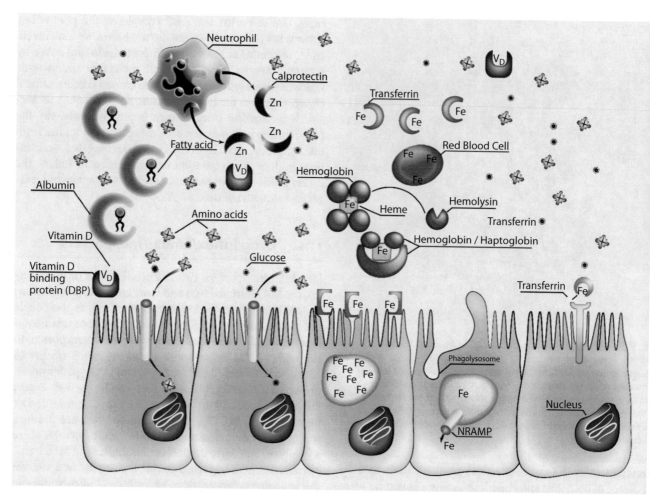

◻ Fig. 11.4 Host nutritional immunity. Pathogenic bacteria have evolved clever ways to acquire critical host nutrients. The host, however, does not make it easy for them, keeping precious nutrients sequestered or low in concentration, a concept sometimes termed nutritional immunity. Shown about are some of the many ways the host limits access to the goodies it needs, strategies that reduce bacteria growth and virulence

oligosaccharides, the host keeps tight control on these nutrients. This concept is referred to as **nutritional immunity** (◻ Fig. 11.4). Like the classic definition of the immune system as something that blocks or kills foreign invaders, nutrient immunity aims to prevent bacterial growth by sequestering nutrients so that pathogens cannot get them. Even if a pathogen is executing its virulence at a local level, by preventing its replication, its systemic dissemination is substantially limited. As a result, this gives the killing part of the immune system time to catch up, mobilize the army, and attack a localized, not sprawling, invader. If pathogenic bacteria overcome nutrient immunity, they may establish a successful infection and grow rapidly via the use of host resources. This concept is termed **metabolovirulence** or **nutritional virulence** (mostly in reference to intracellular growing bacteria). The basic idea is that through the liberation, import, and utilization of host nutrients, the most important and basic needs of the bacterium will have been met. This sets the stage for the rest of virulence. Such nutrients are the building blocks and fuel the synthesis of all other virulence factors. Even more so, they give the pathogen the ability to go from one to two, two to four, and so on.

11.6 Carnivorous Bacteria

Let's start with amino acids. The building blocks of proteins, there are twenty of them, all at some point being used in the translation of mRNA into protein, the catalysts of biology. An average size protein contains most if not all twenty different forms. Humans are auxotrophic for some of the amino acids and must thus acquire them from the environment. In contrast, some pathogenic bacteria can synthesize all twenty, a versatile metabolic weapon. Other pathogens can make most but not all of them. Those they cannot make they must steal from the host. These bacteria must then have evolved transporters dedicated to their import. *B. anthracis*, the causative agent of anthrax and one of the most proficient and fastest growing organisms in mammalian tissues and blood, can make all twenty amino acids, including branched amino acids, which humans cannot make. Yet, despite this synthetic capacity this organism also encodes dozens of putative peptide transporters, including at least five for branched amino acids alone. Bacillus is not the only organism with this arrangement. Many pathogenic bacteria are similar in this regard.

Why?

The answer may lie in the strategy of pathogenic bacteria to "waste not." When challenged, they will spend energy on the production of the biosynthetic enzymes to make them. If convenient to take them from their host with less expenditure of energy, especially if abundant extracellularly, it becomes a preferred option. The objective sometimes is to divide as fast as is metabolically possible. In this case, both import *and* synthesis may be utilized. When one considers pathogenesis in this light, it becomes immediately clear why some pathogens have evolved the ability to do both. Furthermore, depending on the metabolic or environmental state, one or more pathways may be blocked or limited.

The resting concentration of free amino acids in blood is about 1 milligram per 100 milliliters. If we figure the average molecular mass of the amino acids at about 120 daltons, this yields a serum concentration of amino acids at about 100 micromolar, or 0.1 nanomolar, give or take a bit dependent on the amino acid in question and time between meals. Although it will also depend on a source of glucose and other nutrients available, in general, a minimal media with this concentration of amino acids will not support robust growth of pathogenic bacteria even under ideal pH and temperature conditions (the host is anything but ideal). This implies that it would generally be advantageous for pathogenic bacteria to actively liberate *more* amino acids from the host to support their growth. As such, pathogenic bacteria are often armed with a diverse range of secreted proteases that mince host proteins into little, bite-sized, pieces. Free amino acids, di-, tri-, and oligo-peptides are generated in the process. Both ABC (energy from ATP) and MFS (energy from the protein motive force) transporters recognize these peptides and import them into the cell. Once in, they become important sources of nitrogen and carbon and energy and of course free amino acids for protein synthesis. The MFS family members that transport in peptides are also known as **protein dependent oligopeptide transporters** (POTS). These transporters discern different peptides based on their hydrophilicity. Since a proton is coupled to import, the number of protons symported with the peptide often correlates with the number of amino acids in the peptide (*e.g.* two protons for a dipeptide, etc). A number of human bacterial pathogens are attenuated when peptide uptake systems are genetically deleted, including the oligopeptide transport system Opp of *S. aureus* and *L. monocytogenes*, the latter having reduced survival in macrophages.

There are other elegant ways in which virulence can be altered by amino acid uptake. In *C. difficile*, which causes severe intestinal infections, amino acid uptake suppresses sporulation, no doubt a signal that nutrients are replete and growth can continue. Peptide transport in streptococcus regulates adherence and in some enteric bacteria such as salmonella species, it may regulate chemotaxis and expression of the flagellar system. This makes sense given that bacteria may need to move to a new location if nutrients are too low. There is also evidence pathogens upregulate peptide transporters in response to high concentrations of free amino acids or di- and tri-peptides. This is consistent with a pathogenic response whereby the release of host peptides (protease induced) readies the cells to take advantage of available harvest, thereby maximizing their growth potential.

11.7 Carbohydrates as High-Energy Nutrients for Bacteria

Unlike peptides and metals (next section), two tightly sequestered nutrients that are actively liberated from host sources, carbohydrates, are, for the most part, freely and readily abundant, especially glucose. It then comes as no surprise that the eminent bacteriologist Jacob Monod described it as the preferred carbon source for bacteria. Glucose may just be the most important carbon-containing molecule in cellular metabolism. Much of life uses it; the breakdown of glucose in glycolysis provides the energy for cells. Many pathogenic bacteria use glucose as a principal source of carbon and energy. The human host intakes glucose usually as a more complex oligosaccharide, mostly starch from plants and glycogen from animals, but also as lactose (milk), sucrose (plants), fructose (fruits and vegetables) and cellulose (plants). In the intestine, glycolytic enzymes will convert these sugars to glucose which is then absorbed by the intestinal enterocytes directly into blood. Free glucose in blood is delivered to all cell types of the body which themselves have glucose receptors. Glucose is everywhere.

Pathogenic bacteria sense this. Most of their central metabolism is structured around sucking up glucose from the host. There are potentially dozens of different sugar or glucose receptors in the plasma membranes of such bacteria. They are like sponges for the nutrient and if they cannot get it, or a more complex sugar (like glycogen) that can be converted to glucose, they often will struggle to grow. ABC, MFS, and SSF transporters are also able to import glucose or related sugars. But perhaps the most elegant system is the bacterial **phosphoenoltransferase system** (the PEP or PTS). Many enteric bacteria have up to forty different proteins that partake in the PEP transport of sugars with glucose as the primary target. Unlike facilitated diffusion (porins), sodium- or proton-based symport (MFS and SSF etc), and the energy from ATP hydrolysis (ABC transporters), the PEP system uses what is termed group transport. That is, a group of proteins biochemically linked to a process facilitate the import of the glucose. Like other transporters, this system does have a membrane-bound transporter. Unique, however, is that a cytoplasmic domain of the transporter can chemically and physically couple to a series of cytoplasmic enzymes that transfer phosphate amongst their members. The cytoplasmic portion also is linked, through physical interactions, to regulators of transcription – this can control the expression of genes. The transporter itself may be three separate genes that come together in a complex or are a single gene linked as subunits (often termed protein A, B, and C with the C unit being the actual transporter). The A and B proteins or subunits are then bound in the cytoplasm to the histidine containing protein (HPr) which itself interacts with a protein termed enzyme I. This multi-protein complex transfers phosphate from phosphoenolpyruvate (PEP), a product of glycolysis, to the glucose on the surface of the cell bound by protein C. The phosphorylated glucose is then fed into glycolysis and the energy used from its breakdown to power the bacterial cell. The reason the PEP system is so important to bacteria is that the phosphate being transferred through the system is a type of molecular accounting. The more PEP produced the more phosphate can be relayed to glucose for import and thus the more energy units that can be made. If the external glucose becomes low, less PEP is made and thus less phosphate pushed through the chain. The system is balanced with proteins involved in chemotaxis via phosphorelay enzymes and transcriptional modulators binding to the receptor protein C. The state of energy and metabolism is linked to the decision to move or make additional proteins that can adjust to this state.

11.8   Metallometabolism

Vitamins, amino acids, and glucose are all nutrients that bacteria actively try to import. However, most pathogenic bacteria, if challenged, can readily synthesize these metabolites from other building blocks. For the last set of nutrients of importance to a successful infection, synthesis is not an option, for these nutrients are made in the center of stars. This brings us to metals, principally iron, zinc, and manganese but copper and calcium as well. Metals are another one of the factors that has had a profound effect on the evolution of life on Earth. Because of their ability to accept or donate electrons, they have chemical versatility. The range of reactions that comes with incorporating metals in the biological synthesis framework is increased because metals act as cofactors for enzymatic and binding reactions of proteins. Many fundamental process of biology, including DNA synthesis, redox chemistry, signal transduction, and hydrolysis reactions are possible because a metal co-factor facilitates the reaction chemistry. Greater than 10% of all enzymes in bacterial cells use metals as co-factors; and since metals cannot be made by cells but are some of the most abundant atoms on Earth, it is no secret that bacterial cells will need to acquire them from the environment.

When the environment is the host, the obstacles for bacterial growth are great. The term nutrient immunity best fits this paradigm. There may not be a more tightly regulated and controlled bodily nutrient than a metal. The first reason is too much iron is toxic. Its chemistry, through the Fenton reaction, can lead to the production of cell-damaging radicals. But there is no doubt that the host also keeps iron low because it is a bacterial growth restricting strategy. One needs to look no further than the purposeful addition of the general metal chelator EDTA to food to see how effective iron sequestration can be. EDTA keeps food from spoiling at the hands of unrestricted bacterial growth.

The interaction of bacteria with metals has been known since the 1920s and 30s, but the realization of their importance came with the finding that transferrin, a host iron binding protein, restricted bacterial growth shortly thereafter. In this regard, our most complete knowledge comes from the study of bacterial iron intake. Entire volumes have been written on this topic which underscores both the breadth of the topic as well as the fundamental importance of it to bacterial physiology. Although your blood and cells have high levels of total iron (the red color of blood is due to the presence of heme-iron – see below), the concentration of free iron, that soluble and useable ferrous Fe^{2+} iron, is, for lack of a better term, astronomically low. As a result, pathogenic bacteria must work for it. The ways in which pathogenic bacteria acquire metals is a biological masterstroke.

11.8.1   Layer upon Layer upon Layer upon …

The host sequestration of iron is a story of layers upon layers. Most bodily iron is found in the circulation in the form of a porphyrin known as heme. Hemes are necessary for all biology; it is heme that ligates the oxygen for transport and exchange in bodily tissues. More than this though, hemes are shuttles for the transfer of electrons between biological systems. These hemes, termed cytochromes, participate in energy production in the cell. In blood, heme is bound to the oxygen-carrier protein hemoglobin. Made of a tetramer of four globin chains, each globin has at its center a single heme-iron. Oxygen binds here and is eventually released to anoxic tissues; and carbon dioxide taken away for exhalation. The bond between hemoglobin and its heme is very tight. Heme does not readily disassociate from the complex. Locked away at the center of the heme is a single iron atom. This bond is even tighter, almost covalent. For all practical purposes, iron does not fall off from this arrangement. The entire complex of iron in heme and heme in hemoglobin is further locked up inside the protective embrace of a lipid bilayer inside a red blood cell. To access this system, bacteria have to break the mucosal or other barrier, get into a vessel, break a red blood cell, rip the heme from hemoglobin and somehow rip the iron from the heme (□ Fig. 11.5). Even if heme and/or hemoglobin is released from red cells by the actions of bacteria, the host has backup systems to quickly sequester the free nutrient. When hemoglobin is free in the serum, a host protein termed haptoglobin can quickly bind it. This recycles the heme via the reticulendothelial system in the spleen. Should some heme come off hemoglobin, another host protein, hemopexin, will bind the heme, keeping it away from growing bacteria. Consistent with the evolutionary quid pro quo between bacteria and their hosts, several pathogenic bacteria have responded by adapting some of their heme receptors to bind hemopexin or haptoglobin or both, a strategy designed to divert heme from the host and to the pathogen.

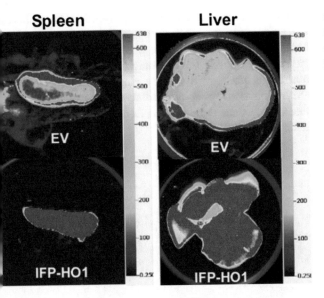

Spleen   **Liver**

■ Fig. 11.5 Imaging heme acquisition during infection. One key nutrient some pathogenic blood-borne bacteria attempt to acquire during infection is heme. Because of its central iron atom, with as much as 80% of the total iron pool, heme is a sought after quantity in the microbial quest for essential metals. Here, murine hosts were infected with an engineered strain of *E. coli* possessing a new type of heme sensor that fluoresces when heme is transported inside the *E. coli* cell. The top image of each panel shows the background flourscence from the spleen and liver of animals infected with a strain that lacks the sensor. The bottom panel shows the fluorescence from a strain that possesses it. Notice the intense red signal in these bottom panels, a clear sign the bacteria are acquiring heme from their hosts during the infection. (Adapted from Maresso et al. (see *suggested readings*) with permission)

11.8.2 Bacterial Metallurgy: Siderophores

Non-heme bodily iron is in transit, in storage, purposefully sequestered, or in use and not bound by porphyrins. The transitory iron comes in the form of host transferrin. This protein binds iron and delivers it to cell receptors for eventual import and use. What iron is not needed by cells is stored in them in the form of the host protein ferritin. A ferritin core can contain thousands of iron atoms in its center. Sequestered iron includes iron locked up by proteins such as lactoferrin in human milk, other secretions, or at the mucosal surface. The main objective of this sequestration is to keep it away from mucosal pathogens. Finally, iron is bound as a co-factor to numerous proteins in cells. This is the active, useable pool and may be less of a source than the others mentioned above.

Regardless of its form, this iron requires bacterial mining. There are two main systems bacterial pathogens use to acquire iron from these sources. The source and form of the iron will determine which bacterial system is used. Most iron in the environment is insoluble, the ferric Fe^{3+} form. This is true for some host sequestration systems as well. In addition to having to somehow pirate the iron from the host, the bacteria also have to keep it soluble. To overcome this challenge, bacteria make organic chelators called **siderophores** ("bearing iron"). Siderophores are synthesized in the cytoplasm

and secreted into the surrounding environment where they scavenge with very high affinity any available iron. The iron-containing siderophore is then captured on the bacterial surface by a cognate siderophore receptor. Siderophores are small (~ 500 daltons) but possess some of the tightest affinities for their iron ligand of any biological interaction. Their importance is evident by the fact that they are often synthesized by a 4–6 gene biosynthetic cluster.

There are many different types and some strains produce more than one type. Pathogens that are artificially made void of their ability to synthesize or import some siderophores are often less virulent. They are very common in intestinal pathogens, no doubt designed to compete against other microbes and the host for scarce iron reserves in the intestinal tract. Some bacteria have even learned to use another bacterium's siderophores to attain iron. They are also known to acquire iron from host proteins like transferrin. The iron-bound siderophore may enter the periplasm via an outer membrane porin and then is captured at the inner membrane by an ABC-type transporter. This transporter consists of a periplasmic binding protein, a permease, and a cytoplasmic subunit that hydrolyses the ATP, which provides energy for the process. The process of transport may be coupled to an energy transducer protein termed Ton. Ton rests in the inner membrane and links the energy from the proton motive force to move the siderophore from the outer to inner membrane. Once imported, the iron may be reduced (converted from Fe^{3+} to Fe^{2+}), which lowers its affinity for the siderophore, leading to its release and increase in solubility. In other cases, it is believed the siderophore is cleaved, releasing the iron. Siderophores are effective, but the host plays its hand against them. Lipocalin is a protein made by the host that can capture the siderophore and prevent the bacterium from acquiring the iron. In turn, bacteria have evolved some siderophores that are resistant to sequestration by lipocalin and its relatives. The arms race continues.

11.8.3 Bacterial Metallurgy: Hemophores

By analogy to siderophore-based chelation of free iron, pathogenic bacteria also make **hemophores**. As the name suggests, hemophores target heme, the most abundant iron present in mammalian blood. Like siderophores, they are secreted into the environment for the ultimate purpose of strongly binding heme. Unlike siderophores, they are proteins, small ones at that, with an average size of about 15–20 kDa. Hemophores are the most distal component in what turns out is a nutrient baton relay, sort of like a track-and-field meet. After a hemolysin has opened a red blood cell and spilled out the hemoglobin, any heme that comes off the globin may be bound by the hemophore. Alternatively, some hemophores bind the hemoglobin and enhance its rate of heme loss. The holo-hemophore, much like the holo-siderophore, can then be recognized by a hemophore receptor on the bacterial surface. Unlike the siderophore, the hemophore is not imported into the cell. Instead, the heme is passed from the hemophore to the receptor. Depending on whether the pathogen is a Gram-negative or positive, the heme is then passed through the periplasm or the cell wall and eventually to the inner or plasma membrane, all the way jumping from heme receptor to heme receptor. There, the heme may be imported into the cell through one of the many families of transporters discussed through this chapter. The most common is an ABC tri-partite transporter similar to the ones used to import iron-bound siderophores. Once the heme enters the cytoplasm, the iron needs to be freed from the porphyrin ring. Since the affinity of the porphyrin for the iron is exceedingly strong, this is accomplished by cleaving the heme ring by a large family of enzymes termed **heme degrading enzymes** or HDEs. The free iron is then incorporated into bacterial proteins as a critical cofactor.

Out of the Box

The Curious Case of Dr. Malcolm Casadaban

The profession of the microbe hunter can be dangerous. Some of us, on a daily basis, work with and are exposed to, the most deadly organisms known to mankind. Precautions are taken. Biosafety level 3 and 4 approaches, complete with engineered labs and "space suits", keep the risk low. At lower biosafety levels (1 and 2), basic personal protective equipment like gloves, lab coats, and masks make work with less virulent organisms safe.

But sometimes nature and the stochastic collide, and with tragic consequence.

Such is the case of the death of Dr. Malcolm Casadaban, a brilliant and pioneering bacterial geneticist working in a laboratory at the University of Chicago. The story highlights the remarkable ability of bacteria to adapt to their environment; in this case, the possibility that the bacterium Dr. Casadaban was working with, *Yersinia Pestis* (the causative agent of the plague), overcame its own genetically-altered deficiency in iron intake via abnormally high levels of iron in the researcher's blood. It's a case of overcoming nutritional immunity much in line with the concepts presented in this chapter.

On September 7th, 2009, Dr. Casadaban had been feeling unwell and decided not to come in for work at his University laboratory. He probably had been feeling unwell since his last day worked on September 4th, and then took the weekend to recover. On September 10th, his general fever and aches persisted and was evaluated at an outpatient clinic for what was presumed to be an upper respiratory infection, possibly the flu. On Sept 13th, his condition worsened and he was rushed by ambulance to the hospital. His breathing was short and heart rate high. A blood smear revealed bacteria and his vitals suggested heart failure; his breathing was getting worse. He was put on antibiotics but despite in intubation and other treatments, he passed about 12 hours after first presentation. That same day, bacterial cultures of his blood yielded evidence of at least two types of bacteria. One of these organisms was ruled out as the likely cause of death because the patient's symptoms were not consistent with the known pathogenesis of that bacterium.

The other strain, however, yielded a different story.

Recognizing that Dr. Casadaban was a researcher that worked with the cause of the plague, that strain was tested and indeed confirmed by PCR to be *Yersinia pestis* – the plague bacterium.

Here is where the story really becomes bizarre. Dr. Casadaban was not working with the fully virulent strain of *Y. pestis*. He was working with a commonly-used attenuated strain termed KIM D27. This strain was derived from a virulent strain of the plague bacteria that was passaged until it generated a deletion in the *pgm* locus. This locus encodes for proteins involved in the uptake and storage of iron and heme. Thus, it is believed that its mechanism of attenuation is due to its inability to efficiently acquire the much-needed iron from the hosts it infects.

On Sept 18th, four days after the death of Dr. Casadaban, university researchers and the CDC confirmed that the strain in Dr. Casadaban's blood was the attenuated strain he had been working with. Further studies at the CDC confirmed that this strain was, by all accounts, still substantially attenuated. Since there is no documented evidence that anyone has ever been infected with this strain, yet alone died from it, it raised the question as to how it grew so well in Dr. Casadaban.

Post-mortem and further analysis of Dr. Casadaban revealed something interesting about his health that likely even he did not know about. He had undiagnosed hemochromatosis. This condition results in abnormally high levels and retention of iron, and, consequently, very high levels of circulating and stored iron amounts in blood and tissues. In Dr. Casadaban's case, about five times the normal level.

Although it cannot be unequivocally proved, it is very likely that Dr. Casadaban's high levels of circulating iron "physiologically complemented" the known attenuation defect of the strain KIM D27. That is, even though this strain cannot efficiently attain iron from its host, and this is the likely reason for its attenuation (and thus relatively safe use by laboratory workers), because of the high levels in his blood, the strain was able to overcome the defect and grow. The result was consistent with symptoms associated with the plague.

This real-world example provides a fascinating, albeit tragic, glimpse into the importance of nutrient uptake during bacterial infection, and the fine balance between what is and is not disease in the host-pathogen interaction. Countless animal studies have also supported this larger point. It also teaches us the importance of safety in the laboratory, and how even with the most detailed knowledge there are circumstances that we are still unaware of that can make even routine work high risk.

The author of this volume knew and worked with Malcolm. He is remembered as a quiet, soft-spoken and kind man whose genetic brilliance was one of the founding contributions to the birth of the molecular biology revolution that gained steam in the late 1980s. He is missed and hopefully always remembered.

1.9 Regulation of Import Processes and Nutrient Use

Metals are double-edged swords. On the one hand, their ability to expand the chemical toolbox of what is possible is of great enzymatic value. On the other hand, low micromolar amounts will prevent bacterial growth and slightly higher levels are toxic. The unused or unoccupied metal poisons biological systems. Too high of one type of metal may overcome the binding constant of another and substitute where it should not. Others, like iron, can stimulate the production of free radicals. Uncontrolled and free range radicals are the bane of biological order. They disrupt membranes, proteins, DNA, just about everything, by freely placing unwanted electrons on these molecules of life. So then how does the bacterium that finds itself awash in newly liberated iron balance its toxicity with its versatility? Bacteria contain a regulatory system that senses the intracellular concentration of iron and reprograms acquisition and uptake systems so that the porridge is just right. The central player in this system is the **ferric uptake regulator** or fur. Fur is a DNA binding repressor. In the presence of sufficient intracellular iron levels, the excess iron is bound by fur. Iron-bound fur has a higher affinity for DNA. A particular 10 base consensus of DNA is preferred as a binding site, sometimes called a **Fur box**, which is analogous in ways to other transcriptional proteins that recognize consensus sequences just upstream from the promoters of the genes they regulate. When bound in this way, fur prevents the binding of RNA polymerase and hence mRNA production for that gene. Genes that house fur boxes in their promoter are those involved in metal homeostasis and includes siderophore/hemophore acquisition systems and membrane-bound transporters. With the relay system decoupled, iron does not come in even if abundant in the extracellular environment. Should the intracellular iron grow low via iron efflux or cell division or simply because there is very little outside to import, Fur too will not be bound by excess iron and lose its affinity for its target DNA. Falling off the promoter, gene transcription can begin, the acquisition and uptake response fully made and engaged, which will eventually lead to iron being imported. When too much iron arrives, the process begins anew. Other metals such as zinc and manganese, are controlled in an analogous manner with Fur-like repressors (Zur and Mur) leading the way. The influx and efflux managed by these central regulators elegantly maintains metallohomeostasis.

11.9.1 Don't Forget Other Metals

The iron paradigm dominates the nutritional immunity narrative, and rightfully so, thus its overemphasis here to use as an example of the regulation of nutrient uptake. Iron is essential in many different ways for so many different pathogens. But the microbe hunter should recognize that other metals are necessary for pathogenic bacteria as well, including manganese and zinc. A common manganese transporter, MntH, is an ABC-type system important for the virulence of the cause of salmonellosis and the plague. The reasons bacteria need manganese are different than those for iron. Manganese concentrations in the serum of mammals is something on the order of 1–10 nM, too low to support growth. There are enzymes involved in DNA replication and oxygen radical detoxification that require manganese as a co-factor for their activity. It is somewhat ironic that one metal (Mn) can be used to protect against the toxic effects of another (Fe), but this is exactly what happens. Specifically, manganese is a co-factor for the widely distributed enzyme superoxide dismutase (SOD). SOD converts oxygen radicals generated by the Fenton reaction (too much iron) into hydrogen peroxide which can be managed by the cell. In this way, Mn protects against iron toxicity. Free radicals are also used by phagocytes to kill engulfed bacteria. In this context, Mn uptake and incorporation into SOD may also protect against killing by macrophages. Too much Mn is also not good for pathogens. Mn resembles Fe in its chemical size and reactivity and as such can be incorporated in the place of Fe as enzyme co-factors. This is termed mis-metallation and can be toxic. Bacterial pathogens harbor Mn exporters to maintain an appropriate balance. The causative agent of a type of bacterial pneumoniae (*S. pneumoniae*) requires Mn export as part of its virulence strategy.

The paradigm for iron most similarly parallels that of zinc. Zinc regulation occurs by a repressor similar to Fur (Zur), Zn is transported into the cell via ABC permease systems, and there are even some siderophores that also chelate zinc (zincophores or more generally **metallophores**). Zn sparing is the concept that other metals can substitute for zinc in biological processes. But one of the more prominent and essential roles for zinc in bacterial pathogens is the incorporation of the metal into metalloproteases. These secreted virulence factors are some of the most potent contributors to a bacterial infection. Zn helps coordinate the chemistry for cleavage of host proteins which both liberates more nutrients, breaks barriers, and disables the immune response. In this regard, zinc is essential for pathogenesis.

The importance of Mn and Zn, like iron, are not lost on the host. To restrict access to these metals, host neutrophils secrete a protein called **calprotectin**. Calprotectin is a potent manganese and zinc chelator. Commonly found in stool samples of humans, its presence is considered a sign of inflammation. Neutrophils also secrete it to stunt staphylococcal growth in infection abscesses, being one of the more prominent nutrient immunity factors protecting against systemic spread of *S. aureus*. Similarly, the macrophage phagolysosome is designed to be a place of bacterial murder. Although some bacteria prevent its formation, for the most part, extracellularly engulfed bacteria will be killed by its highly toxic concentration of free radicals, acidic pH, and lytic enzymes. To ensure that starvation is added to the list of insults in this compartment, macrophage phagosome membranes contain a protein termed **natural resistance-associated macrophage protein 1** (NRAMP1). NRAMP1 actively pumps manganese out of the phagosome. Recall that manganese was an important cofactor in the radical detoxifying activity of SOD. By depleting Mn, the host ensures the inactivation of this bacterial defense mechanism, among other things, in a compartment designed to kill them.

11.10   Nutrient Assimilation Inside Host Cells

The above discussion has focused around the attainment of nutrients in the extracellular environment. However, as we witnessed in ▶ Chap. 8, there are many bacterial pathogens that are facultative or obligate intracellular pathogens. What sources of nutrients do they use? Much less is known about the capture of nutrients by intracellular replicating bacteria. There are technical challenges to studying nutrient acquisition during infection of host cells. Unlike where one can manipulate conditions of broth culture and observe the effect on growth, the conditions inside host cells are difficult to manipulate. The testing of mutant strains for growth and pathogenesis in host cells, as well as the application of sophisticated atomic labeling of nutrient sources, has given us some insight and so we visit the topic here. Above all, it is important to remember that some bacterial pathogens have sought out an intracellular lifestyle because it protects them from the immune system (stealth and Trojan horse idea) as well as provides access to generally higher concentrations of less restricted nutrients. Although host cells are compartmentalized with organelles, for the most part, many nutrients are more accessible here than they are extracellularly. This includes glucose, metals, and fatty acids, all of which must be somewhat free and in good abundance for the host cell itself to readily use them. As such, intracellular pathogenic bacteria have adapted to these barriers to bioavailability. Still, the intracellular compartment is not an open cupboard. When non-intracellular living bacteria are artificially inserted into a host cell, they don't grow well. This means that the ones that have adapted to this environment have specialized ways in which they acquire and metabolize these nutrient pools. By briefly addressing these specialties, we learn that preventing nutrient uptake in intracellular host cells is really an individual endeavor.

11.10.1   Take What You Can

Consideration of a few examples here illustrates the importance of this point. Take *M. tuberculosis*, which we have already discussed is a substantial human pathogen of the lungs and can grow and replicate in lung macrophages.

M. tuberculosis has a unique surface structure unlike either Gram-positive or Gram-negatives rich in complex lipids. When genes involved in the oxidation (and thus breakdown) of fatty acids are deleted, Mtb is attenuated and does not grow well. Interestingly, when similar experiments are performed with enzymes involved in glycolysis, we find these genes are seemingly dispensable. Mtb also possesses transporters and enzymes that can metabolize cholesterol, a fatty acid not present in prokaryotes. It stands to reason then that Mtb has adapted its use of a preferred carbon source as host fatty acids, relying less so on glucose like most extracellular pathogens. Thus, glucose will by synthesized from imported fatty acids using components of the TCA cycle and the offshoot glyoxalate shunt pathways. Another intracellular pathogen, *L. monocytogenes*, does not have a requirement for cholesterol or other host fatty acids. Thus, its primary source of carbon may be different. Interestingly, not only are genes for glycolysis not upregulated during infection, they are not needed for replication in macrophages. However, genes that process glycerol are expressed and when absent, replication is compromised. With listeria we also observe that the pathogen encodes transporters of vitamins and is not able to make its own thiamine and riboflavin. These vitamins are readily available inside mammalian cells though. Here is a case whereby the pathogen has likely diverted energy away from their synthesis because its intracellular niche is rich in them. A similar reliance on glycerol is observed for *S. flexneri*, another intracellular enteric that causes invasive intestinal infections. Related strains of invasive *E. coli* favor glycerol use as well. In contrast, salmonella clearly uses intracellular glucose (and thus runs glycolysis as a primary source of energy) because strains that lack such genes do not replicate well in the salmonella containing vacuole. Salmonella is somewhat of a close cousin of *E. coli* and shigella. The preferred use of glycogen by one set of these pathogens but glucose by another may reflect differences in the host cells (or compartments within host cells) that these pathogens infect; and what they prefer to acquire from the host and metabolize (take Mtb and lipids) reflects the needs of their cell structure. Either way, the specialization of nutrient uptake and metabolism observed for intracellular pathogenic bacteria is not only ripe for future study but presents different challenges in drug development than those for exclusively extracellular bacteria.

Changing their source of energy is one virulence adaptation that has suited intracellular bacterial pathogens. In what may be the most complete and elegant display of metabolo/nutritional virulence to date though, largely because it integrates multiple virulence processes to achieve a singular objective, is the mechanism by which *Legionella pneumophila* acquires amino acids. *L. pneumophila* is the causative agent of Legionnaire's disease. The disease was first described after several deaths occurred from a contingency of American Legion members attending a 1976 conference to celebrate the United States' bicentennial. As we saw in ▶ Chap. 8, Legionella s an intracellular-thriving bacterium that infects human alveolar macrophages. The bacterium is usually contracted via aerosols which originate from a contaminated water source such as air conditioning systems or misters. With symptoms that resemble a bad case of the flu and concomitant pneumonia, the fatality rate approaches 10%. Legionella enters macrophages and prevents the fusion of the lysosome with the phagosome, thereby remodeling the inclusion into a **pathogen containing vacuole** (PCV). Legionella does not have the biosynthetic capacity to make six of the twenty amino acids. This means it must get them from the macrophage cytoplasm. To do this, it first uses the type IV secretion system to secrete a bacterial effector termed Ankyrin B (AnkB). AnkB orchestrates its own farnesylation (a lipid anchor), which redirects it to the PCV membrane. There, it recruits poly-ubiquinated proteins to the host proteasome pathway leading to free peptides and amino acids. These amino acids are then transported into the PCV to feed legionella's craving and relief of its auxotrophy. In this example, we see how remodeling of host cell organelle function and the actions of a secretion system and a secreted effector diverts a normal physiological process to the making of nutrients a pathogen needs for its growth.

The future microbe hunter must not forget, in the face of bacterial toxins, secretion systems, adhesins and all the other prominently studied virulence factors, that, above all, pathogens must eat. When inside you, they eat you. From the elegant strategies bacteria employ to liberate and steal essential nutrients from host sources to the systems that bring these nutrients inside, there is no shortage of new targets for therapeutic development. Given the problems associated with resistance to antibiotics, a topic we approach in ▶ Chap. 16, putting the scientific bullseye on such uptake processes might just be where the microbe hunter should turn next.

Summary of Key Concepts

1. Bacteria are at the mercy of their immediate environment. As such, they have evolved diverse ways to sense and adjust to the nutritional status of the world, utilizing, in some sense as an entire species, just about every known biochemical reaction to turn even the most exotic compounds into a source of energy.

2. Bacteria transport a wide range of key compounds into the cell, most often sugars, vitamins, and amino acids/peptides, but also more exotic molecules like DNA and chelated metal complexes.

3. Regarding metals, they cannot be synthesized. Thus, bacteria absolutely must attain them from their surroundings. For pathogenic bacteria, the surroundings are the host. Thus, these bacteria cleverly thieve such nutrients from your own reserves during infection. Such metals are attained by protein relay systems that transport the metal, most often complexed to a small chemical chelator.

4. The bacterial nutriverse is mostly populated by four main types of transport systems. These groups use the energy from ATP or the proton motive force to move key nutrients into the cell in what would otherwise be a thermodynamically unfavorable process because of their concentration or chemical composition.

5. Bacteria can acquire these resources from host blood, fluids, cells, or tissues, often using secreted or surface bound factors to both liberate and bind them. A deliberate attempt to keep these resources from the bacteria, usually by keeping their concentration low or the nutrient sequestered, is part of a larger type of nutritional immunity designed to keep bacteria from building more of themselves.

6. The challenges bacteria face in acquiring intracellular nutrients from host cells are distinct from those when they are external to host cells. In this context, intracellular bacteria have become quite specialized in using unique host molecules and subverting host pathways to attain what they need.

❓ Expand Your Knowledge

1. Congratulations! Your reputation in your field has earned you the honor of contributing a chapter to a new volume entitled: "Handbook of Bacterial Physiology." The work is meant to be a compact, concise (and quick) guide to all things bacterial, a sort of "Cliff-note" of science. As author, describe the structure, mechanism of action, and function of porin, ABC, and MFS transporters. Be sure to be conservative in your language and number of words, which cannot exceed 500 total.

2. Read ▶ Chap. 16 of this volume on antibiotics. Devise a new antibiotic that targets bacterial hunger via the inhibition of one or more nutrient uptake pathways. Write a short essay on whether you believe it is more or less likely that targeting such a biological process would lead to greater or fewer levels of resistance to this antibiotic, invoking as the central premise your belief that such inhibition would not be bactericidal.

3. Compare and contrast the opportunities and challenges in nutrient uptake from extracellular and intracellular-living bacteria.

Notes

1 = The classification of bacteria on the great tree of life has constantly been revised over the past nearly 300 years since the great taxonomist Carl Linnaeus first proposed ordering life in the early 1700s. Indeed, bacteria were once grouped with plants, a classification just about everyone considers inconsistent with everything we know about these two types of life. Currently, bacteria occupy one of the seven kingdoms of life (the others being Animalia, Fungi, Plantae, Chromista, Protozoa, and Archaea) according to the most recent thorough discussion of this topic by Ruggiero and Kirk (2015).

Suggested Reading

Abu Kwaik Y, Bumann D (2013) Microbial quest for food in vivo: 'nutritional virulence' as an emerging paradigm. Cell Microbiol 15:882–890. https://doi.org/10.1111/cmi.12138

Blanco P et al (2016) Bacterial multidrug efflux pumps: much more than antibiotic resistance determinants. Microorganisms 4. https://doi.org/10.3390/microorganisms4010014

Capdevila DA, Wang J, Giedroc DP (2016) Bacterial strategies to maintain zinc metallostasis at the hostpPathogen interface. J Biol Chem 291:20858–20868. https://doi.org/10.1074/jbc.R116.742023

Centers for Disease Control and Prevention (CDC) (2011) Fatal laboratory-acquired infection with an attenuated Yersinia pestis Strain--Chicago, Illinois, 2009. MMWR Morb Mortal Wkly Rep 60:201–205

Du D, van Veen HW, Murakami S, Pos KM, Luisi BF (2015) Structure, mechanism and cooperation of bacterial multidrug transporters.

Curr Opin Struct Biol 33:76–91. https://doi.org/10.1016/j.sbi.2015.07.015

Eisenreich W, Dandekar T, Heesemann J, Goebel W (2010) Carbon metabolism of intracellular bacterial pathogens and possible links to virulence. Nat Rev Microbiol 8:401–412. https://doi.org/10.1038/nrmicro2351

Flechsig H (2016) Nucleotide-induced conformational dynamics in ABC transporters from structure-based coarse grained modeling. Front Phys 4:3

Garai P, Chandra K, Chakravortty D (2017) Bacterial peptide transporters: messengers of nutrition to virulence. Virulence 8:297–309. https://doi.org/10.1080/21505594.2016.1221025

Law CJ, Maloney PC, Wang DN (2008) Ins and outs of major facilitator superfamily antiporters. Annu Rev Microbiol 62:289–305. https://doi.org/10.1146/annurev.micro.61.080706.093329

Le Bouguénec C, Schouler C (2011) Sugar metabolism, an additional virulence factor in enterobacteria. Int J Med Microbiol 301:1–6. https://doi.org/10.1016/j.ijmm.2010.04.021

Nikaido H (2003) Molecular basis of bacterial outer membrane permeability revisited. Microbiol Mol Biol Rev 67:593–656

Omote H, Hiasa M, Matsumoto T, Otsuka M, Moriyama Y (2006) The MATE proteins as fundamental transporters of metabolic and xenobiotic organic cations. Trends Pharmacol Sci 27:587–593. https://doi.org/10.1016/j.tips.2006.09.001

Palmer LD, Skaar EP (2016) Transition metals and virulence in bacteria. Annu Rev Genet 50:67–91. https://doi.org/10.1146/annurev-genet-120215-035146

Piddock LJ (2006) Clinically relevant chromosomally encoded multidrug resistance efflux pumps in bacteria. Clin Microbiol Rev 19:382–402. https://doi.org/10.1128/CMR.19.2.382-402.2006

Ruggiero MA et al (2015) A higher level classification of all living organisms. PLoS One 10:e0119248. https://doi.org/10.1371/journal.pone.0119248

Siebold C, Flükiger K, Beutler R, Erni B (2001) Carbohydrate transporters of the bacterial phosphoenolpyruvate: sugar phosphotransferase system (PTS). FEBS Lett 504:104–111

11

Biofilms

© Springer Nature Switzerland AG 2019
A. W. Maresso, *Bacterial Virulence*, https://doi.org/10.1007/978-3-030-20464-8_12

Learning Goals

In this chapter, we discuss the idea that some pathogenic bacteria, in addition to their intrinsic virulence, also have the capacity to form organized communities in their host, termed biofilms. Bacterial biofilms are a sizable clustering of bacteria embedded in a sometimes thick extracellular matrix. The steps of biofilm formation are discussed, as are the reasons these structures allow the bacteria to resist the harmful attacks of either the immune system or treatment, notably antibiotics. The host anatomy and conditions that facilitate biofilm formation are framed in the context of the medical issues that fuel them, along with how the film itself forms the foundation for key factors that promote virulence, including bacterial communication and gene transfer. The learner will be well versed in the challenges biofilms present in the bacterial hunter's quest to understand and overcome complex infections.

12.1   Introduction

Human beings are remarkably social animals. We communicate through eye contact, hand gestures, symbols, art, and, most importantly, language. This communication allows us to transmit important information through time and space. Our communication enhances coordination between individuals and groups, may warn of impending danger, and, during times of stress, playful communication can relieve the burden of knowing we live in an imperfect and often ruthless world. A hunting party can coordinate plans for an effective kill. A child can tell a parent they don't feel well. The partitioning of people in society into distinct roles or jobs lowers the overall burden of the total level of work for each individual person. It is also more efficient, energy saving. Natural selection has favored the formation of strong social structures in many species for these reasons. An ant or bee colony, a flock of geese flying in unison, a herd of gazelle – they all group together under certain contexts because the advantages of the division of labor and protection from predators are greater than if the individual went at it alone.

So to it is with pathogenic bacteria. Since the early days of Pasteur and Koch, the microbe hunter often treated bacteria as independent disease-causing entities. Make no mistake, bacteria are selfish and the individual cell is looking out for itself. But we now know that some species, and the list keeps growing, of bacteria also engage in behaviors that are consistent with higher-order social systems we often observe in insects or animals. The advantages are not any different. Bacterial social circles form to enhance communication, to cluster or concentrate nutrients by decreasing the physical space by which they can diffuse, to form protective structures, and to increase their survival by simply being numerous. The objective of this chapter is to learn about bacterial social circles and relate such behavior to their ability to cause disease.

The grouping of dozens to hundreds or even thousands of bacterial cells together is sometimes termed a **microcolony**. When these microcolonies grow in size and are held together by a thick lattice of sticky carbohydrates (and other proteinaceous adhesins) with distinct biological and chemical differences as one pans through the structure the unit can be referred to as a **biofilm**. They are ancient. The fossil record demonstrates evidence of their existence over 3.5 billion years ago. A component of early seas when life first formed, they were likely the precursor to the start of multicellular life. The first recorded human observation of a biofilm, and bacteria for that matter, may have been when Anton Von Leuwenhoek peered under his modified lens' and saw a plaque sample from teeth teeming with little animalcules. For the microbe hunter to understand biofilms, it will be helpful to know how they form, the reasons they form, why they are advantageous, and then tie this into disease.

12.2   The Functions of Biofilms

There are many reasons bacteria may form biofilms (◻ Fig. 12.1). In the context of a host infection, one must consider how a biofilm benefits the bacterial pathogen while in the host microenvironment. Here, we discuss a few key reasons biofilms are advantageous in this context. The first reason is *protection*. A biofilm is a shelter. It is segregated into tiny caverns that house bacterial clusters, just like the individual units of an apartment complex. In an apartment, the rain, wind, and snow does little to alter your living conditions in the apartment; you sleep well in your climate controlled bedroom. The interior of the film can resist a range of environmental insults that would otherwise be very stressful for free-floating cells. This includes osmotic changes that alter the turgor pressure on the cell membrane or resistance to chemical insults including antibiotics and antimicrobial peptides. Inside the biofilm the pH can remain steady and nutrients may concentrate. The inner compartments keep antigens from detection and resist attack by the natural born killers of immune phagocytes. A biofilm can also protect against shear forces generated by currents, such as blood flowing through a vessel or urine through a ureter.

The second reason a biofilm may be beneficial to pathogenic bacteria is as a means to maintain close *communication*. Bacteria in close proximity can communicate more efficiently than if they were separated by great swaths of space, fluid, or tissue. The way bacteria communicate is through the detection of small chemical molecules they secrete, almost like pheromones, in a process described as **quorum sensing**. First reported in studies of marine bacteria in the 1970s, quorum sensing is a way for bacteria to judge the state, often density, of their little community and then make changes based on this state. It often proceeds in three parts, the first of which is the production of small chemicals that diffuse to tightly-packed neighboring cells and act as chemical messengers. In the second stage, the recipient cell senses the chemical and reprograms the expression of its genes in response. The final stage is some adaptation of behavior, the result of gene expression. In the context of a discussion on biofilms, it is commonly thought that quorum

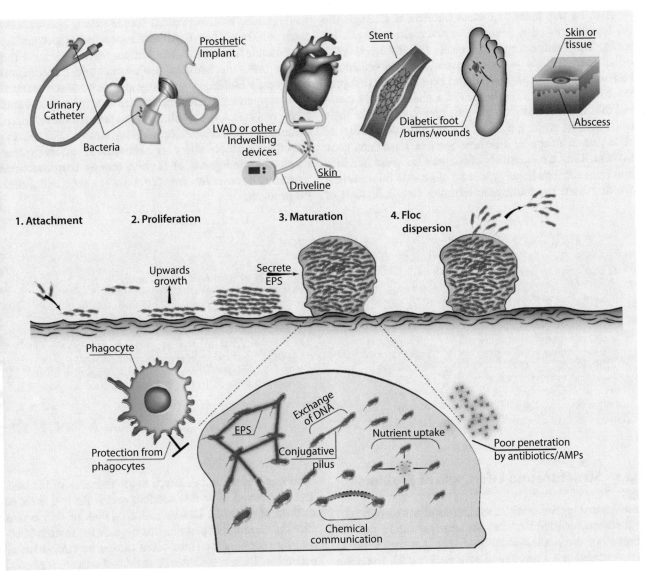

◻ Fig. 12.1 Formation and function of the bacterial biofilm. Bacterial biofilms in hosts present new and different therapeutic challenges. Whether they originate from diseased tissue that promotes their formation or an indwelling devices that serves as a site of attachment and growth, the bacterial biofilm can be generally characterized as having four stages of formation. These include the initial attachment of the pathogenic bacterium to some type of substratum, the proliferation and replication of the organism into a microcolony (usually concomitantly with the secretion of a thick, sticky polymeric polysaccharide or expression of adhesins), the maturation into a large, vertical structure, and finally the release of new cells or aggregates to another location. Biofilms can protect bacteria against immune attack or penetration with antibiotics or antibodies, promote cell-to-cell communication and the exchange of genetic information, and enhance nutrient uptake or the reduction of bacterial metabolism

sensing in concentrated cell populations promotes the formation of biofilms, a kind of signal that says "build a community here." The molecules of communication between bacteria are generally referred to as **inducers** or **autoinducers**, so-named because, at high enough concentrations, they induce bacteria to change gene expression. A prominent class of inducers are the **N-acyl homoserine lactones**. AHLs are structurally composed of a lactone moiety and a string of carbons that may approach a dozen in length. There are many different types of AHLs and they regulate many bacterial processes, but some of the ones important for virulence include biofilm formation, motility, adherence, and capsule production.

Small chemical messengers are not the only way they talk. There are also mechanical and electrical signals that permeate through the community. When combined with the chemical messengers, they represent the language and touch of bacterial interactions. They have as real an outcome to the health and function of the community as do these similar modes of communication for human beings. So little is known about how these signals are sensed, how the sensing coordinates a change in metabolism or behavior, and how this may all influence virulence. Our knowledge of mechanical cues in pathogenesis come from studies that enteric bacteria change their gene expression when they sense the peristalsis or shear forces of the intestinal tract.

A third way biofilms benefit bacteria is through the concept of *proximity*. Being close just makes things a lot easier. The small quorum chemicals can diffuse to each other more readily – so communication is enhanced. Nutrients can be concentrated and kept at levels that promote their import. Adhesins or extracellular matrix material that is needed to glue the cells together is more likely to contact its sticky neighbor. Maybe most substantial of all is that small spatial distances enhance horizontal gene transfer. Thus, a community of bacteria enclosed in a biofilm can exchange important units of genetic information. We discussed the mutagenic tetrasect (the collection of conjugation, transformation, transduction, and de novo mutation) in ▶ Chap. 6. All of these exchange mechanisms are possible in a biofilm. In addition, there is evidence that two of these mechanisms, conjugation and transduction, help shape biofilm community structure. Since many of these elements include genes related to virulence and antibiotic resistance, the biofilm is also a little incubator for the production of resistant or virulent strains. For chronic infections where biofilms are a substantial barrier to treatment, the emergence of mutant strains that overcome treatment or other immune functions is a substantial clinical problem.

Out of the Box

Staphylococcus epidermidis is a resident of the human skin. Many of us are colonized with this organism and know no difference otherwise. We have seen throughout this work of some infections (even epidemics!) that are, seemingly, the result of human medical activity. We eliminate one problem but create another. The current use of the antibiotic clindamycin, and the fortification of our food with certain types of sugars, are major drivers of the dramatic rise in *C. difficile* carriage and infections in the Western world. So too seems to be the case of *S. epidermidis* biofilms, which, for all practical purposes, displays its pathogenic potential almost entirely because of the widespread use of in-dwelling medical devices. This skin microbiome resident turned evil pathogen did not magically inherit this ability. The gene products involved in the formation of its biofilms, including PIA and MSCRAMMs, are the same ones used to efficiently colonize the surface of our skin, just adapted to this new-found niche. The word "opportunism" comes to mind. These opportunist pathogens seemingly grow in frequency each passing year as modern medicine finds ways to keep us alive longer. The microbe hunter, after decades of looking outward for the next pandemic, will now need to look increasingly inward.

12.3   Structure and Life-Cycle of Biofilms

Biofilm making begins with the secretion of an **exo-polymeric substance** (or EPS) that consists largely of sticky carbohydrates but also can include adhesins (such as curli which we encountered in ▶ Chap. 7) and even nucleic acid. The carbohydrates are attachment factors; they stick to almost anything, including host cells or tissues, indwelling devices or other artificial substances, and even other bacterial cells (◘ Figs. 12.2 and 12.3). Whereas the outside of the biofilm is somewhat impenetrable except for small polar molecules, there is evidence of fluid movement and exchange via tunnels that run through the center. The formation of this structure usually occurs when one or a group of bacteria seed themselves on one of these surfaces – simply termed **attachment** - and it is the first step (◘ Fig. 12.4). Once several bacterial cells attach, they may divide and in so doing form a microcolony that will extend in three dimensions upwards and laterally away from the initial site of attachment. This is the **proliferative** phase. The shape of this structure often resembles a tornado or mushroom, or a stadium dome. More EPS is secreted and the structure becomes larger extending upwards as cells divide. This third stage, **maturation**, includes a film or ball-like structure that can grow to a thousand microns in diameter and is anchored to the base by a stalk that links the mushroom to the surface. Here, cells may persist indefinitely, often slowing their metabolism. Finally, it is thought that there is a program by which a portion of this community can shed from this surface and re-attach to another area of the host. This is referred to as floc **seeding** and is likely a directed method of dispersal. Dissemination of flocs of cells occurs after the secretion of proteins that degrade the matrix, infection by phage, or by shear-stress caused by circulation or peristalsis. There is evidence these flocs of cells are very good at initiating a new biofilm at another, nearby location.

12.4   Biofilms and Infections

Bacterial biofilms are a substantial cause of serious human infections. Some of the best examples include the establishment of *Pseudomonas aeruginosa* in the lungs of cystic fibrosis patients. Over the many years they persist in the lungs, these bacteria form hardy biofilms surrounded by thick mucus that is difficult to eradicate. Another common example includes the infection by staphylococcus or streptococcus of the valves of the heart. In this case, it is believed that atherosclerotic plaques or other damage to the lining of the valves or endothelium generates fibrin clots that serves as a landing pad for circulating bacteria. The biofilm will grow, anchored to these clots, and then shed an embolic bolus that is a seed that will plant at another location in the body. Endocarditis is often the result of such biofilms and can lead to a dangerous level of heart dysfunction. Not to be outdone, *E. coli* too can grow into giant biofilms on implants or indwelling devices (also a characteristic of staphylococcus

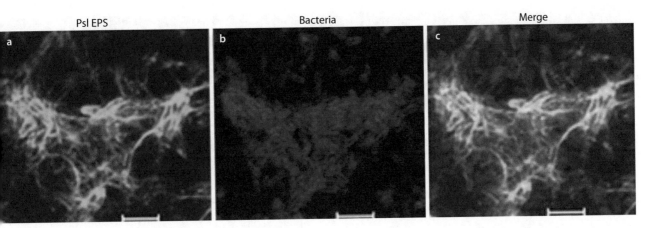

Psl EPS   Bacteria   Merge

Fig. 12.2 Exopolysaccharide (EPS) provides the structure to hold bacterial communities. One of the more important characteristics of biofilms is that their formation is often associated with the secretion of a carbohydrate matrix that acts as a type of "glue" to keep the cells together. In this experiment, the products of the polysaccharide synthesis locus (or Psl), one of the carbohydrate-rich structures important in the formation of biofilms in *P. aeruginosa*, is marked with a fluorescent lectin (panel **a**). Fluorescent *P. aeruginosa* cells are shown in panel **b** and the merge of these two images, shown in panel **c**, demonstrates the complex intertwined mesh both cell and carbohydrates form in the biofilm. (Adapted from Wozniak et al. (see *suggested readings*) under a creative commons license. (▶ https://creativecommons.org/licenses/by/4.0/))

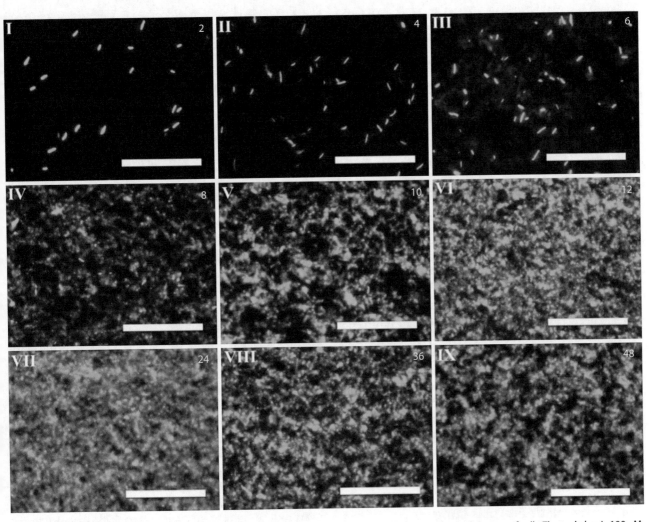

Fig. 12.3 Biofilm growth with time. In this experiment, performed with fluorescent *E. coli* cells, the formation of a biofilm is followed from 2 to 48 hours. Initial adhered cells seem to secrete a substance around them and allows for more cells to gather and grow until eventually the thick structure forms a sheet of clusters of cells. The scale bar is 100 μM. (Adapted from Zhao et al. (see *suggested readings*) under a creative commons license. (▶ https://creativecommons.org/licenses/by/4.0/))

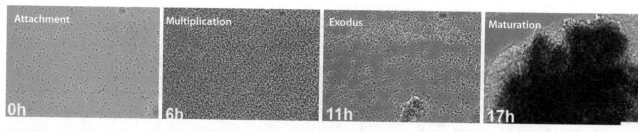

Fig. 12.4 Biofilms can demonstrate predictable but also unexpected properties. Most biofilms form along the lines of those demonstrated in ◻ Fig. 12.1. But complex communities can also demonstrate complex behavior. In this example, a *S. aureus* biofilm begins to first form via attachment to the glass surface and multiplication of the cells into a lawn-like arrangement. By 11 hours, some of the cells have apparently dispersed the field (termed exodus) while others begin to form into a stalk-like structure (lower part of the field) that eventually grows by 17 hours into a giant, mature biofilm. (Adapted from Bayles et al (see *suggested readings*) under a creative commons license. (► https://creativecommons.org/licenses/by-nc-sa/3.0))

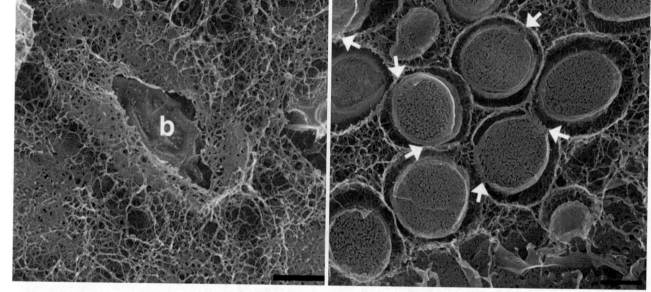

Fig. 12.5 Bacteria in biofilms can be encased in compartments. Freeze-fracture high-resolution electron microscopy allows for the analysis of the unique structures that make up biofilms. In this study, uropathogenic *E. coli* was seen encased in a fibrous network that surrounded the bacterial cells (left panel – the bacterium is marked with a "b"). These fibrous networks connected cells to cells which can be seen in the right panel being encased in compartments that at distinct points touch the bacterial cells (arrows). These networks are supported by or made of many different molecules, possibly including sugars like cellulose, curli and fim adhesins, and even flagellar components. (Adapted from Hultgren et al (see *suggested readings*) under a creative commons license. (► https://creativecommons.org/licenses/by-nc-sa/3.0))

and streptococcus) – ◻ Fig. 12.5. This includes prosthetics, catheters and stents, the surfaces of these devices a seeding point for the growth of the biofilm (◻ Fig. 12.6). Because of the imperviousness of biofilms to antibiotics, which makes them almost impossible to eliminate, these devices, meant to save the life of a patient, in some cases become a source of reoccurring chronic infections. We discuss some of these biofilm-generating infections here to provide real world examples of how pathogenic bacteria use such communities to their advantage, and the difficulties in eradicating them.

12.4.1 The Cystic Fibrosis Lung

We have occasionally in this volume referred to *P. aeruginosa* infections. People who inherit a certain mutation in the CFTR ion transporter demonstrate aberrations in osmotic balance. This is particularly evident in the lung. Such patients, over many years, accumulate mucus in this organ to the point that it blocks proper respiration. Unfortunately, high levels of mucus also trap bacteria, and, since the CF lung cannot clear such mucus readily, these bacteria become a permanent resident of the organ. The sputum of CF patients is noted as having high titers of *P. aeruginosa* that form biofilms of a diameter of about 100 microns. The levels of AHLs are also high, which is consistent with programming towards a biofilm phenotype. While in these structures, the pseudomonads eventually begin to overproduce alginate, an exopolysaccharide that also forms the main structural component of the housing complex. The center of these complexes is impervious to antibiotics (and even oxygen), two conditions that both protect bacteria as

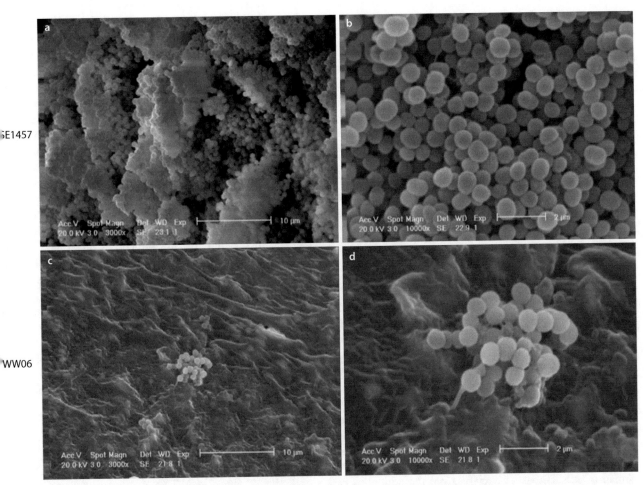

Fig. 12.6 Biofilms on catheters. One of the major problems with in-dwelling devices such as catheters is that they provide a surface by which bacteria can adhere and form biofilms. Panels **a** and **b**: In this experiment, *S. epidermidis* (strain SE1457) was incubated with parts of a central vein catheter and 24 hours later visualized by transmission electron microscopy. Clear biofilms of grape-like bacterial cluster are observed. Panels **c** and **d**: Biofilm formation is dependent on a two-component system termed ArlRS since a strain that lacks this TCS (WW06) forms little to no biofilms. Also in these panels one can observe the surface of the catheter as a series of undulations and ridges that are excellent attachment points for bacteria. (Adapted from Qu et al. (see *suggested readings*) under a creative commons license. (► https://creativecommons.org/licenses/by/4.0/))

well as further drive the production of the polysaccharide. This is a good example of how an underlying mutation in a human gene sows the conditions for the formation of a pathogenic and protected community of bacteria. Over many years, the pathogen may even evolve under these conditions to be more adapted to them, further complicating treatment.

12.4.2 The Diabetic Foot

Another example of an underlying genetic condition that predisposes people to the formation of biofilms is the diabetic foot ulcer. One consequence of chronic diabetes is the loss of nerve function (can't feel pain) and poor circulation, especially to extremities. Such patients are at risk for wounds that heal slowly, especially the foot, and thus are susceptible to infection. The most common organism that colonizes such a wound is *S. aureus* whose combination of toxins and adhesins promotes the expansion and worsening of the wound. Staph biofilms are common and can even be polymicrobial. Despite being exposed and accessible to the physician, such biofilms and wounds are of such depth and complexity that if antibiotics do not improve the condition, amputation of toes or the entire foot are common. Staphylococci in general are proficient in forming biofilms on a number of human sites, including the valves of the heart, shunts, stents, drive-line, and catheters. Their ability to do this stems from the expression of several adhesins that may work together or separately depending on the surface to colonize. This includes the polysaccharide intercellular adhesin (PIA), the biofilm associated protein (BAP), and fibronectin-binding protein (MSCRAMMs – ► Chap. 7). The enzyme coagulase, a common virulence factor in virulent isolates of *S. aureus*, converts host fibrinogen to fibrin. These fibrins accumulate and provide a scaffold or landing pad for the growth of staph biofilms, the afore mentioned adhesins helping drive the aggregation and binding process.

12.4.3   Endocarditis

Cardiac valves are important in separating the chambers of the heart during the exchange of blood between them. Streptococci and staphylococci are able to bind platelets and fibrin on damaged valves mostly because the underlying extracellular matrix is exposed. This makes open landing sites for these bacteria which adhere through there MSCRAMMs. Some streptococcal species encode a fimbrial protein, Fap1, which maintains their presence in biofilms. *S. epidermidis* and *S. aureus* also use PIA for biofilm maintenance. Artificial valves and stents also serve as attachment sites. Since endocarditis is associated with cardiac arrest, these biofilms can be life-threatening.

12.4.4   Other Sites

Other sites of biofilms include catheters, especially in those with loss of bladder function (example, patients with spinal chord injury). Here, *E. coli* and *P. aeruginosa* are the most frequent formers of biofilms. These can be dangerous because *E. coli* in general is a frequent cause of urosepsis (see ► Chap. 13), a condition that may result from the spread of the organism to the blood and other tissues and the accompanying immune response that follows. The gums and teeth are teaming with biofilms. *Streptococcus mutans* is the main culprit here being a significant cause of tooth decay/cavities, but dozens of different streptococcal species inhabit the human mouth. Dispersed bacteria from these biofilms can enter into the intestinal tract or the blood from inflamed gums. Travelling through the circulation, they can land in the heart and contribute to endocarditis as well.

12.5   Tools and Treatments

The study of bacterial biofilms, especially as it pertains to infections, is still in its infancy as a field. There is a dearth of knowledge concerning the genetic programs that control biofilm formation and maturation. Even less is known about the metabolism of bacteria in biofilms. Useful in vitro models have been developed; they include unsophisticated systems such as simply letting a culture sit on the benchtop to continuous flow systems that mimic fluid and shear forces or modified surfaces that facilitate their formation. Animal models have been developed including indwelling devices pre-seeded with biofilms. Rodent models mimic the CF lung and *S. aureus* implants (such as joint replacement) model infections of bone (termed osteomyelitis). Biofilms are often imaged using crystal violet or fluorescence microscopy whereby either the bacteria are detected (often using fluorescence in situ hybridization – FISH) or polysaccharides (the biofilm matrix itself). Manipulation of the focal plane and confocal microscopy allows investigators to probe the depths of the biofilm structure.

Biofilms have been recognized as a medical problem since the late 1960s and as such a number of measures have been taken and developed to eliminate or reduce the likelihood of their occurrence. This includes the development of experimental drugs that are designed to disrupt the biofilm matrix including sugar-cleaving enzymes and metal chelators, as well as the production of biomimetics that compete for or competitively inhibit bacterial adhesins and their interaction with their substrates. Some companies are even designing polymers and plastics that are naturally anti-adhesive or that have a surface that is toxic to bacteria. Phage may have value in dispersing biofilms, while other more radical approaches include preventing quorum sensing. None of these approaches, outside of inert non-sticky surfaces for devices, have gained much traction clinically. With the clear failure of antibiotics to penetrate deep into these biofilms (and their inability to target bacteria in the film that are sometimes metabolically dormant), new approaches to aid those with infections originating from a biofilm will be desperately needed. Some of these approaches may have utility in this regard since they target key features that are needed for the biofilm to maintain its protective properties. In some ways, the traditional line of inquiry when thinking about bacteria as planktonic entities impedes a new mindset that may be needed to solve biofilms. The microbe hunter will have to be open to such paradigm changes as medical advances make new opportunities for bacteria to colonize their unsuspecting hosts.

Summary of Key Concepts

1. Biofilms are ancient. They are the precursors to multicellular organization and group cooperation. This makes them challenging to both study and treat when thinking of their contribution to infection and health.

2. The establishment of biofilms, either on abiotic or biotic surfaces, follows an ordered structural, biological, and genetic framework starting with founding cells adhering to a surface and their communication to form a more organized structure that eventually houses an entire community.

3. Biofilms protect the pathogens they enclose, shielding them from the immune system, antibiotics, and the otherwise harsh environment of the host. As such, they are often difficult to clear from a host and are the source of chronic infections that can have life-threatening consequences.

4. Some medical treatments, patients with underlying genetic disorders, and locations of the body are more susceptible to the formation of biofilms.

5. High-risk patients and medical interventions require new modes of biofilm prevention and treatment that contrast significantly from traditional approaches.

Expand Your Knowledge

1. A problem with the eradication of device-related biofilms in patients is that they are refractory to antibiotics. There are two main reasons for this, one being a lack of penetration into the deepest layers of the film and a second being the tendency for resident bacterial cells to lower their metabolic activity when housed in a film. Outline a new antimicrobial strategy that simultaneously addresses both of these problems. Generate a structured document that introduces the problem, provides the rationale behind your solution, and then methodologically lays out experimentation that will prove or disprove the validity of your approach. Make sure you formulate a hypothesis and clearly articulate the positive and negative controls (or other controls) of the study.

2. N-3-oxo-dodecanoyl homoserine lactone (3OC12-HSL) is a homoserine lactone quorum sensing molecule produced by *P. aeruginosa*. Its production is linked to the expression of many pseudomonas genes, including those involved in virulence in pneumonia and burn-wound infection models in animals. Interestingly, this molecule may also be sensed by our own immune cells, which may become programmed themselves to respond to a bacterial infection, a kind of "cross-kingdom eavesdropping" on bacterial communication pathways. Imagine you are a tough-grading Professor of a Microbiology course at a local college. Formulate an examination question that tests a student's knowledge of how 3OC12-HSL is synthesized, its structure, what it binds to and activates, and how the signal is converted into a biologic response in both pseudomonas and host immune cells. You will need to search Pubmed for published papers on this topic, and read them.

3. Make a storyboard that shows the progression of the formation of a bacterial biofilm. Include at each step the molecular factors, both host and bacterial, that are needed for the execution of that step.

Suggested Reading

Beloin C, Renard S, Ghigo JM, Lebeaux D (2014) Novel approaches to combat bacterial biofilms. Curr Opin Pharmacol 18:61–68. https://doi.org/10.1016/j.coph.2014.09.005

Bjarnsholt T et al (2013) The in vivo biofilm. Trends Microbiol 21:466–474. https://doi.org/10.1016/j.tim.2013.06.002

Fux CA, Costerton JW, Stewart PS, Stoodley P (2005) Survival strategies of infectious biofilms. Trends Microbiol 13:34–40. https://doi.org/10.1016/j.tim.2004.11.010

Hall-Stoodley L, Costerton JW, Stoodley P (2004) Bacterial biofilms: from the natural environment to infectious diseases. Nat Rev Microbiol 2:95–108. https://doi.org/10.1038/nrmicro821

Han Q et al (2017) Removal of foodborne pathogen biofilms by acidic electrolyzed water. Front Microbiol 8:988. https://doi.org/10.3389/fmicb.2017.00988

Hung C et al (2013) Escherichia coli biofilms have an organized and complex extracellular matrix structure. MBio 4:e00645–e00613. https://doi.org/10.1128/mBio.00645-13

Ma L et al (2009) Assembly and development of the Pseudomonas aeruginosa biofilm matrix. PLoS Pathog 5:e1000354. https://doi.org/10.1371/journal.ppat.1000354

Moormeier DE, Bose JL, Horswill AR, Bayles KW (2014) Temporal and stochastic control of Staphylococcus aureus biofilm development. MBio 5:e01341–e01314. https://doi.org/10.1128/mBio.01341-14

Parsek MR, Greenberg EP (2005) Sociomicrobiology: the connections between quorum sensing and biofilms. Trends Microbiol 13:27–33. https://doi.org/10.1016/j.tim.2004.11.007

Parsek MR, Singh PK (2003) Bacterial biofilms: an emerging link to disease pathogenesis. Annu Rev Microbiol 57:677–701. https://doi.org/10.1146/annurev.micro.57.030502.090720

Wu Y et al (2012) The two-component signal transduction system ArlRS regulates Staphylococcus epidermidis biofilm formation in an Ica-dependent manner. PLoS One 7:e40041. https://doi.org/10.1371/journal.pone.0040041

The Human Microbiome

© Springer Nature Switzerland AG 2019
A. W. Maresso, *Bacterial Virulence*, https://doi.org/10.1007/978-3-030-20464-8_13

Learning Goals

In this chapter, we discuss the concept that your body is a living ecosystem of hundreds of different types of bacteria, of which some are opportunists that cause serious infections while others are symbionts and pathobionts that can profoundly affect your health. The location and composition of these communities are highlighted, mostly using the digestive system as a frame of reference, in the context of their balance inside the host, with an unbalanced state being a precursor to pathogen invasion, harmful to the mucosal surface, and ultimately the basis for many acute and chronic diseases. The chapter concludes with a foray into some methods the microbiomist uses to make sense of these complex relationships. The learner will be armed with the foundational knowledge to understand how these relationships may cause disease and the concepts to formulate new reductionist approaches to reveal their mechanistic basis.

13.1 Introduction

The human body is composed of eleven integrated systems that come together to maintain your health and metabolic balance. Each is essential. Remove one and the others will be thrown off, unable to churn efficiently, a state that would promote disease. Each plays its part, contributing an essential function that would be impossible for a single system to execute alone. Take the use of oxygen in the atmosphere, as an example. All know that you must breathe oxygen to stay alive, but why? What we really mean by "oxygen" is atmospheric dioxygen (O_2), two atoms of oxygen linked by a covalent bond. Dioxygen, unlike other gases we breathe (nitrogen and argon), is a highly reactive molecule; it can donate and accept electrons. The flow of electrons along a cell's membrane creates a charge gradient. There is pent up energy in this gradient. Your cells store and convert that energy into a chemical, ATP. All the leftover electrons from this process, which can be deadly if nowhere to go, are absorbed by oxygen. The ATP powers your cells, and you live.

Every breath, your respiratory system facilitates the transfer of oxygen from the outside environment to your blood. Your circulatory system, which carriers your blood, distributes this dissolved oxygen to every cell in the body. Your muscular and skeletal system gives you form so you can move; movement allows you to forage. What you forage is turned into more energy and nutrients for your cells via your digestive system. Your liver converts toxins you take in to harmless byproducts, and your renal system filters these byproducts, readying them for excretion. Your immune system guards it all, your brain controls it all. Should it go well enough, your reproductive system ensures the same processes live on in your progeny.

For the most part, these systems can be observed through the simple dissection of a specimen. The various circulatory or neuronal connections can be traced even by the inexperienced eye and huge groupings of specialized tissues, which we call organs (e.g. heart), can be held in the palm of one's hand. All visible, all tangible. Anatomists and scientists thought we had discovered all there was to know regarding organ systems. But there is a 12th system, recently rediscovered, and it's existence flies in the face of everything we have already proclaimed in this volume about the deadly nature of bacteria.

We are talking about the human microbiome.

13.2 Life Living on Life

The human **microbiome** is the collection of all the bacteria, viruses, fungi, and even protozoa that live in and on your body. By far, its composition is dominated by bacteria. One might argue that you are dominated by bacteria. There are at least as many bacterial cells associated with your body as there are human cells, and some estimates put it as high as 10:1. The chemical reactions your microbiome can carry out on a daily basis would require millions of years for you to evolve. Every day, the simple division of these bacterial cells leads to nine billion new mutations for the several trillions of bacterial cells that are made. The dry weight of all the bacterial cells in and on your body is approximately two kilograms. This is three times as heavy as your heart and about the same weight as your brain. They occupy every niche of your skin, as well as your lungs, urinary tract, and reproductive system. The digestive tract is teaming with them, and it is these bacteria that have the greatest impact on your health. Here, they are an organ within an organ, carrying out reactions needed for your nutritional benefit, stimulating the immune system to mature, and playing the role of an immune system themselves by providing a barrier to the establishment of incoming pathogenic bacteria. Invisible to the eye, but no less significant, the twelfth organ works in segregated parts, in communities and alone, from the skin and various mucosal surfaces, to affect your wellness (◻ Fig. 13.1).

It starts at birth. As you come through the vaginal canal, the bacteria that live on the mucosal surfaces of the vagina touch your cheeks, your nose, and your lips. Some are ingested, survive the passage through the acidic stomach, and find themselves in the intestine. Others are ingested during the first feeding, the nipple of the mother also being colonized with bacteria. The bacteria on the mother's skin make contact with the newborn's skin. The baby's intestinal tract even enhances their capture during passage, being caught in the thick mucus layer that lines these surfaces. The mouth is probably the first colonized; adult human saliva contains up to 10^9 bacteria per milliliter. As bacteria make their way down, the esophagus is next colonized, but at much lower levels (10^4 cells/mL). The stomach represents a major attrition point for bacteria, the harsh acid killing most as they pass through. The mucosa of the stomach is only partially colonized, and often by those bacteria with pathogenic potential, including *H. pylori*, a contributor to ulcers and stomach cancer. Nevertheless, their resiliency abound, about eight different phyla of bacteria are detected in the stomach of healthy people.

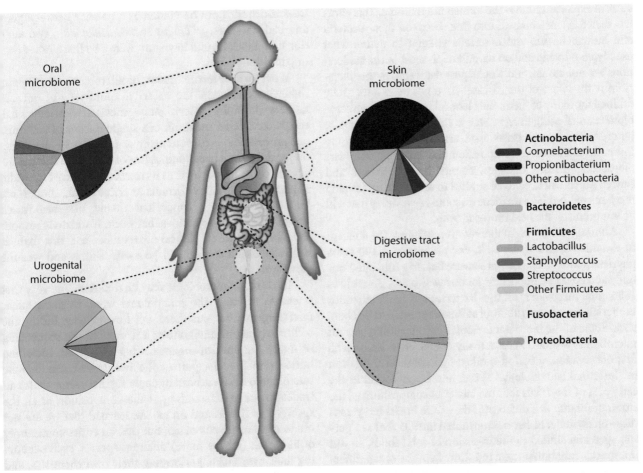

Fig. 13.1 The human microbiome. The human microbiome refers to the collection of microorganisms that live in and on us. Shown below are the relative proportions of bacterial phyla and genera at four locations of the human body, including the mouth, skin, urogenital track, and digestive system. Other areas of the body that also harbor bacteria, but are not indicated here, include the ear canal and respiratory tract. Diseases or conditions associated with the oral microbiome include dental caries and gingivitis. Those associated with the skin microbiome include acne, dermatitis, and psoriasis. Those associated with the urogenital microbiome include yeast infections, UTIs, and vaginosis. Those associated with the microbiome of the digestive tract include invasive infections, inflammatory conditions like Crohn's and IBD, obesity, diabetes, and cancer

Bacteria next encounter the first part of the small intestine, the duodenum and jejunum. The total composition in the early part of the duodenum is low in bacterial numbers, just 10^2–10^5 per gram. Food partially digested by the acid of the stomach is further digested by enzymes and bile, which emulsifies fats. Antimicrobial peptides are secreted here. All of this has a negative effect on the population density. The composition of the microbiome is less diverse, being driven by bacteria that facilitate the metabolism of carbohydrates. Moving further down the small intestine brings us to the ileum. Here, with the acidity of the stomach neutralized and an abundance of complex nutrients reduced to useable forms, both the population numbers and composition of bacteria begins to dramatically increase, reaching 10^8–10^9 organisms per gram. Numerous phyla are present including a healthy dose of not only facultative aerobes but also strict anaerobes.

Next comes the large intestine (colon) and with it the largest collection of diversity and concentration of bacteria. There are greater than 200 genera and perhaps as much as 800 different species. The bacterial population balloons to 10^{12}/gram. Obligate anaerobes dominate. Nutrients, liberated by all the digestive processes upstream, are a-plenty. The high abundance of bacteria makes the interaction with the intestinal epithelium much more frequent. It makes the products that bacteria make much more concentrated. It is not surprising that most diseases of the GI tract occur in the colon, from cancer to inflammation (colitis and Crohn's). It is also not surprising that this is where the benefit of having some of these bacteria also seems to be most evident, from nutrient absorption to vitamin generation to the education of the immune system.

13.3 The Evolution of the Concept of the Human Microbiome

The explosion of studies in the first decade of the twenty-first century that began to systematically sequence, and thus identify, all the bacteria associated with us paved the road for current explorations into the human microbiome. This effort has fueled intense interest into links between these bacteria and human health, and a serious attempt to define what exactly does live in and on us. Although most of the associations are not casual, and Koch's postulates (prove the bacterium is the *cause* of the disease) have not been adequately fulfilled for many of them, the plentiful reports of the microbiome contributing in *some* way to human health cannot be ignored. There now exists firm associations between the intestinal microbiome composition and inflammation, cardiovascular disease, diabetes, obesity, brain function, and cancer. Much will need to be studied to reveal the underlying mechanisms, but here we focus on some key features that will be important as the field moves forward.

Although it may seem like recent revelation, the concept of the microbiome really isn't. For more than a 100 years physicians and scientists were aware bacteria inhabited our body and could be important for our well-being. As early as 1886, the discoverer of the bacterium *E. coli*, Theodor Escherich, noted that the stool of infants contained live bacteria. Some of the more trendy topics encompassing current microbiome studies were actually noted after Escherich's first observation, a period marked by intense investigation in "intestinal bacteriology." Tissier and Logan found in the early part of the 1900s that the bacterial composition of the stools of infants was different if they were breast fed versus those on formula. Fisher demonstrated in 1903 that as a person aged and shifted to the ingestion of solid foods, so did the species inhabiting their intestine. Lembke noted differences between wheat-rich and meat-rich diets as early as 1896. Breast milk, aging, and diet as major drivers of the microbiome have gained recent attention but such observations are more than a 100 years old.

Even the link between the composition and a person's health was heavily debated and took on a fury of belief not too different than what we see today. Noting that the people of Bulgaria have an unusually high number of centennials amongst their population, Élie Metchnikoff, often referred to as the "father of immunity" because of his studies on macrophages, proposed that centennials longevity may be due to their copious consumption of soured milk. This fermented milk, similar to modern yogurt, contained a bacterium we know today as *Lactobacillus bulgaricus*, so-named after the region it was first isolated. Metchnikoff reasoned that the high concentration of bacteria in the intestine lead to "putrefaction" – the leaking of poisons into the body of people. This was believed to be a major driver of many diseases. Physicians often in the first quarter of the twentieth century sought ways to cleanse the intestine of bad bacteria, including prescribing compounds from aspirin to calomel to menthol to their patients. Metchnikoff argued that *L. bulgaricus* in sour milk somehow protected Bulgarians from being poisoned. This extended their life. Although the theory was eventually discarded, elements of it are not too distant from what we believe today about **probiotics**, *i.e.* that good bacteria we ingest may somehow improve our health[1]. So was born the idea that

intestinal health can be viewed as a balance between good and bad microbes. *B. bifidus* and *B. acidophilus*, two additional probiotics found in yogurt, were also first studied during this time period.

What we have learned about the microbiome to this point somewhat challenges the collective mind-view of microbe hunters who study bacterial pathogenesis. Historically, a disease is considered the result of a single infecting bacterium, one process, and even potentially one gene or virulence factor produced by a bacterium. A line of thought of this nature, which uses reductive logic as its intellectual ox cart, provides a simple easy-to-follow formula to arrive at causation. More importantly, it is a conceptual theme that has fueled approaches to make vaccines that work. If a toxin is responsible for a particular clinical observation, and that toxin is neutralized, the disease will go away. This is and was the paradigm.

The human microbiome may be different. The very first scientists to study the microbiome were, in many ways, interested in what was there, not how or why. Riding the technological and methodological wave of the sequencing of many genomes of organisms big and small, including humans, in the first part of the twenty-first century, the microbiome field was born by applying these same tools and trades to the understanding of the composition of all the species that live in and on us. We learned that we are not mono or di or tri-colonized, but that an entire community of hundreds (maybe more) different species, each occupying their own niche, performing their own chemistry, and interacting with their host in their own way, constitutes the paradigm. Here, the thoughts of the microbe hunter must shift to a more holistic way of thinking about biology, rather than the reductionist approach of Koch. It is the interaction of all the moving parts at one time, a dynamic interplay of a *collection* of species, that seemingly drives health or disease. In this worldview, the bacteria, their metabolism, as well as host cells and their metabolism, determine the outcome. Like any ecosystem where all components are connected in some way to others, even perhaps by dozens of degrees of freedom, so too is the microbiome ecosystem. Here, the keyword is balance, or, more accurately, the lack of it, that leads to disease.

13.4 Imbalance and Composition

When the bacterial composition of the microbiota deviates from its normal state, this is **dysbiosis** ("dys" meaning disrupted, "biosis" meaning life). Normal in this case refers to the composition of the community that exists during a healthy state, sometimes referred to as **symbiosis** because the bacterial symbionts of the body are diverse and balanced (◘ Fig. 13.2). But what is normal? What we have come to learn in fact is that normal is unique to each individual. There are no microbiomes exactly the same between two people, at least data to this point suggests there are not. Diet, genetics,

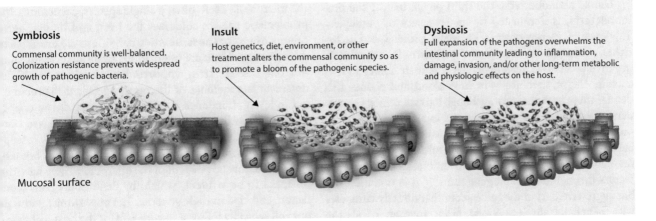

Symbiosis

Commensal community is well-balanced. Colonization resistance prevents widespread growth of pathogenic bacteria.

Insult

Host genetics, diet, environment, or other treatment alters the commensal community so as to promote a bloom of the pathogenic species.

Dysbiosis

Full expansion of the pathogens overwhelms the intestinal community leading to inflammation, damage, invasion, and/or other long-term metabolic and physiologic effects on the host.

Mucosal surface

☐ **Fig. 13.2** Symbiosis, dysbiosis, and disease. A balanced commensal ecosystem is generally considered healthy and confers protection from pathobionts or invasive bacteria via colonization resistance, the concept that commensal organisms outcompete pathogens for an ecological niche. At some point, the host undergoes a trigger or other insult that disrupts the commensal community composition and structure. Such insults may include antibiotic treatment, immunosup- pressive therapy, the onset of a debilitating disease, diet, trauma, or invasion of a pathogen itself (amongst others) which leads to a loss of colonization resistance and expansion of the pathogen or pathobiont population. The net effect, where one or a few species now dominate, is termed dysbiosis and may lead to inflammatory, infectious, or other downstream negative effects on the overall health of the host

race, age, and geographical location, all dramatically affect the composition of the intestinal microbiome, for example. Although more similar than the general population, even the microbiomes of identical twins can be different. In this regard, it is useful to consider normal being what exists when healthy; that is, a state of the composition of the biome that is different from what one may house during healthy times. When the composition deviates from this steady-state, when it becomes dominated by one species or genus, it is at this point that the progression to some type of disease or condition may develop. One challenge the microbe hunter faces in this arena is to precisely define with scientific standards what does and does not constitute balance.

What we have learned about bacterial communities and disease is by far most well developed by examining the bacteria that live in the intestinal tract. Thus, to highlight some of the key biology that underpins the microbiome's relationship to disease, this is the place to start. In this regard, the sequencing of the genomes of bacteria in the gastrointestinal track has revealed that of the kingdom known as bacteria, at least four phyla are routinely observed. These are the bacteroidetes, actinobacteria, proteobacteria, and firmicutes. The **bacteroidetes** are Gram-negative, facultative anaerobic bacilli that also inhabit the skin and are common in soil and water. They are both friend and foe harboring several species that are beneficial to the host as well as those that play the role of pathogen in some capacity. *Bacillus thetaiotaomicron*, for example, is a member of bacteroidetes that aids host energy acquisition by breaking down and fermenting complex carbohydrates. *B. theta*, as it is commonly called, stimulates Paneth cells of the intestinal tract to produce antimicrobial peptides that can destroy bonafide invasive pathogens like *L. monocytogenes*. It stimulates the strengthening of host barriers via mucus production as well. On the flip side is another bacteroidetes member, *Bacillus fragilis* (sometimes called *B. frag*), that harbors virulence factors. *B. fragilis* can secrete proteases that break-down the brush border of the intestinal epithelium. It secretes a toxin, a hallmark of a bacterial pathogen, *B. fragilis* toxin (BFT – a zinc endopeptidase), that cleaves E. cadherin, thereby disrupting the tight junctions between intestinal cells. This may aid *B. fragilis'* spread to the peritoneum from the intestine, where it may form low-oxygen abscesses that can be a source of a serious infection. Indeed, it produces a high-molecular weight polysaccharide capsule that resists complement killing and macrophage phagocytosis. In a sort of paradox, this capsule is also thought to be an antigen that stimulates the production of intestinal T-helper cells, which aids in immunological balance. Here we see the complex role of the microbiome as both helper and hinderance, all dependent on the circumstances involved.

Unlike the bacteroidetes, the **actinobacteria**, for the most part, seem to be beneficial commensals. These Gram-positive, anaerobic bacteria are some of the most important nitrogen fixers of plants and are a prominent part of the soil ecosystem. But their importance to humans has been marked in two main ways. Members of this phylum, especially the streptomyces, make numerous antibiotics that are commonly used to treat infection. It is their ability to stably colonize the gastrointestinal tract within the first few weeks of life that define their most valuable benefit, however. Human breast milk contains many oligosaccharides not naturally digestible by host intestinal cells. A prominent member of the phyla of actinobacteria, that of the genus bifidobacterium (sometimes termed B. fib), can readily digest these human milk sugars, thereby making them more absorbable for the host. B. fib is also one of the main components of yogurt. Its presence in yogurt likely aids in the benefits yogurt imparts to a healthy gut.

Unlike actinobacteria, the third phyla, that of the **proteobacteria**, is dominated by many genera of pathogens. This includes campylobacter, klebsiella, proteus, and escherichia, amongst others. The proteobacteria are Gram-negative facultative anaerobes, but it is their ability to live, actually thrive, aerobically in host blood and tissues that defines them as pathogens. Although a much minor component of the total commensal microbiota, they account for most of the diarrhea-causing and invasive species responsible for food-borne and nosocomial infections. Defined by their ability to acquire resistance to antibiotics and virulence factors through horizontal gene transfer, it is this minority but aggressive part of the microbiota that directly competes with beneficial species. A significant fraction of all the pathogenic mechanisms discussed throughout this volume come directly from this phyla.

The final dominant phyla, the **firmicutes**, are characterized by Gram-positive, anaerobic spore-forming bacteria. Although they are likely the most abundant of all phyla, they are also a mystery, many genera from this class not currently (or with great difficulty) being able to be cultured in the laboratory. They comprise serious pathogens, including the genus clostridia, the cause of severe colon infections, as well as clearly beneficial microbes, such as the genus blautia, which is associated with efficient nutrient absorption, the suppression of virulence factors from diarrhea-causing bacteria, and reduced autoimmunity. Interestingly, the relationship of the firmicutes to bacteroidetes may define susceptibility to obesity.

13.5   Concepts in Causation

Dysbiosis is the basis for infections or inflammatory diseases that originate within the microbiome. Regardless of the composition of the community, there *is* an underlying culprit or cause (or more than one, actually) of the imbalance. There is a tendency to not consider these dysbiotic states as infections … but there are similarities; one or more not-so-friendly bacteria have taken ahold of the community and their metabolism or lifestyle is in conflict with the healthy more balanced state of the host. Here we explore the idea of causation in this context.

13.5.1   Direct Causation

Along these lines, we can now classify infections that arise from within microbiota in two main ways. A **direct infection** is one by which a resident of the microbiome itself directly causes the disease or a pathologic condition. We can view this as consistent with Koch's traditional way of thinking about bacterial pathogenesis. The symptoms or clinical manifestation is the direct result of the virulence properties (toxins, adhesins, etc) made by the member of

the microbiota itself, often a single species. Sometimes, the problematic species colonizes the host, and its long-term presence becomes an issue when conditions are favorable to its expansion. These are often, in the traditional sense, what microbe hunters term **opportunist infections**, or, if the organism is a member of the normal resident microbiome but in lower abundance, a **pathobiont**. They are an opportunist because they take advantage of a compromised state of the host, often lying in waiting, until the host is susceptible, and then strike. They are a pathobiont because although a normal resident of the microbiota, they have the potential to be virulent, which, by definition, stems from factors encoded in their genome. The opportunist pathobiont will typically follow a *two-hit rule* for the host. Hit number one is they must first have the capacity to produce bonafide virulence factors. Hit number two is that the host itself must have an insult or be compromised in some way that opens the door for the pathobiont to take hold (🔲 Fig. 13.3). Depending on how one looks at these two conditions, they can be reversed, but they are both required. The number one risk factor for hit two is a compromised immune system. A compromised immune system is common for dozens of medical conditions, including HIV infection, chemotherapy, transplant, and diabetes and alcoholism. Thus, it is of no surprise that the predominant infections in the developed world are not from bacteria that arise from outside the host, as they have been for most of human history. As civil engineering has improved our living conditions (cleaner water and food for example), the infections of today stem mostly from organisms that live in an on us. They have the capacity to cause disease because of the make-up of their genome, but generally don't unless medical science extends the lifespan beyond what would be considered natural. Because our species will continue to push our lifespan upwards with improvements in technology and medicine, the paradigm of bacterial infections in the future will originate more from those in and less from those out.

One facet of the opportunist pathobiont that is important for disease and inflammation is that this organism will sometimes breach deep into the mucosal and epithelial layers and directly engage the immune system. On the skin, this may involve a normal inhabitant such as *Staphylococcus aureus*, penetrating to the dermis of the skin, causing an abscess, then becoming systemic. In the lungs, it may involve *Streptococcus pneumoniae*, which can live in the upper respiratory tract but invade the deep alveoli, which leads to pneumonia and inflammation. In the gastrointestinal and urinary tract, it may involve *Escherichia coli*, which invade the epithelium of these tracts and sometimes enter the blood. All fall in line with the two-hit model; they are inherently virulent but often cause their infection when the host has become compromised in some way, an important risk factor in this regard being immune-incompetence. Direct microbiota infections are often acute. Horizontal gene transfer of viru-

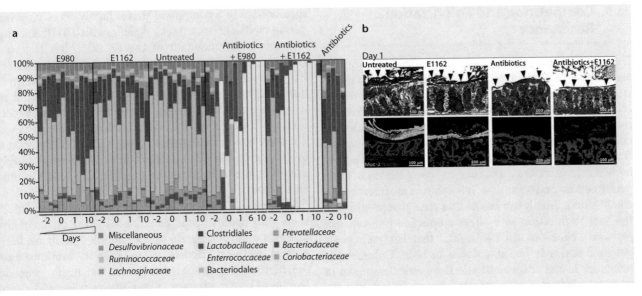

Fig. 13.3 Host "insults" can be powerful stimuli towards destroying the structure of one's microbiome. **a** In this elegant experiment, mice were given either enterococci (*E. faecium*, a growing cause of intestinal and bloodstream infections, using strains E980 or E1162), left untreated, or given enterococci and antibiotics, or antibiotics alone, and the composition of the intestinal microbiome examined. Whereas, antibiotics alone seemed to have dramatic effects on the composition, the combination of antibiotics plus enterococci nearly completely shifted the composition to the invading pathogen. **b** In this panel, we observe that antibiotic treatment completely abrogates the protective mucus barrier (green) that lies between the microbiome and the intestinal epithelial cells (red). Green = anti-muc2 antibody, Red = epithelial cell nuclei. The top panel is a periodic acid-Schiff stain, the mucus layer being highlighted with black arrows. These results illustrate beautifully two of the important concepts in this chapter, namely, that internal or external insults (here antibiotics) can disturb the normal balance of the intestinal ecosystem and second that once disrupted, the loss of colonization resistance opens the door to the invasion by pathogenic microbes. (Adapted from Hendrickx et al (see *suggested readings*) under a creative commons license. (▶ https://creativecommons.org/licenses/by-nc-sa/3.0))

lence factors and antibiotic resistance cassettes are a common element of these types of opportunists as well. When considered in this context, the microbiome itself is a wellspring of these genomic elements and certainly a reservoir for them.

13.5.2 Everything Else…

The above description is in contrast to what we may term an **indirect infection**. These infections do not follow in line with Koch's traditional model of one-pathogen, one-disease thinking. Here, disease does not necessarily result from the actions of one bacterium, but may be due to the collective actions of an entire community. The two-hit effect is also not necessarily a viable explanation either; the underlying players will not be considered true pathogens in the sense of the word, will often lack what the microbe hunter considers bonafide virulence factors (essentially, everything described in this volume to this point), and a compromised immune system or other host insult need not be a trigger for the disease. These infections (if you can call them that), and the clinical manifestation of them, are often chronic, perhaps taking years for the disease, or even a lifetime, to manifest. In the gastrointestinal tract, it may involve a member of the proteobacteria con-

stantly testing the barrier function of the intestinal epithelium, producing low-level invasion that manifests in a type of colitis; but, its ability to do this may wax and wane with the composition of competing microbes, which themselves may be influenced by one's diet or genetics. It may involve the leaching of highly inflammatory bacterial products, such as LPS, across small but relevant breaches in the barrier into the blood, and its deposition into privileged areas not normally accustomed to such highly reactive molecules, causing systemic inflammation that results in arthritis or autoimmunity; but, perhaps the LPS is released in the first place because competing microbes release bacteriocins that kill the bacteria, or a colonizing strain stimulates antimicrobial peptide production that causes the same effect. It may result in the preferential use of one type or none at all (or convert one to the other) of a carbohydrate or fatty acid in the diet, and thus greater adsorption of these calories by the gut epithelium, which trends one towards a more obese rather than lean state, or diabetic or not. None of these effects can be distilled to a simple bacterial toxin or effect (at least to this point); instead, they are the result of a state of bacterial being, often as a community, with host and environmental input, that leads to long-term changes that contribute to chronic human diseases.

13.6   Competition and Colonization Resistance

Direct infection with opportunistic microbiota centers around two prominent factors. One is the ability to gain a stronghold amongst competition with all other commensals, and the second is its correlation with a break-down of the host's immune system. The first is referred to as loss of **colonization resistance**. Colonization resistance is the idea that bonafide pathogens cannot readily colonize areas of the body that have a vibrant and balanced composition of competing commensal organisms. It is a shift in the microbiome composition, usually to a less diverse state, that predisposes the host to infection with either a bonafide non-resident pathogen, or a resident commensal that has pathogenic potential and is in low abundance, or both. Colonization resistance is one of the most effective measures known to prevent an infection, with reports for some enteric invasive species being reduced by factorial 10^5. Often, the commensal population possess a higher level of fitness for the host niche than the incoming pathogen and thus prevents the pathogen from colonizing that niche. The commensal or community may display colonization resistance by several mechanisms. This includes competition for nutrients (prevents growth), competition for host receptors on mucus or cells (prevents attachment), metabolic exclusion (production of fatty acids by some bacteria inhibits the expression of virulence, for example), stimulation of the immune system, strengthening of barriers (inhibits translocation), and direct attack (kills bacteria, such as through the secretion of bacteriocins or use of a type 6 secretion system – see ► Chap. 9).

For the pathogen to gain a stronghold amongst this commensal backdrop, a powerful ecological insult must occur that shifts the composition of the community. In what may be one of the most egregious ironies in modern medicine, the classic example of a loss of colonization resistance is what happens when antibiotics are prescribed. Antibiotics are not specific for one species or even genera of bacteria; instead, they act as broadly sweeping antibacterial agents that can substantially wipe out or suppress major members of the intestinal community. In animal models, some antibiotic treatments reduce the bacterial numbers by as much as six orders of magnitude, used in this context to experimentally "sterilize" the GI tract of resident microbes. In humans, antibiotic treatment is often associated with the onset of diarrhea as a nasty side-effect. The diarrhea stems from the elimination of colonization resistance via the death of protective commensals and the establishment of pathogenic species. This is most evident in the rise of *Clostridium difficile* infections over the past 20 years to an unprecedented level. The antibiotic clindamycin, used to treat various bacterial infections, is metabolized to a compound that is highly effective at targeting intestinal bacteria. *C. difficile*, which itself is a normal low-level inhabitant of the GI tract, but is also a common contaminant of health-care settings, can establish very robust and deadly infections after suppression of native commensals. Here, the very treatment meant to destroy a bacterial pathogen is seen to open an ecological niche to another via the loss of colonization resistance. There are tens of thousands of serious *C. difficile* infection every year in the U.S. alone, an infection almost entirely caused by the widespread use of antibiotics in the health-care setting.

The second external factor important in direct infections with opportunistic pathobionts is the status of the host's immune system. An intact immune system can keep even skilled opportunists at bay. **Primary immunologic deficiencies** are those encoded in the host's genome. Dozens of known primary immunodeficiencies are known. They can be quite severe, including the inability to make functional antibodies, produce T-cells, or macrophages that are compromised for respiratory burst, or a defect in one of the many reactions that lead to an effective complement response. But there are also less catastrophic deficiencies that predispose to infection. Often, the host can compensate with other mechanisms. This includes deficiencies in toll-like signaling, cytokine production, the expression of certain receptors or carbohydrates that favor the binding or invasion of certain pathogens, or the inability to sequester key metals or other nutrients in blood and tissues.

Secondary immunologic deficiencies are not inherently encoded by the host genome; instead, they are induced by dozens of external factors that negatively impact the immune system. Some include trauma, bone marrow transplant, HIV infection, immunosuppressive drugs such as those used for chemotherapy to treat cancer or steroids for pain and inflammation, aging itself, poor nutritional health, and even previous infection. Many opportunists harboring virulence factors are constantly testing the waters, engaged in low-level skirmishes with the immune system that is by far mostly a losing effort from the standpoint of the pathogen. Sometimes though the pathogen wins. A good example is chemotherapy, used in the treatment of cancer. Most chemotherapeutic drugs target rapidly dividing cells including those of hemapoetic origin and, in doing so, reduce the circulating levels of neutrophils substantially (termed neutropenia). Although transient, this period of time is of great concern for physicians treating their cancer patients. Here is where the opportunist is most concerning. If mucosal barriers do not hold up and bacteria get past the many innate systems, the first-responders such as neutrophils may not be at sufficient levels to keep bacteria in check.

13.7 Trisection: The Bacteria, the Host Metabolism, and Immunological Tolerance

When it comes to the microbiome, only a few stones have been over-turned. Emerging from what we do know to this point is that there are two main alterations of host physiology that predisposes the host to changes in health. These two microbiota-induced effects are on host metabolism and host inflammation. Here, there is a clear relationship to human health; even some underlying molecular mechanisms are emerging. Unlike direct microbiota infections, the pathophysiology of these effects involve entire communities. The interactions are more dynamic, and the effects more global and lasting.

13.7.1 Gatekeepers

How can the microbiota effect your metabolism? Well, it persists as gatekeeper, in a way, to the one organ that controls what enters your metabolic pathways. The only way for a human being to naturally acquire exogenous amino acids, lipids, sugars, metals, and other bioactive compounds is through absorption by the digestive tract. Food is ingested, broken down in any of half a dozen different ways as it makes its way through the gastrointestinal tract, and then adsorbed by receptors on the intestinal epithelium. However, before those nutrients even gain access to your hungry cells, they first interact with the complex bacterial microbiota. This means that if these bacteria ingest, metabolize, or otherwise modify these resources before they even have a chance to be seen by host cells, one would expect the composition and bioactivity of the microbiota can alter what the host has access to. "You are what you eat" really is "you are what your microbiota allow you to eat", in some twisted and sometimes sinister ways.

No more is this prevalent than in experiments in obese and lean mice and humans. In obese animals, the overall level of bacteroidetes is low but the phylum of firmicutes is high. If obese animals are given bacteroidetes, they lose weight. If mice with no intestinal microbiota are given any bacteria at all, they gain weight. These trends hold true for obese and lean people that have also been sampled, and, at least in animal model systems, it seems to be inheritable in that the trends follow the species you acquire. The microbiota can affect your ability to access energy from what you ingest. Some complex carbohydrates you eat are only degraded by glycosidases (enzymes that break down sugars) produced by your intestinal bacteria. These sugars can be further fermented by bacteria to short chain fatty acids which are readily absorbed by the intestinal enterocytes and transported to the liver. The body's natural response is to turn these fatty acids into triglycerides that can be stored. At the same time, bacteria in the intestine can down regulate host proteins that activate the action of lipases in adipose tissue. It becomes simple arithmetic at this point. With sugars put in a form by bacteria that can be converted to stored energy (fat), while also being actively suppressed to not use this stored energy, the only way is up (in weight). Obesity is a risk factor for almost every major chronic disease known. Given this logic stream, is it justifiable to call bacterial glycosidases virulence factors? Enteroendocrine cells of the intestine make and secrete the hormones glucagon-like peptides (GLPs). GLPs stimulate the release of insulin which then helps to control the levels of blood glucose. Several bacteria are known to prevent the release of GLPs, or degrade them outright, raising intriguing questions about their role in the pathophysiology of diabetes. Would a vaccine that neutralized the actions of bacterial glycosidases or GLP inhibition protect people from diabetes? These are some of the challenges the next-gen microbe hunter will ponder.

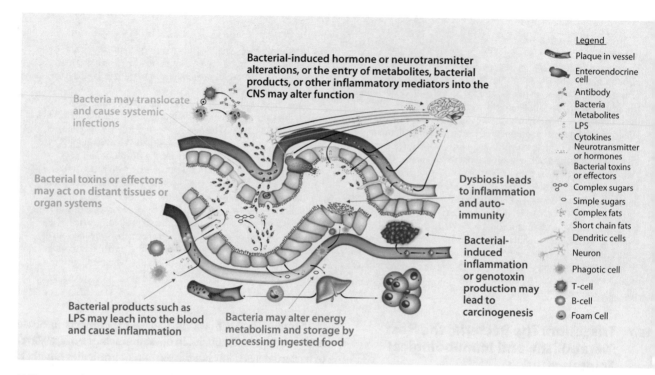

Fig. 13.4   The mucosal bacterial biome and human health

13.7.2 Goldilocks

The second main way the intestinal microbiota contributes to indirect infections, and poor human health, is via its contribution to **immunological imbalance**. The human immune system is a living double-edged sword. The leading edge is used to slice through would be invaders. The back edge, however, can cut the host in the process. With the immune system, it is all about tolerance and balance, a topic we visited in ▶ Chap. 5. Immunological imbalance refers to a diseased state that manifests when the immune response is too heavy or too light. Too much immune system and you have damaging inflammation; the invader is killed but so is the host. Too little and the invader will overtake the host. At mucosal surfaces, this concept is in full effect. Any mucosal surface where there are bacteria presents a tough challenge for the host immune system. When immunological imbalance combines with the virulent properties of would be pathobionts, the result is disease. It differs from a classic direct infection in that the outcome is not binary. Usually, a type of middle ground is reached, and in this middle ground neither is the pathogen cleared nor the inflammation reduced.

To illustrate this point, we can consider localized versus systemic pathologic consequences. A localized immunological imbalance that leads to disease-causing inflammation is illustrated beautifully by the collection of ailments referred to as inflammatory bowel disease, or IBD. IBD encompasses the well-known diseases such as ulcerative colitis and Crohn's, both of which have seen a dramatic rise in incidence over the last 50 years. The etiologic cause and molecular mechanism of these diseases are not known. But what is known is that all three major components (the microbiota, the genetics of the host, and the state of the environment) come together in an undefined way to produce the disease. Since the microbiota is involved, IBD probably should be considered a chronic infection, just not the way we typically think about it. There is a constant give and take between host and microbiota, perhaps partially driven by environmental factors such as the diet, that determines whether the inflammation is high or low and acute versus chronic. Some ways in which bacteria at mucosal surfaces can affect human health are shown in ▢ Fig. 13.4.

13.8 Microbiota Barrier Function

All mucosal surfaces create a barrier to pathogens. They are a barrier to the diffusion of toxic molecules as well. In the intestinal tract, diffusion through the barrier of small molecules that the host needs is highly regulated. The cells lining the barrier may directly take in the molecule, termed **transcytosis**. This is highly specific and usually a receptor on the apical surface lining the lumen recognizes the molecule. The molecule may also go between cells, a **paracellular** route, as we learned for bacteria in our discussion of invasion (▶ Chap. 8). In addition to much desired small molecules like nutrients, bacterial antigens and even virulence factors may be transported and thus brought into close context with the immune system, or worse, may enter the systemic circulation where they can end up almost anywhere in the body. The paracellular route is controlled by the status of the proteins in the tight and adheren's junctions between two adjacent cells. You may recall from our earlier discussion that these functional complexes prevent bacteria and their products from squeezing through. Both the size and charge of small molecules dictate the rates of passage. Molecules selected based on size and not charge may enter systemic circulation via the **leak pathway**. Large solutes and proteins including lipopolysaccharide (but generally not bacteria) can transverse the barrier by this pathway. The converse to this is transport via the **pore pathway**, which typically is more selective and can be biased by the charge of the molecule. The leak and pore pathways, and the underlying biochemistry and cell biology that govern their function, are likely major contributors to any systemic effects the microbiome or its products have on host physiology.

There is also experimental evidence that suggests if the levels and activation state of the junctional complexes are altered, barrier integrity is compromised. If the junctional complexes through either the leak or pore pathway are compromised, microbiota products and antigens may leach through the barrier and into the lamina propria. If too much product leaks or if the products are highly immunogenic, antigen presenting cells may engulf this material and engage immunoregulatory helper T-cells that have previously seen these antigens, thus becoming activated. The T-cells release proinflammatory cytokines, including interferon gamma and tumor necrosis factor (TNF), which can directly act on the epithelial cells of the mucosal surface. For example, TNF, upon binding to the epithelial cell surface, activates an intracellular kinase termed myosin light chain kinase (MLCK). Kinases are known to transmit signals to other proteins via their ability to transfer phosphate – the process called phosphorylation. Once TNF activates MLCK, the kinase can phosphorylate proteins that reside in the cytoplasmic side of the junctional complexes. In this case, the signal results in a rearrangement of the junctional structure to be less tight or restricting. There is a very good reason for this. A lose junction will allow underlying effector cells of the immune system to squeeze between the epithelial cells and enter the lumenal space to engage what they perceive as an invader. This is a normal response meant to defend against bacterial invasion. It is easy to imagine if there is too much antigen getting across how the response can be overblown, thereby allowing junctional complexes to be so open they allow even more antigens of the microbiota to cross – a potentially vicious cycle. We learned in previous chapters of pathogen associated molecular patterns or PAMPs. These highly recognized and immunogenic antigens are inducers of the immune response. If the host itself has an underlying defect in barrier function so that its barrier is more leaky, or has mutations in innate immune recognition molecules that are more sensitive to bacterial antigen, we see how even a slight change in the microbiota to a higher level can result in constant inflammation without ever leading to invasive disease.

There can be homeostasis as well. Some antigens of the microbiota induce the activation of regulatory T-cells. These regulatory cells secrete a different set of cytokines and these cytokines (for example, interleukin 10), turn down the activity of T-cells. Such signals also promote the tightening of junctional complexes, thereby restricting antigen flux which reduces the net amount of the inflammatory signal that enters the lamina propia. Unlike the situation where there is excessive inflammation, here the microbiota counters the effect of the pathobionts, promoting a more immunologically balanced state that does not manifest in inflammation or disease.

13.9 Some Useful Tools of the Microbiomist

The emergence of the study of our body's microbial inhabitants has generated (and required) an all new set of molecular approaches that differ considerably from the more traditional approaches to understanding pathogenesis of the past. The Human Microbiome Project, initiated about 2010, was concerned with the composition of the community – *i.e.* what was on and in our bodies? In the 1970s, the evolutionary biologist Carl Woese described the use of classifying bacteria by the sequence of the bacterial **16s rRNA gene**. This gene changes only slowly over time due to its highly conserved function in DNA protein translation. As such, it represents a kind of molecular clock – the more changes between two bacterial cells, read as mutations in the DNA code, the more likely they have diverged through time from each other. Woese's work with 16s rRNA would eventually allow for the classification of an entirely new kingdom of life, the Archaea, but more recently it has become the keystone method behind the taxonomic classification inherent in the microbiome project. The term applied to such an approach is **phylogenetics**, and classification of a taxa by 16s sequencing is the staple method of determining the composition of our microbiome. The 16s sequence refers to an **amplicon**, that is, a marker gene by which all other comparisons are made in order to place a species in a genus. Since many of the species of microbes that live in and on us are uncultivatable (not able to be grown using traditional broth or plate culture methods) or grow poorly, the use of the sequence of the 16s rRNA amplicon has provided great resolution into the diverse number of different species that actually encompass the microbiome. Sequences that differ by more than 3% are considered a unique **operational taxonomic unit** (or OTU), which, for all practical purposes, means that are likely a different species. To this point, the number and diversity of OTUs in a sample is a quantifiable parameter.

This leads us to one of the more important matters when considering the relationship between the microbiome and human health. As the number of OTUs goes down, so generally does the diversity of the number of species in the sample. A shift in the microbiome to a less diverse state is dysbiosis, as discussed above. A healthy state is one in which the diversity of bacteria, or number of OTUs, is higher. Since diversity is related to the depth of sequencing (*i.e.* some rare microbes may not be represented as well as abundant species and thus may have low to no reads when samples are sequenced), plots of diversity versus the depth of sequencing, termed a **rarefraction curve**, is currently a popular method for determining how "dysbiotic" a sample is from the "healthy" or normal control. Often, for more complex comparisons, a principal **component analysis**, or PCA, may be used. Although not originating from microbiome research, a PCA comparison has become a popular way to mathematically compare a significant number of potentially linked variables into smaller component variables (often two) that are plotted against each other on an X-Y coordinate plane. The spatial distribution of the data can often give clues as to how "related" each individual sample is to the rest of the sample pool or points. In microbiome studies, the presence or absence of taxa may be represented by their spatial distribution under a set of experimental conditions. It allows the investigator to make general conclusions about how large complex data sets cluster as variables change.

Quantitative measures aside, there have also been some stand-out model organisms that have emerged from microbiome studies. The foremost of these, really, is the human being. Unlike many other diseases, whereby to model them invasive procedures or infections are required, this is not necessarily true for microbiome studies. Sampling of the nasal, skin, urogenital, ocular, and even intestinal microbiome is, for the most part, straightforward and of little risk to the subject. Although there are certainly differences between actual intestinal communities and the composition of bacteria in fecal samples (from which most studies are derived), the fecal sample is accepted as generally representative of the state of the digestive biome. When findings in humans need to be more mechanistically verified, the mouse is the turn-to animal. In particular, two versions have been generated, each with unique features that aid in addressing the questions posed. The first is the common use of the **gnotobiotic** or "germ-free" mouse. In this model, pups are reared in specialized sterile environments which prevent their colonization by microorganisms. When the absolute composition of the GI microbiome needs to be controlled, or say the sufficiency of one species needs to be validated for some molecular process or disease linked to that species, using germ-free mice gives the investigator the reductionist tool needed to simplify the experimentation. A second murine model, pioneered by Microbiologist Jeffrey Gordon, includes replacing the murine intestinal microbiome with a human one (at least, as much as one can reasonably do so). This "humanized microbiome mouse" gives the investigator more leverage in testing and generating conclusions that are more physiologically aligned with the human state.

Other models that have been proposed or accepted in bacteriologic research have also gained steam as useful for microbiome studies. This includes the nematode *C. elegans*, which feeds on bacteria, has a simple digestive tract, and is amenable to RNA knockdown techniques (a hallmark of this model in general). The zebrafish too has also been adapted for microbiome research. Their translucent composition is amenable to fluorescence microscopy and bacterial tracking. Three-dimensional human organotypic cultures, first discussed in ▶ Chap. 2, are finding their way into microbiome use, largely due to the fact they are derived from human samples and enclosed. All of these systems have value in different contexts and for the specific research being proposed.

As is true for most experimental systems, the model is only as good as the question being asked.

The microbe hunter faces unprecedented challenges in deciphering the molecular mechanisms by which problematic human biomes contribute to disease. These include the fact that it is a community, as well as that the host metabolism and immune system are usually intertwined in the equation. As the tools to answer the questions become more sophisticated, and the models used approach the human condition, the knowledge of how bacteria behave still has its place and can be of great value.

Summary of Key Points

1. Our bodies are the vessel for a complex ecosystem of bacteria, both in and on us, which contribute to human health either directly or indirectly. This realization, although known for more than a 100 years, has recently captured more attention due to advances in the detection, classification, and analysis of bacterial communities.

2. Species of the biome have been linked to numerous chronic diseases which traditionally have not been thought of as having bacteria as a contributing etiology. This includes obesity, cardiovascular disease, brain function, inflammation (especially in the intestine), and cancer.

3. Specific associations of these diseases with altered states of the microbiome or the presence of one or more species is common. The molecular underpinnings, for the most part, are still to be worked out.

4. The intestinal tract is home to hundreds of species of bacteria, the colon being the most significant reservoir. As such, prominent interactions of bacteria with nutrition and metabolism, as well as the immune system, are expected and even common.

5. The link between intestinal bacteria and health opens the gates for new models of therapeutic modulation using approaches that effect the composition or behavior of bacteria in this environment, including the use of other bacteria (probiotics).

6. Microbiome studies have adapted the use of various statistical methods and other molecular approaches to quantify associations in several key model systems whose technical manipulation allows such studies more feasibility.

❓ Expand Your Knowledge

1. You work for the World Health Organization and are collaborating with the Indian government on a large-scale oral vaccination program to protect children under 5 years of age against rotavirus, a significant cause of childhood diarrhea and malnourishment. You note that sometimes neighboring villages demonstrate gross differences in vaccine efficacy, despite the close geographic

proximity of the villages and intermarriage. Of note, however, is their social traditions which lead to vast differences in their diets, one village being strictly vegan and the other with no limitation in their food choices. Form a hypothesis that may account for their different levels of protection against rotavirus and use some of the techniques and concepts discussed in this chapter to write an experimental plan as to how you will test this hypothesis.

2. As a physician-scientist investigating the etiological cause of stroke, you are examining by histology the molecular integrity of the endothelium (cells lining the walls of arteries) of the brains of deceased stroke patients. When staining 1 day for endothelial antigens, you accidentally use a primary antibody of one of your colleagues who was studying LPS levels in intestinal tissue. To your surprise, the brain samples show distinct patterns of LPS localization around areas of vessel pathology, including a large influx of microglia (brain macrophages) at these sites. Intrigued, you also observe the presence of two notable bacterial toxins, hemolysin and cytotoxic necrotizing factor 1 (CNF1), but no evidence of live bacteria or even bacterial cells. Form a hypothesis as to the etiological origin of stroke in these patients.

3. Read the landmark paper on the Human Microbiome Project ("Structure, function and diversity of the healthy human microbiome", *Nature*, June 2012). Identify four genera present in the human microbiome for which you know little about. Write one paragraph each about prominent bacterial species from each genus covering topics such as its metabolism, cell structure, and associations with any diseases or other microbiologic processes.

Suggested Reading

Anders HJ, Andersen K, Stecher B (2013) The intestinal microbiota, a leaky gut, and abnormal immunity in kidney disease. Kidney Int 83:1010–1016. https://doi.org/10.1038/ki.2012.440

Claesson MJ, Clooney AG, O'Toole PW (2017) A clinician's guide to microbiome analysis. Nat Rev Gastroenterol Hepatol 14:585–595. https://doi.org/10.1038/nrgastro.2017.97

Hendrickx AP et al (2015) Antibiotic-driven dysbiosis mediates intraluminal agglutination and alternative segregation of Enterococcus faecium from the intestinal epithelium. MBio 6:e01346–e01315. https://doi.org/10.1128/mBio.01346-15

Hollister EB, Gao C, Versalovic J (2014) Compositional and functional features of the gastrointestinal microbiome and their effects on human health. Gastroenterology 146:1449–1458. https://doi.org/10.1053/j.gastro.2014.01.052

Kuczynski J et al (2011) Experimental and analytical tools for studying the human microbiome. Nat Rev Genet 13:47–58. https://doi.org/10.1038/nrg3129

Lawley TD, Walker AW (2013) Intestinal colonization resistance. Immunology 138:1–11. https://doi.org/10.1111/j.1365-2567.2012.03616.x

Manichanh C, Borruel N, Casellas F, Guarner F (2012) The gut microbiota in IBD. Nat Rev Gastroenterol Hepatol 9:599–608. https://doi.org/10.1038/nrgastro.2012.152

Marchesi J (2014). The human microbiota and microbiome. Advances in molecular and cellular microbiology. United Kingdom, CAB International. 208

Tuddenham S, Sears CL (2015) The intestinal microbiome and health. Curr Opin Infect Dis 28:464–470. https://doi.org/10.1097/QCO.0000000000000196

Turnbaugh PJ et al (2006) An obesity-associated gut microbiome with increased capacity for energy harvest. Nature 444:1027–1031. https://doi.org/10.1038/nature05414

Turner JR (2009) Intestinal mucosal barrier function in health and disease. Nat Rev Immunol 9:799–809. https://doi.org/10.1038/nri2653

Wexler HM (2007) Bacteroides: the good, the bad, and the nitty-gritty. Clin Microbiol Rev 20:593–621. https://doi.org/10.1128/CMR.00008-07

Note

1 = Probiotic means "for life." This contrasts with "against life" encountered with the term antibiotic. So whereas antibiotics kill bacteria, probiotics mean that bacteria are good for you ("for" biotics). Indeed, many bacteria are important for a healthy body, leading to the formation of an entire 5 billion dollar industry around their sale, addition to yogurt, and consumption. The science behind many of the claims of the virtues of probiotics is murky. In many cases, what is advertised for a probiotic is often inaccurate, or worse, not what is claimed. Only rigorous science will prove or disprove the virtues of these many probiotic strains and combinations as preventative of certain diseases.

Sepsis

© Springer Nature Switzerland AG 2019
A. W. Maresso, *Bacterial Virulence*, https://doi.org/10.1007/978-3-030-20464-8_14

Learning Goals

In this chapter, much of what was learned in the volume to this point will be used to paint a picture of an invading pathogenic bacterium breaking all host defenses, and going systemic. The consequences of this process can be catastrophic for patients, resulting in a complex but highly deadly condition termed sepsis. The disease is framed as an underlying self-perpetuating cycle of immune stimulation and infection, followed by collapse of basic barriers and physiology. The ways in which bacteria, or their products, disseminate are discussed, as are the host or bacterial conditions that promote this dissemination. The learner will become well versed in the holism of the dynamic arrangement of the disease while being able to apply basic concepts from earlier chapters that attest to the underlying mechanisms at play.

14.1   Introduction

» Thane sall thai pass away in haist
   When that thai find na thing but waist

Scottish strategy of defense and desperation against English occupation.

Your amazing self successfully resists countless attacks over your lifetime. No doubt thousands of attempts go unnoticed; every cut, every meal, even every breathe brings danger. The invisible are present but you scarcely notice. They either wither at the impenetrable wall, are ensnarled by mucus traps, or are engulfed and digested by the body's elite units. You move on, working, loving, and living your life without even a hint of most of these microbial assaults. The ones that do escalate to full scale battle may knock you down a bit, confine you to a bed and general malaise, but the duration is short. You recover, vibrantly.

It took eons upon eons to make the almost perfect fortress that preserves the chemistry and biology that propels your living self.

Almost perfect.

When the barriers are breached, the sentinels blinded, and the warriors absent, a common occurrence in the immunocompromised patient, or those in long-term critical care, or even the healthy that may being living without a key immune factor, the final stage in the bacterial invasion strategy is to globalize. Having planted the flag at the initial site of infection, bacteria seek to expand to other areas of the body. For the host, these areas are critically important. For the bacterium, they represent new areas of colonization and growth. The mucosal surface is accustomed to mortar and fire; like a demilitarized zone between two long-standing warring nations, there are casualties here. It seems a part of daily life. Inflammation is common. Our bodies trade this danger for tubular access to the outside world. Tubes take in energy and they dispel wastes, and both are necessary for higher-order organisms.

But bacteria are not supposed to be in the liver. They are not to intrude on the brain's domain either. When they move past the mucosal surface deeper into the tissue, they encounter the circulation. Bacteria ride the systemic circulation like a subway to Eden. They find capillaries which widen to arterioles which become vessels and are carried to new pastures. Eventually, the reverse process ensues – vessel to arteriole to capillary – until they touch individual organ cells or the surrounding extracellular matrix far from where their journey began. During the transit, they may reprogram their gene expression. The challenges in the blood are different than those at the mucosal surface. Here, they contend with complement that destroys their membranes. They contend with greater levels of phagocytes that can eat them outright. Bacteria produce a capsule to resist the complement, or secrete toxins to disarm the phagocytes. The nutrient sources change as well. A low iron state induces the regulators of virulence to make new transporters to scavenge what little resources are available. High-affinity receptors are placed at the surface, sucking up nutrients. Siderophores are secreted to lock down essential metals. Stress response proteins ward off free radicals and changes in osmolarity. Bacteria are in full combat. At their call now are the many powerful strategies described throughout this text. The vascular subway brings them to new tissues, and new tissues bring new opportunities and challenges. More adhesins may be synthesized to ensure the bacterium binds to a particular organ. Organ or new tissue colonization brings more nutrients; growth may accelerate. The genes for biofilm formation may turn on, leading to a fortified microcolony, maybe even a biofilm. New bacteria break-off these garrisons and enter the subway; they deposit in another organ, the process repeats. In just a few hours these new niches become saturated but their division does not. What phagocytes there are act with courage. They circulate to the site and take in as many as the bacterial cells as they can. The bacteria may resist engulfment or prevent lysosomal maturation using secretion systems and other effectors to de-arm these processes. More bacteria brings more secreted toxins, their concentration growing. Now, phagocytes at very distant sites become casualties, the blood consumed by floating land mines that bring death inside of life. The rate of division begins to exceed what can be killed by the immune system. The toxins hit bystander cells in other tissues and organs. The host cells implode, or explode, releasing molecules that drive inflammation to even higher levels.

Soon, a much more dire issue arises. Critical host cells, those of organs, begin to feel the effects of war. Whereas before only the mucosal epithelium could withstand the death of a few epithelial cells, the defenses of the cells of the kidneys, liver, heart, and others are not as equipped. They start to lose their metabolic function, working less optimally. In the meantime, the levels of bacterial antigen builds, tripping so many innate wires the host effectively becomes confused. For Gram-negative bacteria, pathogen corpses shed lipopolysaccharide. For Gram-positives, cell wall fragments like techoic acid are released. DNA spills out from the bacterial cytoplasm. Other bacterial antigens – toxins, adhesins, outer membrane vesicles – also flood the blood and tissues. All these PAMPs, factors we discussed in early chapters, are carried throughout the body, binding to their pattern recognition receptors, the tolls and nods. Major rearrangements in host cell physiology occurs and the immune response grows to a maximum. This leads to more collateral damage, seemingly now endless and perpetual, and the cascade amplifies.

With no other option, your body commits to scorched-earth tactics. The breach has left no alternative but to throw everything and anything at the invader. The levels of cytokines and interleukins skyrocket, so do circulating immune cells. Fever and chills ensue and the person begins to feel weak and tired. The all-out assault escalates. Collateral damage, once a top priority to prevent harm to self, becomes the rule rather than the exception. The combination of toxic bacterial products and now toxic host products lay waste to the body's physiologic functions. So much damage results that the blood clotting system can't repair the holes fast enough. Fibrin, the main clotting factor, forms small clots that block small arterioles. This prevents the blood from bathing the cells of critical organs, which in turn leads to a low oxygenation state of the tissues in that organ. These cells slowly begin to asphyxiate, strangulated from within.

The lack of oxygen brings a lack of energy. The kidneys, already damaged from all the toxic compounds being filtered from the blood, lose their purification function. Very little urine is generated, and what urine is made, is bloody, full of floating clots caught in the glomerulus net. The heart loses output, each pump bringing less and less power, its cardiac myocytes losing performance because of death from afar. Blood pressure drops, thereby amplifying the already hypoxic condition in organs. Whole cells now begin to die, starved of the energy to maintain even the most basic of functions. The patient passes into delirium and incoherence, unable to oxygenate the brain. The command center loses executive control, no longer able to regulate the systems of the body. Without leadership, mutiny ensues.

Still, the invaders grow and divide and so do their poisons. Still the host fires its own lands, a last resort for a creature in complete despair. The cycle continues.

This is sepsis.

Only the technology and advancements in modern medicine can save the patient. Antibiotics are given to target the bacterial invader. Fluids are administered and osmotic balance is a priority. A respirator mechanically oxygenates tissues and drugs are given to break and prevents clots. Dialysis supplants kidney function and hormones stimulate cardiac output. In 70% of the cases, these supportive interventions prevail, but it may take weeks to months before the patient can leave the hospital. In 30% of the cases, the bacterium chews and spits out the antibiotics and the body is thrown into multi-organ failure. This patient will not survive, or, if they do, they may be permanently damaged (◘ Fig. 14.1).

14.2 Impact and Risk Factors

There may not be a more underappreciated, and ill-defined, disease of humans than sepsis. Approximately 10% of all intensive care hospitalizations in the U.S. are for sepsis. This totals between 1 and 1.5 million cases per year, according to the Centers for Disease Control. Due to poor reporting, the global incidence is not established but lower estimates have it at no less than 20 million a year. For the roughly one million U.S. residents that endure a stint with sepsis, weeks to months in the hospital will cost an average of 20,000 dollars per person, a total loss of 24 billion a year. This does not include lost wages.

Largely a disease of the chronically ill, sepsis is the result of the unchecked ravage of privileged spaces. Physicians have done a wonderful job classifying the disease based on clinical assessment (◘ Fig. 14.2). We also understand some of the risk-factors for the disease, one being some underlying dysfunction of immunity, another being in an intensive care unit, still another being chronically ill with comorbidities. An immune dysfunction may be completely unknown to the host. A person may be born with a deficiency in the production of a type of immune cell or lack an innate immune response at the mucosal surface; there are dozens of known mutations in immune function and probably that many and more that are unknown. People may also acquire a disease that as part of its pathophysiology leads to immunosuppression. HIV infection and the resulting loss of T-cell function is a good example. These errors or conditions are a weak link in the immunity chain that lead to its eventual failure to fully protect. Systemic infections have an element of stochasticity to them. A seemingly healthy child or adult with an underlying defect in immunity may cut themselves. If a bacterium with just the right composition of virulence factors enters the wound, a deadly infection may result.

That said, a common risk factor is **medical-induced immunodeficiency**. Here, treatment for another condition leads to a reduced ability of the immune system to combat the bacterial invader. Although the term "immunodeficiency" implies that the entire immune system may be lost, it often is not. Some common examples of risk-factors for loss of the complete function of the immune system include chemotherapy (used to treat cancer), bone marrow transplantation, or drug-induced immunosuppression (because of an overactive immune system). Most of the nearly two million cases of cancer in the U.S. every year will result in some form of chemotherapy. Many chemotherapies work by poisoning any cells that divide rapidly, a feature of cancerous cells. Many cell types of the body also divide rapidly as part of their normal cell cycle, including cells of the immune lineage in the bone marrow that give rise to all the mature cells of the immune system. The temporary absence of circulating immune cells, in particular, neutrophils, opens a window of attack by which pathogenic microorganisms can colonize and invade. This period of time is of immense concern for physicians caring for such patients. An important point

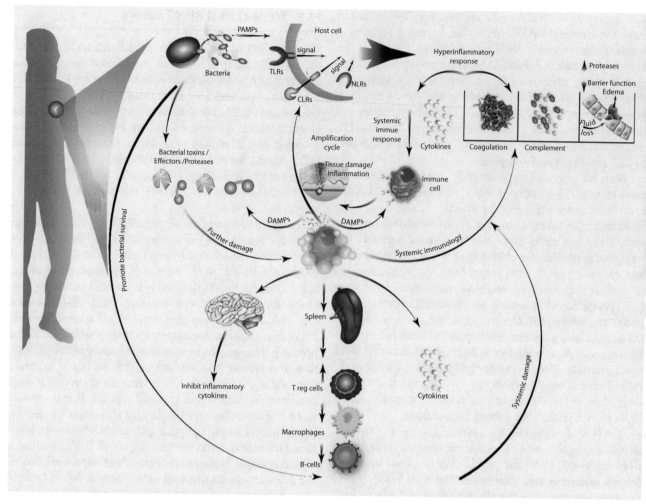

Fig. 14.1 The complexity, and vicious circle, of bacterial sepsis. Sepsis is a complex disease with multiple intersecting pathologies, organ systems, and molecular processes that culminates in a vicious circle with seemingly no beginning or end. Bacterial pathogen associated molecular patterns (PAMPs) are recognized by the host's innate immune system which triggers an inflammatory response. This response can promote coagulation, barrier loss, and excessive immune cell activation that can damage tissues. Damaged tissues in turn release damage associated molecular patterns (DAMPs) that further stimulate the innate immune response and immune cell activation. Concomitantly, bacterial toxins, effectors or other molecules accentuate the release of DAMPs which themselves drive the inflammatory response even higher, leading to more tissue damage. Major organ systems (e.g. the brain) react by down-modulating the immune system, which in turn promotes bacterial survival, which in turn leads to the release of more DAMPs and PAMPs, while other organ systems (e.g. the spleen) continues the development of immune lineages to combat the infection

though is that whereas the circulating special ops warriors may be transiently lost in these cases, the innate immune system is often not. It can still sound the alarm of the invaders and ramp up other inflammatory processes, and these can contribute to the systemic scorched earth tactics that can define sepsis.

Sepsis is also characterized by a wide swath of general symptoms and often unknown point of origin. It rides on the back of other ailments or complications and may be masked by them. There are dozens of symptoms and indications, few of which are exclusive to sepsis, as we see in ☐ Fig. 14.2. A full one-third of all sepsis patients are **culture-negative**; that is, a sample of their blood analyzed using traditional microbiology techniques does not result in the identification of a bacterial species as the invading culprit. It may be the infection is not in the blood or that the species responsible is not able to be cultivated, or that products of the bacteria itself (secreted toxins or LPS from dead bacteria) are inducing the condition. Like an enemy constructed of shadows, no tangible target is identified for treatment. In cases when a bacteria is detected, they commonly include staphylococci from the skin or nares, escherichia, klebsiella, or enterococci from the intestinal tract, and pseudomonas and acinetobactera from the lungs. The infections are often, but not always, drug-resistant. In some cases, antibiotics are not effective, or only the most cytotoxic of antibiotics show some efficacy. These cases rely on **supportive therapy** (hydration, oxygen, dialysis, etc) for survival. There is no cure for sepsis in the sense that one drug eliminates the disease. Hundreds of different "silver bullet" approaches to

General	Inflammatory	Hemodynamic	Organ-dysfunction	Tissue-perfusion
• Fever (>38.3) • Hypothermia (<36) • Heart rate > 90 min^{-1} or 2 SD above normal value for age • Tachypnea • Altered mental status • Significant edema or positive fluid balance (>20 mL/kg over 24 hrs) • Hyperglycemia in absence of diabetes	• Leukocytosis (WBC count > 12,000 μL^{-1}) • Leukopenia (WBC count < 4,000 μL^{-1}) • Normal WBC count with > 10% immature forms • Plasma C-reactive protein (CRP) > 2 SD above normal • Plasma procalcitonin > 2 SD above normal	• Arterial hypotension (SBP < 90 mm Hg, MAP < 70, or an SBP decrease > 40 mm Hg in adults; or < 2 SD below normal for age) • Svo_2 > 70% • Cardiac index > 3.5 L· min^{-1}·M^{-23}	• Arterial hypoxemia (PaO$_2$ / F$_{IO2}$ < 300) • Acute oliguria (urine output < 0.5 mL· kg^{-1}·hr^{-1} or 45 mmol/L for at least 2 hrs) • Creatinine increase > 0.5 mg/dL • Coagulation abnormalities (INT > 1.5 or aPTT > 60 sec) • Ileus (absent bowel sounds) • Thrombocytopenia (platelet count < 100,000 μL^{-1}) • Hyperbilirubinemia (plasma total bilirubin, > 4 mg/dL [68 μmol/L])	• Hyperlactatemia (>1 mmol/L) • Decreased capillary refill or mottling

Fig. 14.2 Criteria for the diagnosis and classification of sepsis. Severe sepsis includes sepsis plus organ dysfunction. Septic shock includes sepsis plus either hypotension refractory to intravenous fluids or hyperlactatemia. (Guidelines are adapted from the work of Ramsay and the International Sepsis Definitions Conference and van der Poll et al. (see *Suggested Readings*))

vaccinate (a prophylaxis) or reduce symptoms of the failing state of the body in clinical trials have not been convincing. Supportive therapy and medical/public education about the symptoms of sepsis have significantly lowered mortality. At the moment, these are the best options for reducing the overall incidence and mortality.

Out of the Box

To this point, these little "box" sessions have been about thinking about the science of the chapter. Here, we are going to change things a bit. Sepsis has been called the "silent killer." It is silent for many reasons but principal amongst them is that the disease gets almost no national attention. Let's consider some facts published by the Sepsis Alliance which are backed by science. Every 2 min, a person dies from sepsis in the U.S. This will lead to about 258,000 per year, more than breast cancer and HIV combined. About 42,000 kids will develop sepsis this year; about 1.6 million people in total in the U.S. Worldwide, it is 26 million. Sepsis is the leading cause of death in those hospitalized. In the U.S. alone, sepsis costs the economy 24 billion dollars a year.

Yet, only about half of all adults have heard of sepsis.

How can this be? Sepsis is a complicated disease. It is hard to diagnose, sometimes the etiology is unclear, and most of all it is the most sick, vulnerable, and elderly that acquire the disease. Yet, science and medicine, often seen as repositories of the truth, also suffers from the same political forces and fads that govern all human activities. There is very little monetary support for the study of sepsis compared to other, more highly profiled diseases. These diseases have powerful political allies lobbying on their behalf. The microbe hunter must also learn that in addition to molecules and toxins and invasion, etc., their challenges include education and awareness and fighting for what is fair and right.

14.3 Stages of Sepsis

Sepsis is defined as a disease of progressive stages. Each stage brings its own challenges. Attempts have been made to define them according to clinical criteria. The **first stage** in sepsis is dominated by symptoms generated by the immune response to an actual or perceived infection. Termed **systemic inflammatory response syndrome** (**SIRS**), symptoms include increased rate of breathing and heart beat with either an elevated or very low temperature and an elevated or very low white blood cell count. If SIRS is present and a blood culture or other tests demonstrate there is an active infection, the diagnosis of sepsis is made. Depending on the level of organ dysfunction that follows, the condition may progress to **severe sepsis** or **septic shock**. Prolonged septic shock can lead to **multi-organ failure**, which is the major cause of death in sepsis patients. ◻ Figure 14.2 lists some of the symptoms of sepsis and septic shock. Although useful, exclusive reliance on these parameters for the construction of a treatment plan should take into account all available diagnostic information since the disease is characterized by its many twists from conformity.

14.4 Source of Sepsis

The general consensus is that sepsis originates with an infection. This makes determining the source of bacterial infection important in the resolution of the disease. It is from this source that the bacteria orchestrate their attack. Although sepsis or bacteremia can arise in theory from any bodily site where bacteria can live or grow, most of the time only a handful of areas are of concern. These include the gastrointestinal, urinary, and respiratory tracts – all mucosal surfaces that are in almost constant contact with microorganisms. It includes the skin, with its ecosystem of colonized bacteria, which is the likely source for sepsis originating from wounds. These include lacerations or punctures but also surgical openings. Finally, in-dwelling devices such as catheters, pacemakers, drive lines or prosthetics can also be point sources of infection. Successful resolution of the disease must include healing or treatment of the source, especially if the individual is immunocompromised, and barrier function must be restored. Of these locations, the lung and/or gastrointestinal tract are considered the most common sources of most sepsis cases. Being both colonized with potentially pathogenic organisms and near to the mucosal/blood interface, these source sites account for most cases.

14.4.1 Mechanisms of Invasion

As we discussed in ▶ Chap. 13, the gastrointestinal tract is colonized by hundreds, perhaps up to a thousand, different species of bacteria. The vast majority of these bacteria are incapable of causing a systemic infection. There are two main reasons for this. First, the blood is an oxygenated environment and many of the intestinal species are anaerobes, the gut being a low-oxygen environment. They simply cannot perform functional metabolic processes in blood and thus do not thrive. Another reason is they are not enriched in the virulence factors needed to scale host defenses and survive the immune onslaught. This includes adhesins to interact with the mucosa, invasins or proteases to break barriers, nutrient acquisition systems to grow rapidly, and toxins and effectors to disable the multi-faceted host response that will seek to destroy them. Those that do possess these factors are often facultative anaerobes; they can be metabolically active in low or high oxygen environments. They also possess the stealth-like quality of existing as residents of the intestinal tract without even a whisper of suspicion or symptom. Such bacteria are often termed **opportunists**, or more recently **pathobionts** – terms used to signify that they have pathogenic potential but such fury only is manifested if correlated with the status and environment of the host.

A host that undergoes chemotherapy may have many of their defenses suppressed. An opportunist, armed with the genetic capacity of virulence, can leverage this terrain to disseminate from the original site of colonization. For all the attention given to bacteria in the intestinal tract, it is quite astounding that only about a dozen or less have any real ability to become systemic and induce sepsis. For those that do, a defining feature as occupants of the intestinal mucosa is somehow being able to move through this barrier. This process is termed **translocation**, whereby the bacterium "translocates" from the intestinal lumen to the blood. The resulting condition is referred to as gut-derived sepsis due to the origin of the infecting bacterium. Translocation can be active, that is, the virulence properties of the bacterium facilitate its movement through the mucosa. This may include the destruction of mucus via the secretion of mucinases, the adherence to the epithelium via adhesins, and either invasion into the host cells (with exit on the reverse side – termed **transcellular or transcytotic translocation**) or movement between cells after destruction of host cell junctions (termed **paracellular translocation**). Alternatively, the bacterium may obliterate the epithelium with toxins, thus generating their own portal for exit. In this case, pathology may be observable as an ulcer or intense inflammation. **Passive translocation**, on the other hand, results from some type of destruction of the host barrier and epithelium, either by trauma or by medical treatment including medication. Chemotherapy, for example, is a medication that can thin the mucus barrier by destroying the rapidly dividing cells of the intestinal epithelium. Surgery or trauma, for instance, may result in ulcers or other perforations in the intestinal wall. These conditions predispose the host to having intestinal pathobionts break out of their luminal niche and gain access to systemic circulation. These mechanisms are summarized in ◻ Fig. 14.3.

Sepsis that originates from the bladder is termed **urosepsis** and, unlike the GI tract, results from an active infection of the urinary system. Urinary tract infections are common in females, accounting for approximately 7–8 million infections per year in the U.S. alone. The most common cause, as is true for **gut-derived sepsis**, is E. coli, followed closely by proteus and klebsiella species. They are also residents of the intestinal tract. It is mainly accepted that these organisms enter via the vagina and ascend to the urethra and eventually the bladder. It is the bladder which then becomes colonized and a source of repeated or reoccurring infections. This is because the bacteria, mainly E. coli, that infect the bladder due so by invading the bladder epithelium. They reside in an inclusion body termed an **intracellular bacterial community** or **IBC** (because it often contains more than one), which itself becomes a kind of protective cocoon that is refractory to antibiotics and detection by the immune system. Here we see another example of bacteria co-opting a strategy to avoid detection and establishing a niche until conditions are favorable for spread. It is not known how bacteria in the bladder access the blood; but their persistent location in the bladder epithelium brings them that much closer to the circulation such that, when

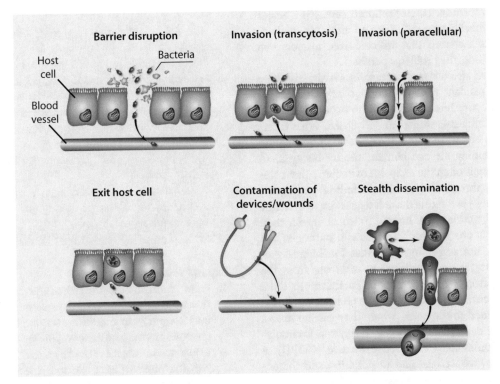

Barrier disruption   **Invasion (transcytosis)**   **Invasion (paracellular)**

Host cell

Bacteria

Blood vessel

Exit host cell   **Contamination of devices/wounds**   **Stealth dissemination**

Fig. 14.3 The ways bacteria cause systemic infections. Infection-induced sepsis is associated with the movement of bacteria, or their products, from a site of localized infection to systemic tissues, blood, and organs. The presence of bacteria at such sites can trigger massive inflammation and, when combined with harmful proteins or molecules that the bacteria produce, overwhelms host physiology and balance

compromised, they likely seed into the arteriole subway and disseminate.

Sepsis can also originate from medical procedures or implanted devices, a type of **device-associated sepsis**. There are two main points of entry or infection in these cases. The first includes the fact that there must be a medically-induced **breach** of the skin and barrier epithelium. This includes surgical openings but also natural openings through which a medical device inserts into the body (a catheter is a great example). Although the physician does their best to make sure the site is sterile, or near sterile, bacteria are everywhere and they cannot be seen. Theoretically, one organism can cause an infection but in reality many are usually needed. Surgical procedures most often proceed through an incision in the skin. The skin is teaming with different bacteria, including pathogenic members of the staphylococci and streptococci. Although the skin is rubbed with an agent that kills bacteria, it is an undulating organ with crevices and oils that can protect bacteria. Some even live below or in the dermis, in glands, which are not accessible to the topical application. Instruments used in the procedure, the surgeon's hands, and even the air itself can bring a founder cell. Often times the weakened state of the patient makes it more difficult for the infection to be contained. If closed and left untreated, the founder may grow to a colony and eventually break free into the blood. In the case of in-dwelling devices, including catheters, pacemakers, drive-lines, or even IVs, the port itself may be the point by which bacteria enter, either through the cannel in the device or at the point in the skin where it is inserted.

The second complicating factor is structure; namely, anything that is foreign that is inserted into the body can either be contaminated, or worse – serve as a structure to attach and breed more pathogenic bacteria. In the case of prosthetics, the technology often replaces an internal human part, such as a joint and thus becomes sealed inside the body. If the prosthetic is not sterile, the bacteria are sealed with it and may permanently infect the site in the absence of treatment. For catheters or lines that continuously enter the body, the device itself may become a site of bacterial attachment. Recall that although bacteria have evolved adhesins to interact with host components, the host counters with strategies that resist adherence, including hiding receptors, sending out soluble decoys, or building a layered mucosa. This is not true for plastics and other materials that make up the devices. They often contain etched or rough surfaces that bacteria readily can bind and in doing so provide a platform by which to grow without all the harmful insults that a host surface may bring. In addition, these devices often have nobs, crevices, or caves that effectively serve as a shelter for the attached bacterium, shielding them from the flow of blood or circulating immune cells. In these medical devices turned Trojan horses the bacteria replicate to the point they can form a biofilm. The biofilm itself generates additional security including being impenetrable to antimicrobial peptides, phagocytes, or antibiotics. The biofilm will also serve as a source of bacterial budding, leaching new founders into the surrounding tissue or worse the circulation. Device-induced sepsis is a major problem in the health-care industry and although we have learned to make materials that are colonized less or even cytotoxic to bacteria, the problems persist.

The lungs are also a source organ for sepsis. The lung does harbor a resident microbiome, but its exact role in defining a true ecosystem with long-term occupiers, unlike the intestine, is still being studied and explored. What is certain is that this organ interfaces with the surrounding air, and the surrounding air can contain deadly bacteria. In addition, the lung is often the recipient of bacteria that colonize our nares, throat, and tonsils, including pathogenic streptococci. These two facets make it a gateway to systemic circulation, and, with a more limited mucosal barrier than the GI tract, it is one in which a successful pathogen can transverse. It is not surprising than that the highest frequency of sepsis cases are believed to originate from the lung, especially from active pneumonia. Furthermore, there is strong evidence that pathobionts in the GI tract can translocate via the blood to the lungs, where they can serve as a source organ for continuous entry into the systemic circulation. Chronic pulmonary obstructive disease (COPD), a disease caused by tobacco use and air pollution and characterized by poor oxygenation of blood and high rates of pneumonia, is a leading killer of people world-wide. People with COPD often can progress to sepsis. Those with COPD can acquire bacterial pneumonia. Cystic fibrosis patients are also substantially colonized by high levels of pathogenic bacteria. For COPD and CF patients, species of klebsiella and pseudomonas are common.

The microbe hunter, aware of these source organs, can use such knowledge to prevent them from being breeding grounds for the wave of dissemination that may follow. Each bacterium in its own way harbors molecular factors that allow it to escape these source barriers, or imbed on a medical device. The understanding of these mechanisms, much of which have been discussed throughout this volume, will lead to preventative or treatment options that limit the emergence of this mysterious, but deadly, disease.

Summary of Key Concepts

1. Sepsis is a complicated human disease often induced by the systemic spread of bacteria but sometimes with unknown etiology.
2. Its main clinical feature is the global breakdown of balance and host physiology (manifested in many ways) and, in the most severe cases, the breakdown of organ function.
3. The molecular hallmark of sepsis is associated with overt immunological imbalance likely driven by bacterial PAMPs and host DAMPs that contribute to a vicious cycle of stimulation and overblown response to a bacteria invader.
4. There are many conditions that are risk-factors for the disease, including being chronically ill with another condition, a suppressed immune system, or the presence of an underlying immunological defect in the host.
5. Bacterial dissemination can begin from several source organs, as well as in-dwelling devices or other medical procedures.

❓ Expand Your Knowledge

1. From your reading of the source environments of the human body that promote the systemic infection of bacteria, and your knowledge acquired from past chapters on bacterial adhesins, design a strategy that would prevent sepsis caused by bacteria from the skin, the intestinal tract, and an in-dwelling device.
2. Read ▶ Chap. 10 on bacterial toxins. Pick two of these toxins and explain how their activity may contribute to the self-perpetuating cycle of host damage outline in ◻ Fig. 14.1.
3. Organize a whiteboard session around a description of a systemic bacterial infection, from start to sepsis. Incorporate knowledge from previous chapters in this description, including those dealing with effectors, secretion systems, and bacterial invasion. Write a 10-question quiz that you can administer to participates after the end of session being sure to touch on the answers to the questions in your demonstration.

Suggested Reading

Angus DC, van der Poll T (2013) Severe sepsis and septic shock. N Engl J Med 369:2063. https://doi.org/10.1056/NEJMc1312359

de Jong HK, van der Poll T, Wiersinga WJ (2010) The systemic pro-inflammatory response in sepsis. J Innate Immun 2:422–430. https://doi.org/10.1159/000316286

Reinhart K, Bauer M, Riedemann NC, Hartog CS (2012) New approaches to sepsis: molecular diagnostics and biomarkers. Clin Microbiol Rev 25:609–634. https://doi.org/10.1128/CMR.00016-12

Stearns-Kurosawa DJ, Osuchowski MF, Valentine C, Kurosawa S, Remick DG (2011) The pathogenesis of sepsis. Annu Rev Pathol 6:19–48. https://doi.org/10.1146/annurev-pathol-011110-130327

Bacterial Vaccines and the Challenges Ahead

© Springer Nature Switzerland AG 2019
A. W. Maresso, *Bacterial Virulence*, https://doi.org/10.1007/978-3-030-20464-8_15

Learning Goals

In this chapter, the learner is introduced to the history of, and process behind, the discovery and making of vaccines against bacterial diseases. This includes the types of formulations that have been constructed and the current guiding principles used to make safe and efficacious vaccines, including the selection and discovery of antigens and the process for their preparation and testing in animal models and people. The text also includes a discussion of approved adjuvants, salient features of current vaccines, and an introduction into the challenges vaccinologists face in the future.

15.1 Introduction and History

15.1.1 *Vaccinae* Triumphant!

Edward Jenner is credited as being the father of modern vaccinology. His inoculation of the 8-year old boy James Phipps in May of 1796 with cowpox as an attempt to protect against human smallpox is recognized as the seminal event in creation of this procedure, probably because it was well documented by a later publication of Jenner. Others, such as the farmer Benjamin Jesty and the English physician John Fewster, were noted to have made similar observations years before Jenner's experiments. Even before this, the practice of variolation, scarring the arm with samples of smallpox from a recently infected individual, was practiced for perhaps centuries before these documented incidents, especially in the Far East. It was a dangerous procedure; a sizable fraction of those variolated would actually contract full-blown disease and die. The practice was outlawed in Europe. In Jenner's time, Germ Theory was still immature. It would take Koch and Pasteur and their mentees to work it out a 100 years later. Jenner's important contribution was the realization that a *related* but less serious cause of a pox-like disease in another host might still retain protection from the primary disease in humans, but without the risk. He inoculated others besides Phipps, and they were also protected. As such, this was the first systematic attempt at assessing this new procedure of "vaccination", and it followed principles that would become standard in medicine.

15.1.2 Make It Scientific

Smallpox is caused by a virus. We have to wait 85 years after this landmark event before there came a controlled study of a bacterial vaccine. Fast-forward from Jenner to a small town outside of Paris and the great French Microbiologist Louis Pasteur. Building off some observations during the vaccination of chickens against the fowl cholera virus (at that time, virus was the general term given to a disease of transmission; the actual pathogen in this case was a bacterium later named *Pasteurella multocida*, in honor of Pasteur). The maestro himself staged a public demonstration of vaccination using sheep. His audacity as a showman is evident in this example.

As bold a scientist as he was, he also knew how to set the stage so he would receive the credit! Twenty five animals received a modified (either killed or partially attenuated) version of *B. anthracis* (the cause of anthrax – at that time, farm animals were often struck dead with this brutal disease) and another twenty five receiving nothing but the inoculation. About a month later, Pasteur infected all the animals with live *B. anthracis*. In a remarkable demonstration of the effectiveness of the procedure, all twenty five vaccinated animals lived. All twenty five not receiving the vaccine died. Here, we see two additional improvements on the concept of vaccination. First, that the modification of the agent to make it less virulent can safeguard recipients from the original disease while also inducing immunity. Second, that the experiment was well controlled. Pasteur vaccinated a test *and* a control group, each with enough animals per group to make the interpretation of the results unambiguous. In reference to Jenner's work, the inoculant was termed by Pasteur "vaccine"; and the process, "vaccination", the word being derived from the name of *Variolae vaccinae* which Jenner ascribed to the cowpox disease.

The scientific community caught on quickly and other vaccine attempts soon followed. In the late 1890s vaccines against the causative agents of the plague, typhoid and cholera, all bacterial diseases, were made and tested. Pasteur, and many of his trainees, travelled the world bringing the results and ideas to academic and medical circles. These were live attenuated or killed preparations. On or about 1908, French Microbiologist Albert Calmette, in charge of a small satellite colony of the Pasteur Institute in Lille France, was struck by the high levels of tuberculosis (*Mycobacterium tuberculosis*) in the city. Accidentally culturing the related *Mycobacterium bovis* on beef extract with his veterinary assistant Camille Guerin, and applying principles established by both Jenner (use a related organism) and Pasteur (repeated culturing to attenuate), they succeeded in establishing an avirulent strain – after more than 13 years of (interrupted) culturing! This strain, known as BCG (bacillus-Calmette-Guerin), is still used today, despite its limited efficacy, as the only vaccine for *M. tuberculosis* widely approved by regulatory agencies. It reduces disease symptoms and prevents mycobacterial dissemination, but immunity is not long-lived and it may not protect against latent disease. More than one billion people have had the BCG vaccine. In 1924, culture supernatants from the cause of diphtheria (*C. diptheriae*), which were known since the early part of the century to contain toxic activity, were treated by the French biologist Gaston Ramon with formaldehyde in an attempt to detoxify the toxic activity but retain its immunogenicity. It worked and protected against lethal diphtheria, thus adding another triumphant scientific advance to the concept of vaccinology; namely, that molecules produced by the organism, if treated to remove the poisonous effect, themselves can be vaccines. To this day, formaldehyde is used as the inactivating agent in the highly effective, safe, and U.S. FDA-approved vaccines against diphtheria. A similar story played out for a vaccine for tetanus (lockjaw, caused by *Clostridium tetani*) and a toxoid inactivated toxin preparation) was made in the late 1920s. In the 1930s, formalin-inactivated pertussis was tested and used, thereby providing protection against *Bordetella pertussis* infection (whooping cough). By this time, basic correlates of immunity, such as whether neutralizing antibodies to toxin activity developed, were in full swing, and animal models were routinely used to assess vaccine efficacy. Scientists could now examine whether vaccines made of just supernatants or mostly toxins could generate immune responses and stop disease. World War II would slow things down in the 1940s but the 50s through the 60s brought improvements in the vaccines to prevent tetanus, pertussis, and diphtheria, often driven by improvements in the preparation and purification of bacterial material used in the formulation. Largely toxigenic diseases (that is, the symptoms of the infection are in part due to a toxin the organism makes), vaccine strategies that use inactivated toxin-containing preparations continue to this day. Nearly everyone in the U.S. is given a vaccine that combines the toxins from these three diseases.

15.1.3 Make Them Different

In the 1970s, it was recognized that toxin-only approaches to vaccination were not universally applicable to all bacteria that cause diseases in humans. Some bacteria do not produce a toxin that is responsible for the symptoms of the disease, or they produce many different types of toxins which can complicate things because one has to pick the right ones in the vaccine formulation. Some of these bacteria colonize our body, often asymptomatically, having adapted to avoiding our immune system. This includes capsulated opportunistic bacteria that may produce dozens of different surface polysaccharide variants that act as an antigenic smokescreen. Thus was born the strategy of making a vaccine from purified capsule variants from the most represented human strains to achieve broad protection against pathogenic serogroups. The result: we now have licensed vaccines against capsulated *Haemophilus influenza*, meningococcus (*Neisseria meningitidis*), and pneumonococcus (*Streptococcus pneumoniae*). Various improvements have been made along the way with the addition of more capsule variants or protein conjugates to drive antibody production. Collectively, these vaccines tackled some of the most dangerous childhood diseases.

Attention could now be turned to other types of infections, especially of more neglected diseases of the developing world, where water and food-borne illness remains a significant cause of childhood mortality. As such, the 1980s and 1990s brought many advances in tackling diseases like cholera (*V. cholerae*) and typhoid (*Salmonella enterica*) with both polysaccharide and toxin vaccines approved for human use. The 1990s brought the application of genomics, and the sequencing of whole organisms, to vaccinology. Now, vaccine targets could be identified by in silico methods to identify surface or secreted virulence factors or antigens that were more frequent in pathogenic strains – so called reverse genetics. Advances in protein expression and purification technologies facilitated the testing of hundreds of different antigens for dozens of different infections in relevant animal models. In addition, efforts continued to improve currently licensed vaccines, especially the conjugated polysaccharide versions, as well as the pre-clinical development of many bacterial species whose vaccine creation had been hard to come by. The story of vaccine success, the vast bulk coming over the past 100 years of human history, is remarkable. Perhaps no other technological intervention, civil engineering and antibiotics aside, has had a greater impact on human health. Conservative estimates have it that an additional 10 years have been added to human life expectancy. Various worldwide health organizations have put the number at more than 1.5 million children saved every year because of vaccination (◘ Fig. 15.1). Still, the challenges ahead are formidable. We discuss the gaps, and how we might fill them, below. In addition, the last decade has brought doubts about the safety and effectiveness of vaccination, and many common infections are still left without a clear path for an approved vaccine.

15.2 The Types of Vaccines

15.2.1 No Stone Unturned

There are three main types of bacterial vaccines. Two types have been approved for human use. They are classified by the composition of the vaccine, that is, what the actual antigen or immunity-inducing component is. The first type is a **cell-based vaccine**. Cell-based vaccines can either be live bacterial cells that are attenuated or bacterial cells that have been killed by either heat or the addition of chemicals. This type of vaccine was common in the first 50 years of bacterial vaccinology. It is still used today but generally there has been a move away from these vaccines as technologies at identifying and isolating antigens have improved. The main advantage of a cell-based vaccine is, frankly, that it contains the bacterium in its entirety as the immunity-inducing component, or **immunogen**. This is how nature intended our body to encounter the pathogen, more or less in its whole form. From this form, many **antigens**, the portion of the pathogen that the body directs the immune response against, are present. As such, both B- and T-cell responses are common with broader immunity; and because the vaccine encompasses the entire bacterial cell, many antigens are also present. This increases the total breadth of antigens the body can develop immunity against. It may also lead to diverse responses generated against the same antigen, thereby making the breadth and specificity **multivalent**. Like a well-balanced stock portfolio, the immune system can distribute its response across many of the antigens present in cell-based formulation. The BCG tuberculosis vaccine is a good example of a cell-based vaccine.

The downside to a cell-based vaccine is several fold. For live formulations, there is the risk that an infection may develop from the vaccine itself. This violates the "do no harm" principle of medicine and generally this risk is the primary

15

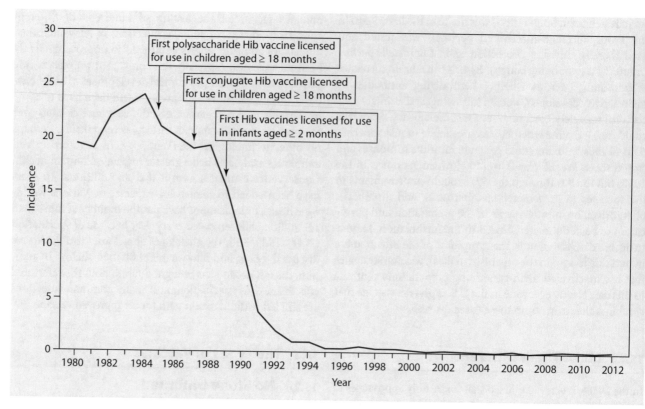

◻ Fig. 15.1 The remarkable effectiveness of vaccination: the haemophilus example. Estimated annual incidence* of invasive Haemophilus influenzae type b (Hib) disease in children aged <5 years — United States, 1980–2012. Sources: 1980–1997: National Bacterial Meningitis Reporting System and National Notifiable Diseases Surveillance (NNDSS) data; Adams WG, Deaver KA, Cochi SL et al (1993) Decline of childhood Haemophilus influenzae Type b (Hib) disease in the Hib vaccine era. *JAMA* 269:221–226; CDC (1996) Progress toward elimination of Haemophilus influenzae type b disease among infants and children—United States, 1987–1995. *MMWR* 45:901–906; CDC (1998) Progress toward elimination of Haemophilus influenzae type b disease among infants and children—United States, 1987–1997. *MMWR* 47:993–8. 1998–2009: NNDSS and Active Bacterial Core Surveillance (ABCs) data. 2010–2012: ABCs cases estimated to the U.S. population. * Per 100,000 population. (Reproduced from Messonnier et al (see *suggested readings*))

reason why many have moved away from such approaches, unless there is no other option. The inactivation of the bacterial cells in the vaccine (heat or chemicals) may overcome this problem but it may also reduce the immune response. Conversely, too little attenuation may lead to adverse reactions either at the vaccine site or systemically. Because one is dealing with a complex cell with a dynamic biology, the making of such formulations on a consistent basis is more challenging than if only a single antigen was chosen as the vaccine component. There is also concern that the cell has not been totally inactivated or that there is a contaminating species that is indistinguishable from the target pathogen that itself is pathogenic. In general, only in the absence of a better alternative are cell-based vaccines used. The trend in most cases is to take a reductionist approach and simplify the vaccine to only those antigens that provide the best protection.

15.2.2 Intelligent and Targeted

This leads us to the second type of vaccine – the **subunit vaccine**. This vaccine does not have whole bacterial cells, although it may be composed of cell components or fragments. Examples of subunit vaccines include those that have the outer capsular polysaccharide as the antigen, a cell-free supernatant from the bacterium that was grown in culture, or contains one or more bacterial proteins. The advantages of a subunit vaccine are straightforward. They center around safety and consistency. Because there are no cells, there is little chance the vaccine will result in an infection. The components of the vaccine are attained using a standardized process with strict adherence to methodology that is reproducible. This ensures consistency and provides confidence that the vaccine contains exactly what it is intended to contain. In the cases of cell-free supernatants, whatever is secreted by the bacterium while growing is what will go into the vaccine. Examples of approved human vaccines of this nature include the acellular pertussis vaccine and the vaccine against anthrax. In these two cases, the dominant antigen secreted in the culture medium are two secreted toxins, pertussis and anthrax toxin, respectively, and protection is primarily driven by the immune response to these two antigens. But, it is quite possible other components in these formulations contribute to or enhance the immunogenicity or efficacy of the vaccine. Because of their somewhat undefined nature (other bacterial proteins present), the possibility or adverse reactions would seemingly be higher than if a single component was present. Like cell-based vaccines, acellular culture supernatants are tolerated mostly in the absence of a more defined alternative. A similar arrangement occurs with the purification of capsular polysaccharide from the approved vaccines described below. They also originate from the pathogen, and, as such, there is the possibility harmful substances can co-purify with the target immunogen.

It is clear that the experts and probably also the public would prefer for all vaccines to be subunit vaccines, and at that, only contain the minimal number of antigens (highly purified) that elicit the necessary immune response needed for complete protection. Even more so, if the antigen is produced in a heterologous host (genetically engineered and inactivated toxin produced in *E. coli*, for example), this eliminates the need to purify the antigen from the pathogen and safeguards against any and all toxicity that may result from the toxin or protein itself. The purification of the cell-binding fragment of cholera toxin (used to protect against cholera) is a good example. Because it contains only a part of the toxin needed for binding to the host cell, it is more safe and defined. Advancements in protein purification and genetic engineering (so you can "mutate out" the toxic part but retain the antigenicity) make this possible. What subunit vaccines gain in safety and consistency, however, they may lose in immunogenicity. For example, to drive a better T-cell response against the capsular polysaccharide, it was determined they needed to be chemically conjugated to proteins. Companies have ingeniously used already proven protein toxins (such as diphtheria toxin) as the conjugating factor. Some single antigen vaccines may only activate one aspect of immunity (example opsonophagocytosis versus neutralization of virulence factors) or because they only have one component they do not cover strains that lack that component. This is a common problem in the formation of vaccines against opportunistic pathogens that use multiple virulence mechanisms to cause disease.

15.2.3 Code It, Make It

The final type of vaccine is a **DNA-based vaccine**. In this vaccine type, DNA that encodes an immunogenic antigen is delivered into the host using either a viral vector, plasmid, or other carrier system. When the DNA enters host cells, the antigen is made and the host mounts an immune response, especially if the antigen is seen as "foreign" because it contains a pathogen associated molecular pattern (PAMP). There are currently no DNA vaccines approved for human use but their efficacy and safety has been demonstrated for a number of pathogens in animal models of infection.

15.3 Concepts in Vaccine Design

One of the objectives of this volume is to educate the young Microbiologist, the next-gen microbe hunter, about the often sinister ways pathogenic bacteria overcome the human immune system. The hope is that this knowledge will be used to stimulate creative ways to prevent the diseases they cause. Perhaps the single most cost effective way to do this is through vaccination. Yet, despite 100 years of fervent work on this front, only six vaccine targeting bacterial pathogens are routinely given to people in the U.S, with three of these more or less optional (Fig. 15.2). Another three (against *M. tuberculosis*, *V. cholerae*, and *S. enterica*) are approved but almost never administered, mostly because the incidence of these diseases in developed nations is low. They are administered more commonly in other countries where these infections are endemic. There are more than two dozen different and common bacterial diseases with no vaccine and, collectively, take the lives of millions of people worldwide. Even with BCG, over two million people still succumb to *M. tuberculosis* infection alone yearly. What principles should the eager microbe hunter use in their quest against vaccine-based protection against bacterial diseases? One guiding principle is the rule of "S."

15.3.1 "S" Stands for Safety

For most new medical developments and investigational medicines, safety is a top priority. Outside of the obvious reason that we should not be comfortable with the loss of an innocent life as a result of vaccination, the liability that companies inherent in their testing of a vaccine on human subjects is great. Even the slightest bad press or adverse reactions can cause biotech to jitter, regardless of whether it is justified or not. If toxins are the immunogen, the toxin activity should be inactivated either by chemical or genetic means. If another type of protein effector is the immunogen, the activity of the protein should not interfere with normal human physiology. The immunogen needs to be sufficiently distinct from host proteins so there is no autoimmunity. This is especially important for bacteria that inhabit our gastrointestinal tract (which can lead to colitis if an immune response targets them) or if the antigen resembles the sugars on the surface of our neurons (which can cause autoimmunity to the tissues and cells of the nervous system). Both of these scenarios have been observed in experimental bacterial vaccines.

Due to their inconsistency and potential risk for actual infection, attempts should be made to move away from live, attenuated vaccines unless the risks do not out-weight the global burden of the disease with no other feasible option. Animal studies examining the effect of the antigens on their health, preferably multiple models/different species, should be used. The exact components of the formulation should, when appropriate, be determined and all ingredients should be carefully chosen and justified for inclusion. It goes without saying that each vaccine needs to be tested in the typical three-tiered clinical trial system to test human vaccines. This occurs in the first phase, which focuses on safety and delivery. In addition, and now more than ever, the target population (age, gender, geographic location, etc) needs to be carefully considered. What may be highly effective in one population may not be in another.

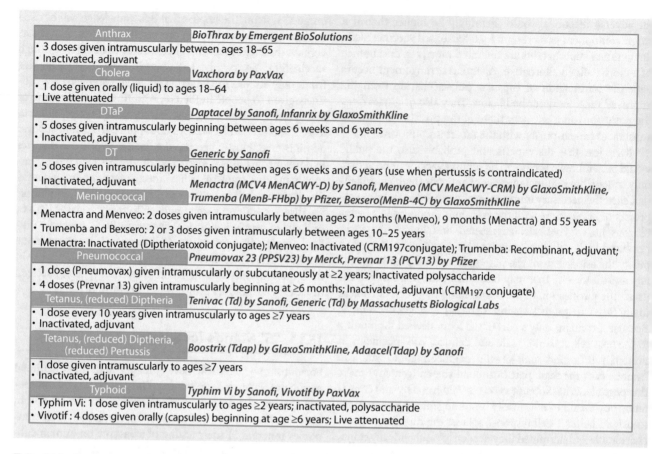

Anthrax	***BioThrax by Emergent BioSolutions***
• 3 doses given intramuscularly between ages 18–65 • Inactivated, adjuvant	
Cholera	***Vaxchora by PaxVax***
• 1 dose given orally (liquid) to ages 18–64 • Live attenuated	
DTaP	***Daptacel by Sanofi, Infanrix by GlaxoSmithKline***
• 5 doses given intramuscularly beginning between ages 6 weeks and 6 years • Inactivated, adjuvant	
DT	***Generic by Sanofi***
• 5 doses given intramuscularly beginning between ages 6 weeks and 6 years (use when pertussis is contraindicated) • Inactivated, adjuvant	
Meningococcal	***Menactra (MCV4 MenACWY-D) by Sanofi, Menveo (MCV MeACWY-CRM) by GlaxoSmithKline, Trumenba (MenB-FHbp) by Pfizer, Bexsero(MenB-4C) by GlaxoSmithKline***
• Menactra and Menveo: 2 doses given intramuscularly between ages 2 months (Menveo), 9 months (Menactra) and 55 years • Trumenba and Bexsero: 2 or 3 doses given intramuscularly between ages 10–25 years • Menactra: Inactivated (Diptheriatoxoid conjugate); Menveo: Inactivated (CRM197conjugate); Trumenba: Recombinant, adjuvant;	
Pneumococcal	***Pneumovax 23 (PPSV23) by Merck, Prevnar 13 (PCV13) by Pfizer***
• 1 dose (Pneumovax) given intramuscularly or subcutaneously at ≥2 years; Inactivated polysaccharide • 4 doses (Prevnar 13) given intramuscularly beginning at ≥6 months; Inactivated, adjuvant (CRM$_{197}$ conjugate)	
Tetanus, (reduced) Diptheria	***Tenivac (Td) by Sanofi, Generic (Td) by Massachusetts Biological Labs***
• 1 dose every 10 years given intramuscularly to ages ≥7 years • Inactivated, adjuvant	
Tetanus, (reduced) Diptheria, (reduced) Pertussis	***Boostrix (Tdap) by GlaxoSmithKline, Adaacel(Tdap) by Sanofi***
• 1 dose given intramuscularly to ages ≥7 years • Inactivated, adjuvant	
Typhoid	***Typhim Vi by Sanofi, Vivotif by PaxVax***
• Typhim Vi: 1 dose given intramuscularly to ages ≥2 years; inactivated, polysaccharide • Vivotif : 4 doses given orally (capsules) beginning at age ≥6 years; Live attenuated	

◻ Fig. 15.2 Current approved vaccines (U.S.)

15.3.2 "S" Stands for Success

That is, the vaccine must work. As above with safety, the effectiveness of any vaccine should first be assessed in an animal model of infection. Dose, number of boosts, duration of protection, and if possible, the mechanism of protection (humoral versus cell-mediated or both – see ► Chaps. 4 and 5) should be assessed. The vaccine should protect against the most common circulating strains of the target bacterial species and, if the bacterium causes multiple distinct types of pathology (say meningitis in one case but a urinary tract infection in another), a good vaccine is one in which all diseases from that species are covered. The vaccine should induce immunological memory that lasts for multiple years and, if not, proof should be provided that a booster dose restores protection. The ideal vaccine provides complete protection in the target human population; realistically, though, this is rarely achieved. In its absence, the degree of protection should be measured versus the cost to produce and administer. A vaccine that reduces mortality or hospital stays by a factor of one-half may save billions of dollars in lost economy and productivity. Finally, a good vaccine induces **herd immunity** and reduces the level of circulating pathogen in the human population to a level that makes it unlikely that an unvaccinated individual will be exposed. This may include preventing transmission of the pathogen across the population but, in the most ideal sense, it also means the elimination of humans as being a reservoir for chronic colonization.

An important part of the success of a vaccine is to choose the right antigen. The antigen should not direct the immune response to target host proteins. This will result in autoimmunity, manifested in symptoms associated with arthritis and inflammation. In addition, the antigen should not be toxic itself. This means bacterial protein toxins should be inactivated. Other antigens, such as adhesins, should not bind to host tissues. Polysaccharides should not resemble the carbohydrate on native tissues, etc. Antigens that direct an immune response to neutralize the activity of toxin/effector/adhesion/capsule, or direct the opsonophagocytosis of the pathogen, or antigens that direct killer T-cells to the pathogen, are good candidates for vaccine development.

The antigen should also be expressed by the pathogen during infection, and the pathogen should not be able to downregulate or modify the antigen to avoid detection *without* losing pathogenicity in the process. One of the successful characteristics of bacteria that avoid the immune system is that many of their antigens are like fighter-plane chaff. This bacterial chaff may misdirect the immune system so that other virulence properties are left untouched. The antigen can also undergo variation such that no one immune response locks the pathogen down, a scenario we encountered in ► Chap. 7. Some virulence factors with these properties include capsule and various adhesins or other surface roteins. If a bacterial factor is the choice of an antigen for a accine, it is necessary that the most frequent or important ersions of that antigen be tested for broad protection against ll the strains that have this antigen. The antigen should also e expressed during key stages during the infection.

The antigen should not direct an attack against beneficial members of our own microbiota. These members live at our mucosal interface, including the GI tract, nasal passages, ear, skin, urinary/genital tracts and others. Not only may these microbes stimulate our immune system and provide colonization resistance (and so getting rid of them would predispose us to infection), but the immune response against them s likely to induce inflammation at these surfaces, which can also weaken barriers.

Finally, the antigen should induce long-lasting immunological memory. Any antigen that protects for only a few months or years runs the risk of losing public support. People that get the vaccination but acquire an infection after the immunity wanes will view the vaccine as being unsuccessful. Plus, one relies on the rigor and responsibility of the patient to come back at frequent intervals for boosts. One characteristic of vaccines currently approved for human use is that one or a few boosters induces long-term immunity. The intervals between boosts can be ten or more years, and some provide life-long immunity with a single or few boosts. Such boosts can be timed with key entry points into school or the workforce, thus generating a kind of societal or cultural sticky note that becomes part of our collective memory. If the vaccine requires frequent boosts (say yearly), it is unlikely the patient will on a consistent basis remain vaccinated.

15.3.3 "S" Is for Scalable

That is, the vaccine must be able to be mass produced in a timely manner, be cost-effective so the manufacturing company has incentive to make it, and not be cost-prohibitive so that patients do not allow finances to influence their decision to take the vaccine. In addition, the vaccine should not be so complicated that its production cannot be replicated consistently across the world by different people at different geographic locations. The difficult science of finding and testing good antigen candidates aside, these barriers prevent vaccines from entering the market. Simply put, vaccines have traditionally followed the 10-10-10 parameter; they take 10 years to test and develop at about ten million per year a cost, and only about 10% make it to phase 3 clinical trials. We might have more vaccines on the market if there was more emphasis on overcoming these challenges.

15.3.4 "S" Is for Storage

The final "S" is *Storage*. Vaccines need to have a long-shelf life so that more can be made than are needed and any surplus can be put into storage to meet later demands. This is especially true for vaccines that target infrequent bacterial infections that may cause outbreaks every few years or vaccines made in case of an emergency (a bioterrorism event, etc.). Storage encompasses more than timing; it also refers to what is in the vaccine. Is it free of proteases that can degrade the components? Are stabilizers added? If so, are they safe? The public has been increasingly concerned with added ingredients and their effect on the health of their children. The ingredients added to the vaccine not only have to extend the shelf life but they must also be safe at the levels present in the vaccine. If possible, the ideal vaccine is one that can be stored without the need for temperature control, especially if the vaccine targets diseases prevalent in poor countries. Keeping the costs of energy use low should be a sought-after goal as well.

15.4 The Vaccine Development Process

15.4.1 It's the Immunogen!

In the wild west of early vaccine development, whole cells or their supernatants were used as vaccines, often times without knowing the protective antigen. Today, the process of making a vaccine is more complicated, but for all the right reasons (◘ Fig. 15.3). Antigen identification now benefits from advances in molecular biology. The most useful may be "omics" technologies. Genomics yields the sequence of the pathogen, as well as numerous strains of that pathogen, which allows for comparative genomics to identify possible virulence factors that are common between them. If these factors are present in commensals, they may not be chosen as an antigen for development. Since advances in computational approaches have informed about what constitutes functional protein domains, we often can also identify other useful features, such as if a protein is displayed on the bacterial surface, secreted, or retained in the cytoplasm. Antigens that are surface exposed are desired; they often interact with the host (thus their neutralization might be beneficial) and they may also direct antibodies, macrophages, or T-cells to the pathogen. But there is more to selecting an antigen on purely sequence grounds. It is helpful to also know a little about the biology of the protein of interest, when it is made, and if it is important enough for the disease. Proteomics and transcriptomics may inform when it is made and at what levels. These approaches can determine if the antigen is expressed during the infection or disease. Mechanistic studies can then assess the function of the target immunogen. Molecular biology techniques can be used to render the immunogen safe by changing amino acids that may lead to toxic effects to those that render the immunogen harmless. Biochemical techniques can be employed to also inactivate the target or couple it to another molecule that enhances its immunogenicity. The function of all immunogens in currently approved U.S. and European vaccines are either known or we have a solid idea of their function. If the immunogen can be purified, a 3-dimensional structure may aid in vaccine design. If not, making strains of bacteria that lack

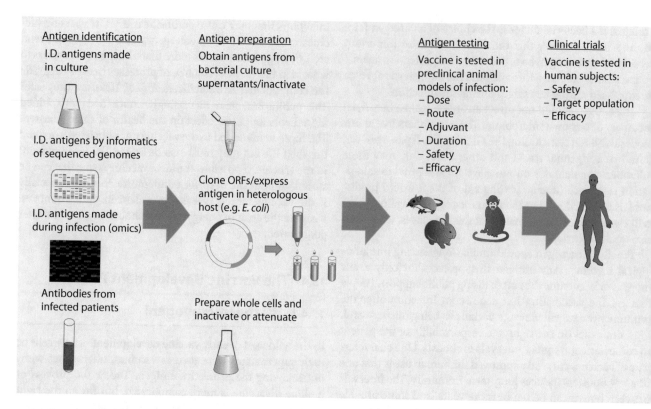

◻ **Fig. 15.3** The stages of vaccine development. Vaccine development can be divided into four distinct stages. In the first stage, various techniques are used to identify bacterial antigens that may constitute a safe and effective vaccine. This may include mining sequenced genomes for surface proteins or otherwise secreted effectors or toxins, identifying antibodies reactive to bacterial proteins from patient's sera, identifying antigens made during infection, or the use of bacterial products or bacteria themselves grown in culture. In stage 2, the antigen is prepared by either purifying it or inactivating it or both. Proteins expressed in heterologous hosts may yield high levels of immunogens after purification. In the third stage, the putative immunogen is tested for efficacy, often varying the adjuvant, dose, and route, in a suitable animal model of infection. In the final stage, what is learned from the animal studies is applied to a series of clinical trials in humans

15

the proposed immunogen and testing them in relevant animal models of infection will not only inform on function but also importance. Should a proposed immunogen be dispensable for disease, it may not be a good vaccine candidate unless its presence allows the immune system to hone in on the pathogen. In those individuals that have survived an infection, their serum may contain antibodies to the pathogen's antigens. These antibodies can be screened for their reactivity to a lysate or a supernatant of the bacterium grown in culture. Routine Western blots, ELISAs and pull-down assays all can aid in antigen identification using sera from infected patients. These antibodies may be the reason why the patient survived as well, thus bringing the process one step closer to acquiring an effective vaccine.

conjugated to a soluble carrier protein. Non-proteinacious antigens like capsular polysaccharide may need to be coupled to protein carriers, but for different reasons. This method has been found to improve immunogenicity. The batch will need to be scaled and the process of production standardized as well. If the antigen can be reduced to a specific subunit of the protein, and that domain alone purified, this is desirable for many of the reasons discussed above. Many studies have also shown that small peptides harboring the relevant immunological epitope are also effective. This minimalist approach might be safe but should be weighed against productive efficacy as sometimes minimal epitopes do not induce the most robust of an immune response.

15.4.2 … and It's the Design

Once the immunogen is chosen, an experimental program has to be developed that revolves around testing the immunogen for safety and efficacy. Different purification methods of the immunogen may be tested, and, once settled, may be shortened and made consistent. The immunogen may be insoluble and purified under denaturing conditions, or

15.4.3 Validation

Next, the vaccine should be tested using an appropriate animal model that best mimics not only the infection pathophysiology but also is an accepted representation of the immune response desired. The advantage of an animal model is that the dose of antigen, the route of delivery, the number of boosts, and the duration between post-vaccination challenge (best at different doses of pathogen), can all be varied nd the data used to decide the most optimal formulation nd parameters to achieve maximum protection when even- ually scaled to humans. Efficacy can be measured in many vays. The most well accepted is a reduction or elimination of ymptoms associated with the infection. A disease index core, which quantifies the health of the animals, should be ised. The lethal dose 50 and mean time to death with and vithout vaccination would ideally be performed (see ► Chap. 2 for a description of these procedures). If the ani- mals are protected by the vaccine, some experiments should oe performed to determine how long they are protected, as vell as post-vaccination challenges occurring months to per- haps a year after vaccination if feasible. Post-challenge nec- ropsies on the animals should assess the levels of bacteria in the major organs and blood (most especially the target organ or tissue that is part of the pathophysiology) and a histologi- cal analysis of said tissues looking for any pathology or immune cell infiltration. As much serum as possible should oe collected. This will aid in determining if antibodies are produced against the immunogen, whether these antibodies induce opsonophagocytosis of the pathogens when co-incu- bated in culture with macrophages, or if they induce other immunity (neutralization of function, etc.). Blood should be drawn and serum isolated to assess the levels all major cyto- kines and chemokines. Blood chemistry can be measured; this, and the latter analysis can also be carried out on small quantities of blood before, during, and after vaccination and boosters. An approach like this will inform on liver and kid- ney biomarkers of health as well as other important measure- ments related to overall bodily balance and health. One of the standard measures of antibody-based efficacy is if the trans- fer of antibodies to a naïve animal that has been infected will protect against infection. This is termed **passive immuniza- tion**. If possible, and often needed for acceptance by regula- tory agencies, efficacy should be demonstrated in another animal model (maybe even a third), the last one often being a species of non-human primate. This is meant to get as close to a human immune assessment as possible before clinical trials are started.

15.4.4 The Real McCoy

Following successful demonstration of safety and efficacy in animal studies, the evaluation of the vaccine moves to the human-testing stage. In the U.S., which is often cited as a model system for clinical testing, this stage is further divided into three phases. In **phase I**, the emphasis focuses on first learning if the vaccine is safe. A small group of individuals, usually less than one-hundred, are recruited as participants. This population is healthy. They will not be evaluated for pro- tection against the disease in question. Instead, using the animal studies as a guide, the dose is human-adjusted and the vaccine given by the same route as in the pre-clinical studies. The participants are often staggered and rolled out slowly. Adverse reactions are monitored both at the site of inocula- tion and systemically. Local changes may include swelling,

redness, and pain. More systemic reactions include fever, nausea, vomiting, aches, pains and general malaise. If boost- ers are given, the same assessment is used through the vac- cine regimen. Blood may be drawn and the degree of antibody production against the antigen in the experimental vaccine determined. If the basis of the vaccine is neutralization of an antigen or stimulation of a phagocytic response, these may also be assessed in appropriate in vitro assays. The staggered administration of the vaccine allows the study leaders to halt the study if early participants show ill effects.

If there are no adverse reactions or they are mild, and an immune response is detected, the vaccine may progress to **phase II** human trials. During this phase, safety is still the top concern; however, now the safety is evaluated in the target population. In most cases, this population either has the dis- ease or is susceptible to it. In the case of a vaccine, the target participants are those most likely to get the infection. For example, the currently approved meningococcal vaccine tar- gets young adults before they enter middle/high school and again before they enter college. These populations are at higher risk for meningitis. Target populations for bacterial vaccines may include infants to 2 years old, the elderly (>65), pregnant women, or those at risk for cancer or being immu- nocompromised. They may also include groups that engage in an occupation or have a genetic predisposition that puts them at higher vulnerability than their peers. Soldiers vacci- nated against anthrax disease are an example of the latter, an attempt to protect them from a bioweapon attack.

Once the vaccine is deemed safe in the target population, it can proceed to **phase III** – testing its ability to protect against the actual disease or infection and a much larger scale. It is probably true to say that at this stage is when most vaccines fail. Here, the target population is vaccinated and followed, often for many years, until one can make a conclu- sion about the frequency of the infection in the test (vacci- nated) versus the placebo (unvaccinated) groups. All the same measurements as above are applied; safety, immuno- logical correlates, etc., but this time determined alongside infection rates (sometimes termed incidence), morbidity (how sick they get), and mortality (whether they live or die). The data will be analyzed and statistical comparisons made between test and control groups. Should the vaccine prove effective, a government body (in the U.S. it is the Food and Drug Administration) will review all the data from every study and a panel of experts will decide if the vaccine will be approved and licensed for routine human use.

15.5 The Importance of Adjuvants

The discussion to this point has centered almost entirely around the prospective antigen and the chosen immunogen. We talked about the qualities of a good antigen, including discovery, purification, and evaluation. What we have so far ignored is that a good vaccine often is adjuvated. The word **adjuvant** comes from the latin word adjuvare, "to help." An adjuvant is something added to the vaccine formulation that helps the immune system generate a strong, long-lasting response to that antigen. To understand why an adjuvant helps, one must understand that vaccination is a somewhat unnatural process. The immune system, in general, did not evolve to interact with only one or a few pathogen components in the absence of the rest of the organism; and, infections do not readily begin via the subcutaneous delivery of a single virulence factor without the accompanying pathogen, for example. Many virulence factors lack inherent antigenicity, perhaps evolution developed them this way to go unnoticed by our cellular alarms. An adjuvant "tricks" the host into thinking an active infection – pathogen and all – just entered the body. Adjuvants mainly function by providing **pathogen associated molecular patterns** (PAMPs) to the formulation. These are recognized by host cells and activate the innate arm of immunity. The innate arm will then send signals for phagocytic cells like dendritic cells to investigate the area and take samples back for processing. It is commonly believed that a robust stimulation of the innate immune system during the time of vaccination is key to the maintenance of an equally robust long term cellular and humoral response. Because of this, the microbe hunter interested in the development of vaccines should carefully consider the appropriate adjuvant to use during pre-clinical development. Such considerations go hand in hand with dose and boosts, both being important in stimulating the immune system to achieve higher immunological responses (Fig. 15.4).

The most common adjuvant used in animal research during the pre-clinical testing of a vaccine is called **Freund's complete adjuvant**, or CFA. Named after its developer, the immunologist Jules Freund, CFA is composed of killed mycobacteria. It stimulates a potent innate immune response that includes the production of interleukins and enhanced uptake of antigens by dendritic cells. This drives a strong antibody and T-cell response to the pathogen. All of this likely stems from mycobacterial PAMPs. CFA, however, is not approved for use in humans because of associated toxicity; it simply is too strong of an adjuvant. The only approved adjuvant in bacterial vaccines in the U.S. are those that are made of various **aluminum salts**, including salts of potassium ($AlKO_4$), phosphate ($AlPO_4$), and hydroxide $Al(OH)_3$. The common name for this adjuvant is alum and it was first found to boost immunity with the diphtheria vaccine developed in the 1920s and 1930s. Because aluminum is a ubiquitous metal found in just about every component of our environment, it is generally regarded as safe in the low amounts used in many bacterial vaccines. Interestingly, the exact mechanism by which this simple formulation sensitizes our immune system is not known. Theories range from it increasing the stability of the vaccine at the site of inoculation to it promoting the uptake of the antigen by antigen presenting cells. Nevertheless, alum is used in dozens of worldwide approved vaccines.

Work over the past 25 years has led to the development of new, and from a developmental perspective, exciting, adjuvants. Perhaps equal to finding new bacterial antigens to use in a vaccine is the choice of an adjuvant that directs the

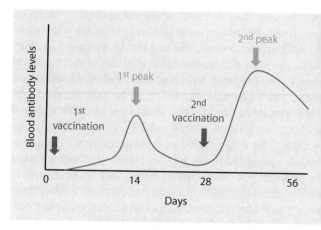

Fig. 15.4 Common vaccination schedule and response. After the primary inoculation with an immunogen, antibodies can be detected at high levels about 14 days later. In many cases, immunity begins to wane shortly thereafter unless a second vaccination, termed a boost, is given. Typically, in experimental studies of a vaccine, this second vaccination occurs on or about day 28. A second antibody increase is observed that typically is both higher in magnitude and duration than the first. Immunity may still wane but at a lower rate. Third and more boosts can be given after this period to maintain high levels of circulating antibodies. These responses can go even higher if paired with stimulating adjuvants

immune system down the desired response for that particular pathogen. This is particularly true for the dichotomy that exists between directing an immune response against extracellular and intracellular bacteria. Alum, for instance, is known to stimulate a strong humoral antibody response in contrast to a T-cell mode of immunity. A T-cell response would be needed to recognize host cells infected with intracellular bacteria. Thus, another adjuvant will be needed to direct this arm of immunity. The adjuvant and the antigen have to be carefully balanced in producing the type of immunity needed without too many adverse reactions that come with overstimulation of the immune system. A balance between the two is probably the best vaccine to develop; too much reactivity and even if the vaccine works, the public outcry might limit acceptance. Too little reactivity and the vaccine may not be protective.

Other adjuvants besides aluminum salts are being used in approved viral vaccines. Perhaps the best example is **MF59**, one of the adjuvants in the seasonal flu vaccine. The stimulating component is squalene, a 30-carbon fatty acid isolated from shark livers that is also found in many tissues of the human body. Like every adjuvant, the exact mechanism of stimulation is not worked out but it has been observed to promote the presentation of antigen to immune cells in the lymph nodes. Another adjuvant is **monophosphoryl lipid A**, which is derived from the lipopolysaccharide of salmonella. As such, it is a stimulator of toll-like receptor 4, the LPS receptor. This adjuvant has been successfully used in the hepatitis vaccines, generating a Th1 response. Another promising adjuvant in development is bacterial DNA, commonly referred to as **CpG**. CpG is an unmethylated oligonucleotide that is recognized by toll-like receptor 9 (and thus can be onsidered a PAMP). The C and Gs refer to cytosine and guanosine as a dinucleotide, respectively. Bacterial DNA is recognized by the immune system as foreign, and the key specificity determinant seems to be that it is largely unmethylated (our host DNA is heavily methylated). CpG stimulates potent B-cell responses since TLR9 is a major receptor on this immune cell type. As such, Th1-cell driven responses with strong antibody production is a key feature. For those bacterial vaccines requiring high neutralizing or opsonophagocytic antibodies, CpG may be an adjuvant of choice. In support of this is the finding in several animal models that neutralizing antibodies to anthrax toxin, when the anthrax vaccine adsorbed (AVA) is mixed with CpG, improve by up to 10-fold in levels. We see in these examples that one of the most effective, but probably least discussed, ways a microbe hunter can work to prevent bacterial diseases is by careful and further development of adjuvants.

15.6 The High Ground: Current Approved Bacterial Vaccines

15.6.1 May the Children Breathe Again

Many have toiled away tirelessly in the lab and clinic to bring the world protective vaccines. The experience of learning what does and does not work has been invaluable to the makers of newer formulations. In the U.S., there are six routinely licensed and used bacterial vaccines: tetanus, diphtheria, pertussis, meningitis caused by neisseria, pneumonia caused by streptococcus, and pneumonia and meningitis caused by haemophilus. Three of these (tetanus, diphtheria, and pertussis) are covered by one vaccine, referred to as DTaP. The "D" refers to diphtheria, "T" tetanus, and "aP" acellular pertussis. The upper case letter indicates that the formulation is an inactivated toxoid. In fact, the mechanism of vaccine efficacy for all three is likely through the neutralization of diphtheria, tetanus, and pertussis toxins (see ▶ Chap. 10 for a description of these toxins). Diptheria is caused by the Gram-positive bacterium *Corynebacterium diptheriae*. The disease is characterized by an intensely sore and swollen throat. The inflammation is so bad that death can be caused by the inability to breathe from an occluded trachea. For the first 20 or so years of the twentieth century, it is estimated there were 200,000 cases/year in the U.S. alone, mostly in children. After introduction of early versions of the diphtheria vaccine, less than ~ 10,000/year cases were reported. The vaccine is made by treating culture supernatants containing diphtheria toxin with formalin, which inactivates the toxin, and then adsorbing this material to aluminum salts (alum).

Bordetella pertussis is the cause of whooping cough. Like diphtheria, it is primarily an infection of the upper respiratory tract. Intense coughing fits are common and the concomitant intake of air becomes labored, leading to the characteristic "whoop" sound. The cough likely expels droplets of *B. pertussis* that are inhaled by the next unlucky recipient. In the 1930s, there were about 200,000 infections per year with a death rate of 2%. A whole cell vaccine was developed in the 1940s, but was replaced with an inactivated acellular vaccine of culture supernatants shortly thereafter. From the 1950s to the 1990s, less than 20,000 cases were reported, with the lowest cases just a few thousand in the 1960s. Worldwide incidence also declined substantially following widespread vaccination. Lately, the frequency of the disease is on the rise with a recent peak in 2012 of nearly 50,000 cases in the U.S. Still, once a widespread scourge of children, it is now mostly isolated to sporadic cases in parts of the world where vaccination is not common. The current pertussis vaccine takes a three-pronged approach. In addition to containing the toxin, it also contains the proteins pertactin and filamentous hemagglutinin (FHA). Pertactin is an outer membrane protein that likely is important for binding to lung epithelial cells. FHA binds to ciliated cells of the trachea. A five-member vaccine with two more additional adhesins is also effective in humans. The multi-faceted targeting of several important virulence factors, of which one is very important (pertussis toxin), allows for a highly efficacious vaccine. It also demonstrates that this approach, the sort of swiss-army knife blocking of multiple virulence pathways, might just be a template for future vaccine development.

15.6.2 May They Have Motion

Tetanus or "lock jaw" is a disease caused by the Gram-positive anaerobe *Clostridium tetani*. It is a highly fatal disease with mortality between 50% and 90% following intoxication. To the best of our knowledge, the disease is entirely attributable to a single protein toxin, tetanus toxin, that acts as a zinc endopeptidase cleaving key neuronal proteins that are important for the control of action potentials. It is considered one of the most potent toxins in the world. Emil von Behring demonstrated in the 1890s that "antitoxin" (which was antibody) could protect from intoxication. This work was the foundational basis for the development of a tetanus toxoid in the 1920s and its eventual incorporation with the diphtheria and pertussis vaccine thereafter. Vaccination with the inactivated toxin is one of the most effective vaccines known to humanity resulting in almost complete protection against the disease.

The DTP vaccine ranks up there with penicillin in the positive impact it has had on the health of humankind. In use for nearly 80 years now, there is no more consistently administered, safe, trusted, and widely protective vaccine than the diphtheria, tetanus, and pertussis combinatorial vaccine. Children receive this vaccine at 2, 4, and 6 months after birth with additional boosters around age 2 and 6 years old. It is recommended for pregnant mothers so that newborns acquire maternal antibodies. The elderly also receive it. Built on the back of much basic research performed before the 1940s, then with constant tinkering of the formulation thereafter, the DTP vaccine remains the standard by which all developmental vaccines are judged.

15.6.3 May They Think Again

Streptococcus pneumoniae (also referred to as pneumococcus) is a leading cause of bacterial pneumoniae, especially in very young children. It may also be the most common cause of ear infections in the world (estimates suggest at least 20 million a year in the U.S. alone) and invasive forms cause a life-threatening meningitis with a case mortality of about 15%. Conservative estimates suggest that in developing countries where vaccination rates are lower, the organism may be responsible for more than one million deaths per year. Most of these are likely pneumonia since lower respiratory infections are a top five cause of death in young children globally. Approximately 3 of every 10 infections are with strains resistant to commonly used antibiotics, including penicillin and erythromycin. The elderly are also at risk as are those with HIV or an otherwise immunocompromised state. Like other problematic bacteria discussed in this chapter, *S. pneumoniae* colonizes the nasal passages of its human host. Transmission probably occurs through saliva and cough droplets.

A pneumonococcus vaccine is licensed in many countries and is highly effective at providing protection against infection. Like diphtheria, pertussis and tetanus, diseases in which a single prominent virulence factor is a major player in the pathogenesis, *S. pneumoniae* also relies heavily on a single virulence component. It's not a toxin. This virulence factor is the polysaccharide capsule, which protects pneumonococcus against phagocytosis and complement. Non-encapsulated strains are substantially less harmful and not often observed in infected patients. Nearly 100 different capsule types are described in this organism, but, fortunately, it has been found that many of the most frequent types can be captured with less than 25% of the total capsule types. Vaccine studies performed by the U.S. military substantiated the use of capsule as a major immunogen. Since then, various capsular polysaccharide-based vaccines have emerged and been approved over the years, each new iteration adding more and more capsule types to the vaccine (from 7 to now 23). To enhance the immune response, there are versions of the vaccine where capsule is conjugated to a protein carrier (conjugated polysaccharide vaccines). It is generally believed the major mechanism of protection is via antibodies that bind to the surface capsule, leading to an avalanche of opsonophagocytic activity against the bacterial version of a force field. Current recommendations are that a 13-capsule type conjugate vaccine be given to young children at 2, 4, and 6 months with another boost about a year later. The elderly are given a 23-type un-conjugated vaccine. The efficacy of the vaccine is demonstrated by a halving of all cases of *S. pneumoniae* infection, regardless of resistance, since 2000.

The success of vaccines targeting bacterial diseases of the upper respiratory tract continues with the currently approved vaccines against *Haemophilus influenziae*. Mistakenly thought to be the cause of an outbreak of flu in the late 1890s (this was before the flu was proven to be a viral disease), influenza was affixed to its name. The invasive forms are a potent gobbler of the iron-containing compound heme (thus the "haem" loving fixture). *H. influenziae* causes life threatening pneumonia and meningitis. Far less menacing but much more frequent, it also is a common cause of ear infections in children. A Gram-negative bacillus that is a superb colonizer of the human respiratory mucosal surfaces as much as 8 in 10 people may be carriers of the organism. Disease is multi-factorial and depends on the type of strain, host genetics, and medical status. The development of the *H. influenza* vaccine is another testament to the use of protein carriers to enhance the immune response, especially in the most vulnerable populations (children in this case). Because invasive forms of the organism (which cause pneumonia and meningitis) are often associated with a polysaccharide capsule (similar to pneumonococcus and neisseria), the capsule was targeted as the primary immunogen. Six capsular variants were recognized with one, type B, associated with most infections.

Vaccines containing the capsule were developed in the 1970s and 1980s but setbacks occurred because the immunity was short-lived. The recognition that the capsule conjugated to a protein carrier (particularly tetanus or diphtheria toxin) resulted in significant improvement in long-term immunity and antibody responses. Although several versions are available, there is now a vaccine that encompasses antigens against *H. influenziae* capsule, diphtheria, pertussis, tetanus, and even polio in a single formulation. Boosters are necessary but complete protection from all five diseases, with a single formulation, is possible. The development of the *H. influenziae* capsular conjugate not only established capsule as a bonafide vaccine antigen for bacteria that use them as part of their virulence arsenal, it also demonstrated that protein carriers added to the formulation (especially if they are already proven to be effective against other bacterial infections, for example, tetanus toxin) is a clever way to enhance immunity with fewer boosts. Although the *H. influenza* vaccine has lowered the worldwide incidence of deaths from this pathogen, challenges do remain. A non-typeable version, that is, one without a capsule, can colonize human hosts and, unlike *S. pneumoniae* whose loss of capsule renders the organism wimpy, capsule-less heamophilus can still cause infections, albeit they are not as invasive. Vaccine candidates against non-typeable heamophilus include protein targets such as Hap (haemophilus adhesin), Hif (haemophilus fimbriae) and various outer membrane proteins such as the lipoprotein P6 (whose antibodies in children correlate with protection). Thus, next generation versions may include both capsular and non-capsular antigens to provide near universal protection against this dangerous pathobiont.

Medical science has done a wonderful job focusing its efforts at reducing bacterial meningitis in children and young adults. The haemophilus and pneumonococcal vaccines both target this deadly invasive condition. The trifecta on the subject is complete with consideration of the vaccine for *Neisseria meningitidis*, which was developed in the 1950s and 1960s and first licensed in the 1970s. Various improved versions offering stronger immunity or more coverage of strains has continued to this day. In the United States, a licensed vaccine overs four of the most prevalent serotypes. A separate licensed vaccine covers another serotype whose epitopes resemble human antigens and thus required more development. *N. meningitidis* is a Gram-negative pathogen that can colonize the human respiratory tract in about 10% of the population. Like haemophilus and pneumonococcus, its dominant pathogenic feature seems to be its polysaccharide capsule, which inhibits phagocytosis. At least 13 capsular serotypes have been recognized, which seem to distribute by their geographic location. This property represents a challenge to universal vaccination attempts as each vaccine will need to cover the serotypes present in that region.

The main concern with this organism is bacterial meningitis, which, in about 10% of the cases, is fatal. Another 10–20% of those infected live but suffer long-term sequelae including neurological or musculoskeletal issues related to invasive penetration of the bacterium during disease. Antibiotics are thought to be effective in about two third of all cases; in those where antibiotics do not help, the consequences are often devastating. Worldwide, there are about 300,000 cases (U.S. ~ 3000) but these are likely underestimates. A hallmark of the organism is its ability to start epidemics every few years in certain parts of the world, especially Africa. During these episodes, tens of thousands of people may contract the disease in a short period of time. An epidemic in Africa in 1996 approached 200,000 cases. They highlight the need to anticipate these waves and appropriately time vaccination efforts around their expected seasonal arrival. Several neisseria vaccines are licensed and used throughout the world. Most of them contain one or more capsular polysaccharides conjugated to a protein carrier. In the U.S., the vaccine is recommended for pre-teens (usually before they enter middle school – age 11–12) and a boost for older teens (at the middle of high school or before they enter college – age 16–17). Young children and older adults may also receive the vaccine if they are at a higher risk for meningococcal infection, including the immunocompromised. The vaccine may be given to children younger than pre-teens in parts of the world where epidemics may occur. The timing of the vaccine is designed around teens entering high-cluster environments (such as college dorms) where the spread of the bacterium is more likely. Being primarily exchanged via saliva, one can envision how giving it before the teenage years is a logical time period for vaccination.

Out of the Box

Fear and unfounded accusations can be a powerful anti-vaccination force. In 1998, GlaxoSmithKline introduced the vaccine LYMErix™ which was approved by the FDA in the same year. Approval was granted after the vaccine successfully completed two clinical trials for efficacy against *Borrelia burgdorferi* infection, the causative agent of Lyme Disease. The disease is chronically debilitating, characterized by soreness and muscle aches, arthritis and fever for months. Treatment involves long-term antibiotic use. The clinical trials evaluated over 10,000 volunteers. The result: three injections led to 76–92% efficacy in preventing Lyme Disease. The vaccine is comprised of the outer surface protein A, often abbreviated OspA. In 1999, 1 year after FDA approval, 1.5 million doses were administered in the Northeastern United States. Interestingly, the mechanism of protection seems to prevent the transmission of the spirochete from tick to bitten host.

But the success of the vaccine was to be short-lived. In 1998, the same year as vaccine approval, a paper published in the journal *The Lancet* claimed to link the MMR (measles, mumps, and rubella) vaccine to autism. The paper was eventually retracted and the CDC investigated the causal link between vaccination and autism,

finding no evidence of any. But the popular press that the paper generated helped fuel a growing anti-vaccination movement. Two years later, a study published in hamsters suggested that the Lyme vaccine caused arthritis. This paper was also highlighted by the press, which fueled more suspicion of vaccination, and in particular, vaccination with LYMErix. Several people came forward claiming that the vaccine caused their arthritis. The FDA reviewed 1.4 million cases of those vaccinated and found only 59 incidents of reported arthritis, none of them conclusively linked to the vaccine. Nevertheless, the negative press and the growing anti-vaccination sentiment led to an astounding drop of 1.5 million vaccinated in 1999 to only 10,000 in 2002. Due to the low demand for the vaccine following the negative media, the company discontinued the vaccine. Consequently, there continues to be 25,000 confirmed cases of Lyme Disease each year with another 15,000–30,000 suspected cases. Oddly enough, your dog can still be vaccinated against the disease. This case highlights the tenuous nature of even the most successful medical intervention ever created – the vaccine – and highlights the challenges that the microbe hunter faces in the continuation and further development of vaccination programs.

15.7 The Bottom of the Hill: The Difficult Climb Ahead

The success of vaccinating against several deadly childhood diseases has, at the least, saved millions of lives. At the best, it will save hundreds of millions more. These early successes, now worldwide with the administration of programs, represent the cornerstone of medical achievement. As far as we have come, it may be we only have taken the first heave up the mountain ahead. There is still a sizable list of organisms that cause harmful or deadly diseases in humans for which there is no vaccine. Why? We touch on some of the more impactful of them here.

One idea is that many of these bacteria are a part of our microbiome. *E. coli*, two species of streptococcus, *H. pylori*, *P. aeruginosa*, and *S. aureus* all have planted a flag on Planet Human. We are one of their reservoirs. This raises the interesting notion that one of the reasons there is no vaccine is because they are adapted to us. They also have pleiotropic virulence mechanisms. These bacteria often contain multiple toxins with malleable genomes and can mix and match virulence factors by horizontal gene transfer. Another observation is where they colonize: mucosal surfaces. Many bacterial infections are acute and mainly infect blood or soft-tissue. The first time they infect is the only time they infect (think *C. tetani* and immunity developed against tetanus toxin). This concept does not apply for some of the bacteria for which there is no vaccine. Unlike their infrequent bacterial counterparts, these microbiome inhabitants hide in our nooks and crannies, in mucus and with other bacteria, and at mucosal surfaces. They are also adapted to disguise themselves, and are thus not detected. Finally, some of the bacteria on this list present challenges for a different reason. This includes that they are intracellular dwelling bacteria whose main challenge is they hide in our cells. Below, we highlight the challenges of making vaccines against the Most-Wanted of bacterial pathogens.

15.7.1 *E. coli*

Escherichia coli is the Houdini of pathogenic bacteria. This Janus-faced organism colonizes our GI tract. There, it is an infrequent member of the total intestinal community, playing discreet amongst more abundant beneficial commensals. *E. coli* makes vitamins we use, may prevent the colonization by pathogens, and may assist in immune maturation. It can also, on a dime, acquire pathogenicity islands, antibiotic resistance determinants, or other virulence factors that morph it from playful symbiont to harmful pathogen. This mix and match virulence makes vaccine design challenging. In fact, this is the primary reason why *E. coli* causes such a broad range of clinical symptoms and pathology. As if being a quasi-species with a pan-genome larger than its own core genome was not enough of a problem, its surface is also riddled with at least 200 different serologically distinct O-antigen structures, dozens of flagellar variants and an antigenically diverse capsule. Most of the pathogenic forms that cause meningitis display a capsule similar in structure to the B capsule of neisseria, which itself bears resemblance to sugars present in fetal brain tissue. More than half of its genome is shared with so-called "commensal" strains. In fact, what it means to be a "commensal" in this species is not really defined; and, as stated above, many of these commensals are a horizontal gene transfer event away from being a pathogen.

The selection of the immunogen in this organism must be handled with great care. Antigens present in commensals may lead to colitis. O-antigen and capsule vaccines have proven effective in animal models, and much work has also been performed developing surface proteins as vaccines (e.g., the adhesin and pilus tip protein FimH). The latter factor, important for urinary tract infections (by far the most dominant, up to eight million in the U.S. alone), progressed to clinical trials, as well as a whole cell vaccine, but were discontinued. The development of a vaccine is further complicated by the fact that some *E. coli* pathotypes can disseminate from the GI tract to the blood but remain extracellular, others are invasive and can hide in epithelial cells, and others never leave the GI tract and only cause diarrheal-like disease. A universal bullet against all these possibilities may not be attainable, or, if it is, it will focus on common mechanism related to a few key virulence determinants, being either adhesins, virulence factors, or O- and K-surface antigens, or a combination thereof, that can be added into one formulation. If universal protection does not seem achievable, an alternate strategy is to delineate each type of *E. coli* infection from the others, identify high risk groups for that infection and vaccinate these individuals using only the virulence factors important for that particular infection.

15.7.2 *P. aeruginosa*

Similar obstacles for vaccine development are also present for a similar pathogen, *Pseudomonas aeruginosa* (Pa). Like *E. coli*, this organism harbors many distinct virulence mechanisms, including O-antigen and LPS surface structures, secreted toxins delivered by specialized secretion systems, iron uptake systems, adhesins, and the production of an exopolysaccharide termed alginate. A number of patient populations are at high risk for *P. aeruginosa* infections; burn victims, those with cystic fibrosis, and the immunocompromised (often cancer patients receiving chemotherapy). The combination of challenging patient populations and the multitude of virulence strategies has led some leaders in this area to describe the generation of a safe and effective Pa vaccine the "long and winding road." There is some hope though.

Alginate is a substance made by *P. aeruginosa* in the lungs of cystic fibrosis (CF) patients. Rodent models have demonstrated that antibodies to this substance can safeguard against lethal infection, and some CF patients that do not suffer from such infections have antibodies against alginate. However, effective opsonizing antibodies do not seem to be commonly produced in humans, especially if they have already been exposed to Pa and made other anti-alginate antibodies. This particular example highlights one of the issues associated with vaccination against pathobionts. The body may already have been exposed to these inhabitants and generated many antibodies against different antigens, diffusing the response. Progress was made with a vaccine consisting of flagellar components, so much in fact that it went to clinical trials and showed some efficacy. The effort was discontinued with little available notice, a not-to-all uncommon occurrence in vaccine trials. Here we see another problem; vaccines don't always fail because of biological or medical reasons. Many of them include a shortage of monies, a change in investigator or company direction, or public outcry. Without sustained funding, large patient cohorts, or the will to continue, even trials with solid results are difficult to maintain. LPS O-antigen based vaccines have also been successful in animal models, and burn and cancer patients in trials. The caveats for these studies were that only those serotypes that constituted the vaccine were targeted while in other patient cohorts (cystic fibrosis) there was limited or no efficacy. Vaccines constructed of lipopolysaccharide components also raise concerns about safety.

5.7.3 S. aureus

The number one cause of Gram-positive bacteremia in critical care settings is *Staphylococcus aureus*. It is a common culprit of endocarditis, skin abscesses, and invasive bloodstream infections that can be deadly, but, like *E. coli*, it can infect nearly every tissue of the body. Horizontal gene transfer is common, mixing and matching virulence factors, and Sa is often multidrug resistant. All of these present significant challenges. Of great concern though is that about 30% of humans are chronically colonized, the location being the nasal passages and skin. Sa's presence at these surfaces mean the organism is largely kept away from the main assault of the systemic immune system, which would imply a mucosal vaccine is desired. No mucosal vaccine has been approved in the U.S. for any bacterial pathogen. This is an area with a great lack of knowledge. *E. coli* and *P. aeruginosa* also are mucosal inhabitants. *S. aureus* is also adept at blocking measures the immune system uses to get rid of it, including sucking up antibodies with protein decoys, immunological confusion via antigenic variation of capsule structures, and potent toxins that disable special-ops leukocytes.

"Staph" as it is called is a master of adherence. It uses the host's extracellular matrix (collagen, fibronectin, etc) as a landing pad through the display of surface adhesins termed **MSCRAMMs** (microbial cell surface components recognizing adhesive matrix molecules), which we discussed in ▶ Chap. 7. The host receptors include fibronectin-, fibrinogen-, and collagen-binding proteins. Fibrinogen-binding proteins include clumping factor A and B (CfA and CfB). Vaccination with these proteins protects against invasive disease, and passive immunity also seems possible. Similar studies have been performed with the collagen-binding protein (Cna) and fibronectin-binding protein (FnBps), which have shown efficacy against invasive disease and experimental arthritis, respectively. These targets have not moved into clinical trials.

Other recombinant protein approaches to vaccination have utilized nutrient transporters, including a creative and novel attempt to use a specialized iron transport domain (V710) as immunogen. After showing strong efficacy and safety in animal models, the vaccine progressed through several clinical trials until it was discontinued for unexplained adverse reactions in a patient cohort. Inactivated forms of some of the staphylococcal toxins have also been used with positive results observed for passive immunization studies, suggesting antibodies to the toxins can brunt pathogenesis. Non-protein based vaccines, for example capsular polysaccharide, stemming from the precedent of neisseria and pneumococcus, were also evaluated when conjugated to a protein carrier. Phase I and II clinical trials indicated the vaccine was safe but associated with modest increases in antibodies to the target antigens. This vaccine consisted of only two capsular variants. The similarities between *S. aureus* and *S. pneumoniae* (for which there is a licensed vaccine) makes one wonder whether a staph vaccine should take heed from the capsular vaccine success of pneumococcus. Perhaps a capsular vaccine encompassing most serotypes combined with a protein carrier (iron transporter, adhesin, or secreted toxin) would be a clever way to target multiple virulence strategies of this pathogen.

15.7.4 H. pylori

The global burden of *Helicobacter pylori* infection rivals, if not exceeds, that of *M. tuberculosis*. A vaccine for *H. pylori* is a top priority. Yet, unlike tuberculosis, there are no approved formulations and progress has been slowed by many obstacles. *H. pylori* was the first bacterium demonstrated to cause cancer (cancer of the stomach – gastric cancer – a recognition that earned the Nobel prize). This disease takes years to develop and is associated with the chronic colonization of the mucosa of the stomach. Once colonized, clearance of the bacterium requires strong antibiotics and other drugs over a long term. Even then it may not work. Gastritis and ulcers are acute symptoms, the product of the organism damaging the stomach mucosa and the harsh acid making contact with the tender epithelium. Vaccine studies have not been lacking. No less than six animal models, not including humans, have been used to test various immunogens for efficacy. Mucosal vaccines of the intestinal, oral, nasal, and rectal routes have shown positive results. Human patients make antibodies to major *H. pylori* virulence factors. Some of these include urease, an enzyme that breaks down urea in the stomach, and CagA, a secreted effector that modulates the actin cytoskeleton. Urease was even the subject of a human trial, as was an *H. pylori* whole cell vaccine. Modest results were attained with some adverse reactions, likely from the protein stabilizer included in the formulation. Known for stimulating a Th1-type immune response, driven by the production of mucosal IL-12, the T-cells primed for *H. pylori* antigens declare all-out war on a mucosal battlefield littered with them. The result is inflammation that, over the long run, leads to the major symptoms of these infections, including cancer. The *H. pylori* example is one where we see the need to reach that fulcrum of balance between immunogenicity and safety; stimulating the wrong or too intense an immune response in those that are chronically colonized may do more harm than good.

15.7.5 S. pyogenes

We discussed how several licensed vaccines have focused on childhood diseases. An area where these efforts have fallen short for children include the lack of vaccines for Group A and B streptococcus. Let's first begin with *Streptococcus pyogenes*, otherwise known as Group A Streptococcus (GAS). Worldwide estimates include about 300,000 yearly deaths from GAS and close to 35 million total infections. These are likely underestimates. Many of these infections occur in children and young adults. It can cause rheumatic fever (damage of the heart) in older individuals, especially pregnant women. We know much about the immune response to GAS from the careful studies of Rebecca Lancefield and her colleagues in the 1930s. From this work we learned that a dominant feature of GAS is its ability to produce the M protein, a surface protein that uses its inherent variability in its N terminal domain to deflect opsonophagocytic antibodies, along with short-circuiting a key component of the complement cascade. No doubt a defensive strategy evolved to undercut two major arms of our immune response, the M protein has been sought as the top candidate immunogen for GAS vaccine development. Taking a page from the approaches used to develop capsule-based vaccines, current efforts have focused on building an immunogen that contains as many representative M protein peptide serotypes covering circulating strains. In Western countries, this is achieved by fusing polypeptides in tandem to form a 26-valent M protein construct. The vaccine, however, does not cover other frequent types in other parts of the world. This was overcome by extending the M type valency to 30. Vaccination with many M types does generate opsonophagocytic antibodies against the strains having these M types, and, as such, there have been, and continue to be, extensive clinical studies of their efficacy.

Other approaches have targeted the conserved region of the M protein as a vaccine. The strategy here is that since most strains have this region highly conserved, broad efficacy against most strains can be achieved. Clinical trials using this region of the M protein are also ongoing. The main concern with GAS epitopes is that they may also induce an immune response against host tissues, especially in the heart. This may be a main driver of rheumatic fever in those colonized with GAS. Thus, all vaccine attempts against GAS should take special precaution to assess for these symptoms in animal and human trials.

15.7.6 *S. agalactiae*

What GAS is to adolescents, Group B Streptococcus (GBS), or *Streptococcus agalactiae*, is to newborns. GBS is the top infectious disease risk to neonates, resulting in invasive infections of meningitis, pneumoniae, and bloodstream infections or neonatal sepsis. The issue is two-fold; first, nearly one-third of all women are colonized with GBS, primarily in the urogenital tract. This means infants are exposed to GBS as they pass through the birth canal. Second, the infant has an underdeveloped immune system and thus is not as equipped to handle an invasive pathogen such as GBS. Most vaccine efforts have focused on the development of a capsular polysaccharide immunogen, a major virulence factor that resists phagocytosis. There are at least 10 antigenic types of capsule, with about half causing most of the infections in people. Given the risk to newborns, vaccination plans have centered around inducing antibody-based immunity in the mother that can be transferred to child in utero. There is evidence that such antibodies can protect against the most invasive GBS. As such, several clinical trials were initiated and some are still ongoing that are evaluating capsular polysaccharide types conjugated to CRM (the inactivated diphtheria toxin

carrier also used in the capsular vaccines for pneumococcu and neisseria). There is optimism such an approach will be feasible. Challenges still remain, including the notion that effective screening of expectant mothers for GBS has reduced the incidence of neonate infection from 4–20 fold in the last 20 years, as well as that GBS remains sensitive to penicillin with those testing positive being administered the antibiotic to lower transmission rates. The developers of a vaccine will have to consider that these simple measures have also been effective at reducing infections.

15.8 Vaccination Against Intracellular Bacteria

The invasion and parasitism of host cells by intracellular bacteria is a marvel of pathogen evolution, and bravery. Straight into the heat of the fire, they risk it all. It may be worth it. By hiding inside host cells, bacteria act like viruses. This means their antigens may be shielded from detection and almost certainly shielded from antibodies. The current licensed U.S. vaccines, for the most part, all rely on strong Th2 B-cell antibody responses for protection. These antibodies likely neutralize toxin or capsule and brunt the strong positive impact these factors have on virulence. B-cell responses have little effect on intracellular bacteria unless the pathogen is undergoing extracellular transit, either hopping to a new host cell or at the initial stages of infection when it is searching for its Trojan horse host. Alum, the adjuvant in many of approved vaccines, is also known for driving humoral responses. The challenge is really two-fold. First, the vaccine formulation must contain an antigen (s) and adjuvant that drive the presentation of the antigen to T-cells and second, the infected host cell must be able to display that antigen on its surface so readied T-cells can pick the bad from the good apples.

The above challenges are personified by chlamydia species, which here serves as an example of the challenges for vaccine development for intracellular bacteria. Chlamydia are obligate intracellular Gram-negatives that infect a diverse range of mammals. Two subspecies are important for human infections. *Chlamydia trachomatis* causes ocular infections. In the developing world, it is a leading cause of blindness. Other serovars of this species cause infections of the genitalia. They are associated with infertility and ectopic pregnancy, and, as such, are classified as a sexually transmitted disease. *Chlamydia pneumoniae* causes bronchitis and pneumonia. Chronic infection is possible and may not be readily treatable with antibiotics. There is no vaccine. As mentioned above, intracellular bacteria often hide themselves and their antigens from the immune system by infecting host cells. Chlamydia is a master of this process; in addition to residing in reticulate bodies in the host phagosome, generally safe, when they bud off to infect new cells they are also encapsulated. These bubbles are like an air freshener spray for a stinky home; they cover up the true insidious nature of the pathogen, making it unrecognizable by antibodies. To make matters worse for the host, chlamydia shuts down the display f antigens on the surface of MHC. It also hides its cards. here is evidence only a single chlamydial protein localizes to he host cell cytoplasm. Without much to choose from, the ormal innate immune mechanism of breaking down the athogen with a proteasome and displaying antigenic pep-ides on the host cell surface is infrequent. Amazingly, this rotein, termed CPAF, is a protease that actually chops up ost proteins responsible for the expression of the MHC omplex on the surface!

That said, sometimes the host does win out and the phago-ome directs the degradation of chlamydia antigens. In these nstances, the best displayed antigen is a major outer mem-rane protein termed MOMP. MOMP is highly variable in mino acid sequence in certain regions, probably to again onfuse the immune system, but certain regions of the vari-ble region seem to lead to more neutralizing antibodies than others. In vitro T-cell selection methods using MOMP, anti-gen presenting cells, and T cells from infected patients (a reenactment of what happens during normal immunity in the spleen), has confirmed that cell-based immunity against chla-mydia is possible. These cytotoxic T-cells kill chlamydia-infected cells in culture, a finding that suggests MOMP should be developed as a possible antigen in a new vaccine. Clinical trials of whole-cell inactivated chlamydia have been attempted and do produce a verifiable immune response, but the immu-nity is weak and short-lived. Purified MOMP-like antigens mixed with newer adjuvants that direct a T-cell response may represent a more feasible solution to the chlamydia vaccine problem. Other promising antigens for a vaccine include the use of polymorphic membrane proteins and genetically atten-uated whole-cell forms (now made possible by advances in chlamydia reverse genetics development). The evaluation of MOMP antigens in human clinical trials is ongoing. In sum-mary, identifying T-cell epitopes from patients that have cleared these infections may be a path forward for the devel-opment of vaccines against intracellular bacteria. It is also clear that cell infection assays that identify bacterial proteins that are localized to the host cell phagosome or cytoplasm may also be candidates since they may be more likely pro-cessed as peptides on MHC receptors. Whole-cell vaccines using inactivated intracellular pathogens that drive both B and T-cell responses also offer the prospect of ramping up the immune response to a diverse set of proteins that might not otherwise be abundant during natural immunity.

15.9 Ideological Barriers

We end this chapter with an example of a new threat to solv-ing humanity's bacterial crisis, that of ideology. Unlike the challenges we have already discussed, where the solutions will ultimately arise from rigorous science and careful medi-cine, this new foe is undeterred by discourse of reason. Its energy is fear, a pipeline of it channeled through a parent's love of their children and their relentless will to protect them from an encroaching worldview. Its messengers deceitfully manipulate the gifts and persuasion of science for their own

cause, preying upon those that respect these gifts but have not been taught to properly interpret or use them. This takes us to Lyme disease and *Borellia burgdorferi*, the fastidious spirochete that causes it, and how quickly promise turns to poison in today's vaccination culture. *B. burgdorferi* infects its human host from a tick that is feeding on that host. The tick is its arthropod vector, which is widespread throughout the world. Other borellia species are the cause of a related disease termed relapsing fever. This malady is characterized by a very high fever that can resolve on its own but then reap-pear. It is treatable with antibiotics, as is Lyme-disease, but long term sequelae from the infection can remain. The num-ber of confirmed cases of Lyme-disease in the U.S. is about 20,000 per year. This is no doubt a substantial underestimate as most cases go unreported, are asymptomatic, or are assumed to be another disease, particularly autoimmune dis-orders. There are >10 genospecies of borellia with hundreds of different subspecies or strains. These strains may vary con-siderably in their genomic content, a finding that may com-plicate attempts at a universal vaccine. They may contain up to 6–10 different plasmids with the content differing between strains. Two of the dominant antigens developed as immuno-gens include the Vmp-like sequence expressed (VlsE) factors, a lipoprotein with such antigenic variation in its variable domain that upwards of a million different types are thought to be possible. Another antigen is one of the outer surface proteins (or OSPs), of which there are at least six, of which one (OspA) has been the target of significant vaccine devel-opment. Animal studies have demonstrated borellia super-natants can protect against infection, and passive transfer protection to recombinant Osp proteins is possible, but only if antibodies are present before the bite by the tick. This raises the interesting hypothesis that efficacious antibodies against an arthropod-born disease like Lyme occur by acting inside or at the tick interface. In fact, some Osps are not expressed in the animal host, which further supports this contention.

The efficacy of OspA in animal studies led to its develop-ment in phase I-III clinical trials. Efficacy after a third boost was substantial; asymptomatic seroconversion rates reached nearly all the recipients. LYME$_{rix}$^{tm} was approved by the U.S. FDA in 1999, but poor sales, largely due to fears the vac-cine caused arthritis in a limited number of recipients (which were not substantiated), led GlaxoSmithKline to pull it from the market 3 years later. The vaccine remains unused (see "out of the box" earlier in this chapter). The Lyme vaccine story highlights the many challenges, including those not scientific, facing the microbe hunter of the future. In addition to astute detectives searching for the best and safest antigen, the microbe hunter will also need to be an educator. It is not just cases like this that raise the level of concern, recent pushback for use of the measles vaccine, mostly over false claims that it causes autism, led to reductions in its use in some communi-ties, especially where parents are allowed to opt-out of vacci-nation. Fueled by naïve celebrities with no scientific training, and in some cases politicians appealing to a fringe base of sup-porters, the false information spreads. The microbe hunter, once only a finder of truth, now must also become its defender.

Summary of Key Concepts

1. Vaccination has had a profound positive impact on human health. It is a cost-effective and nearly universal form of preventative healthcare that strengthens the human immune system against pathogen invaders.

2. Bacterial vaccines can be comprised of attenuated but live bacterial cells, killed cells, inactivated bacterial cultured supernatants, or purified or partially purified bacterial components, including secreted toxins or surface polysaccharides. The latter components are currently found in commonly licensed vaccines.

3. Ideal bacterial vaccines should be safe, efficacious, scalable, and store well.

4. Vaccine construction begins with the discovery of bacterial antigens that generate a robust immune response that targets a key bacterial process (or processes). Candidate antigens undergo a rigorous testing process that begins with the demonstration of success in relevant animal models and the progression through phase I-III clinical trials.

5. Adjuvants are a substance or substances added to a bacterial component that stimulates that components antigenicity, or propensity to form a robust immune response. Some adjuvants can direct the immune response to be either more antibody-mediated or cellular-mediated.

6. Most of the world's bacterial diseases do not have a vaccine approved for human use. There are many challenges that lie ahead, including the development of vaccines for bacteria that reside within our biome and those that prefer or require an intracellular lifestyle.

❓ Expand Your Knowledge

1. The first fourteen chapters of this work provides the knowledge necessary to understand the major underpinnings of bacterial virulence. Based upon your reading of this chapter, and those preceding it, choose a sensible strategy (or strategies) for the construction of an immunogen from at least three different problematic bacterial species for which there currently is no approved vaccine.

2. As Project Manager of Novartis' vaccine design and evaluation unit, your objective is to make a capsule-based vaccine against *E. coli*. Describe what will be needed for this vaccine to be approved by regulatory agencies and how your vaccine will be universally effective.

3. Compare the composition of the vaccines meant to protect patients against pertussis, diphtheria, tetanus, haemophilus, pneumonococcus, and meningococcus. Share with your peers and instructor two important findings may be relevant for future vaccine design.

Suggested Reading

Bode C, Zhao G, Steinhagen F, Kinjo T, Klinman DM (2011) CpG DNA as a vaccine adjuvant. Expert Rev Vaccines 10:499–511. https://doi.org/10.1586/erv.10.174

Briere EC et al (2014) Prevention and control of haemophilus influenzae type b disease: recommendations of the advisory committee on immunization practices (ACIP). MMWR Recomm Rep 63:1–14

Brock T (1961) Milestones in Microbiology. Thomas Brock; Prentice-Hall International

Di Pasquale A, Preiss S, Tavares Da Silva F, Garçon N (2015) Vaccine adjuvants: from 1920 to 2015 and beyond. Vaccines (Basel) 3:320–343 https://doi.org/10.3390/vaccines3020320

Excler JL, Kim JH (2016) Accelerating the development of a group A Streptococcus vaccine: an urgent public health need. Clin Exp Vaccine Res 5:101–107. https://doi.org/10.7774/cevr.2016.5.2.101

Girard MP, Preziosi MP, Aguado MT, Kieny MP (2006) A review of vaccine research and development: meningococcal disease. Vaccine 24:4692–4700. https://doi.org/10.1016/j.vaccine.2006.03.034

Griffiths KL, Khader SA (2014) Novel vaccine approaches for protection against intracellular pathogens. Curr Opin Immunol 28:58–63. https://doi.org/10.1016/j.coi.2014.02.003

Lambrecht BN, Kool M, Willart MA, Hammad H (2009) Mechanism of action of clinically approved adjuvants. Curr Opin Immunol 21:23–29. https://doi.org/10.1016/j.coi.2009.01.004

Leininger E et al (1991) Pertactin, an Arg-Gly-Asp-containing Bordetella pertussis surface protein that promotes adherence of mammalian cells. Proc Natl Acad Sci U S A 88:345–349

Nuccitelli A, Rinaudo CD, Maione D (2015) Group B Streptococcus vaccine: state of the art. Ther Adv Vaccines 3:76–90. https://doi.org/10.1177/2051013615579869

Plotkin S (2014) History of vaccination. Proc Natl Acad Sci U S A 111:12283–12287. https://doi.org/10.1073/pnas.1400472111

Poolman JT, Hallander HO (2007) Acellular pertussis vaccines and the role of pertactin and fimbriae. Expert Rev Vaccines 6:47–56. https://doi.org/10.1586/14760584.6.1.47

Priebe GP, Goldberg JB (2014) Vaccines for Pseudomonas aeruginosa: a long and winding road. Expert Rev Vaccines 13:507–519. https://doi.org/10.1586/14760584.2014.890053

Tan SY, Kwok E (2012) Albert Calmette (1863–1933): originator of the BCG vaccine. Singapore Med J 53:433–434

Tritto E, Mosca F, De Gregorio E (2009) Mechanism of action of licensed vaccine adjuvants. Vaccine 27:3331–3334. https://doi.org/10.1016/j.vaccine.2009.01.084

Antibiotics ... and Their Destruction

© Springer Nature Switzerland AG 2019
A. W. Maresso, *Bacterial Virulence*, https://doi.org/10.1007/978-3-030-20464-8_16

Learning Goals

In this chapter, the learner is exposed to the history, structures and molecular mechanism of action of the major classes of clinically-used antibiotics. This includes those antibiotics which inhibit cell wall, DNA, and/or protein synthesis, as well as those that disrupt membrane function. The creative ways in which bacteria counter the action of antibiotics, including efflux, modification of target, or destruction of drug, are discussed. Future avenues for the development of new antibacterial measures are highlighted. The learner will be well-versed in the arms race between pathogenic bacteria and chemical antibiotics and the steps to be taken in the future for humanity to stay ahead.

16.1 Introduction

Antibiotic literally means "against life." In truth, antibiotics target a narrow range of species that exist on Earth and almost all of it is invisible to our eyes. Since the first cellular life replicated and evolved greater abilities to inhabit new niches of our early planet, prokaryotic organisms have been engaging in chemical warfare. When we think of the word "bacteria", the connotation tends to group all of them as alike, maybe on the same side. They are far from this. Bacteria engage in competition, constantly, and the battles they wage for space and sustenance are fierce. Furthermore, other species of life have recognized that bacteria are a threat too. Accordingly, they have built their own chemical weapons against them. Much cytoplasm has been spilled in the eons leading to this point, but in doing so, it has generated another problem. The modern revolution in the use of antibiotics as medicines to treat bacterial infections, a 30 billion dollar-a-year industry, is almost entirely built of what nature has already constructed. This industry, though, is now in great distress, shrinking under the threat of resistance and the inability to make new drugs that keep pace. Here, we discuss the successes and losses of this struggle so the microbe hunter can learn from past mistakes and create a brighter therapeutic future.

16.2 What Are Antibiotics and What Do they Effect?

How are antibiotics against life? Broadly, antibiotics perform one of two main activities. They can stop bacteria from growing, in which case they are called **bacteriostatic**; or they can outright kill them, in which case they are called **bactericidal**. Bacteriostatic antibiotics work by inhibiting a key step in the physiology of the bacterium, leading to the inability to divide. They don't often die from this event, but they can't execute fully on their pathogenic potential. Since pathogenesis is related to the levels of the organism at the infection site, preventing their levels from increasing, perhaps allowing the immune system time to catch up, is an effective way to treat bacterial infections. This contrast with bactericidal antibiotics. The end point here is death with substantial reduction in the overall burden of bacteria expected. There is some belief that bactericidal antibiotics, which lack a life or death selective pressure, might lead to lower levels of antibiotic resistance, a topic we get into below. The line between static and cidal is often blurred since many antibiotics do a little of both depending on their concentration.

When considering how antibiotics are against bacterial life, the key word is synthesis. All antibiotics, in one way or another, stop the synthesis of biomolecules important for the production of key molecules. There are four main synthetic pathways that antibiotics target. One of them is the making of new **polymers of nucleic acid**, DNA or RNA. These antibiotics prevent the replication of these molecules and, in doing so, prevent the production of daughter cells. We will learn more about the specific mechanism behind this inhibition but suffice it to say that these antibiotics disrupt the function of the enzymes that untie the DNA during its duplication. A second way antibiotics work is by **stopping the production of one of the four nucleosides** that are used to construct DNA. This too inhibits DNA synthesis but at a more upstream step, the production of folate, which is a biosynthetic intermediate in the pathway to make thymidine. Targeting DNA synthesis is exceptionally clever. Striking right at the heart of what allows cells to divide, this class of antibiotics is widely employed in the chemical warfare microbes use against each other.

DNA synthesis inhibition is one thing, **protein synthesis inhibition** is another. This is the third major way antibiotics stop bacteria. Since protein production is a constant part of any cell's needs, preventing its ability to make new proteins is an effective way to halt or kill them. This class of antibiotics does so by targeting the complex needed to translate the RNA message into a linear polypeptide, the ribosome complex. The fourth pathway antibiotics can inhibit is the selective targeting of the **production of the building blocks of the cell wall**. In both Gram-positive (external cell wall) and Gram-negative (cell wall lies between the outer and inner membranes) bacteria, the cell wall helps maintain the form or structure of the bacterial cell, kind of like a skeleton does for vertebrates (see ▶ Chap. 2). The cell wall is the consummate example of a structure composed of repeating and orderly building blocks – like bricks in a wall. Some antibiotics can interfere with the addition of new bricks such that the structure collapses, and the cell with it. Finally, antibiotics can **disrupt the bacterial membrane**. All of these are discussed below, with ◻ Fig. 16.1 summarizing the cellular functions antibiotics inhibit.

16.3 Inhibition of Protein Synthesis

Protein synthesis in bacteria occurs with the coordinated action of key cellular players. This includes messenger RNA, which relays the information from the DNA code to the pro-

Fig. 16.1 The actions of
ntibiotics. In general, most
mmonly used antibiotics
rget four distinct bacterial
rocesses. These include the
hibition of protein synthesis,
e inhibition of DNA or RNA
nthesis, the inhibition of cell
all synthesis, or the disruption
f the membrane. Not shown,
ut also important for one class
f antibiotics, is the inhibition of
late biosynthesis

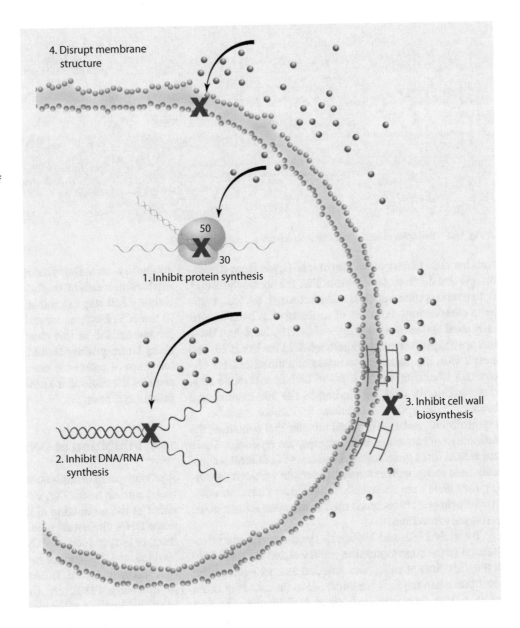

tein translation machinery, and the machinery itself, which includes two ribosomal subunits (50S and 30S). These two key factors come together like a sandwich with the 50S and 30S enclosing the mRNA. The 50S slice peels back a bit and allows transfer RNAs (tRNAs), each charged with an amino acid, to enter the complex and land on its appropriate three-letter codon on the mRNA template. The ribosome complex scans the mRNA, one codon at a time, and inserts the next tRNA loaded with an amino acid into the complex. As it does this, each amino acid is joined to the previous one and the polypeptide chain grows. This is called the **peptidyl-transferase reaction**. The process is often initiated in bacteria with a formylated methionine tRNA, termed initiation, and ends when a protein release factor cleaves the polypeptide after the ribosome scans a termination codon. In this complex, the site on the mRNA that interacts with the ribosome and the growing polypeptide chain is termed the **P**

site. The incoming tRNA carrying the amino acid to be added to the polypeptide chain lies in the **A site**. Antibiotics can react with the A or P sites on the 30S subunit in a way that prevents either the incoming tRNA from properly landing on the complex or the new amino acid from being properly joined to the growing polypeptide; *i.e.*, inhibit the peptidyltransferase reaction.

There are several classes of antibiotics that target protein synthesis in bacteria (◘ Fig. 16.2). The first class was uncovered in the 1940s, produced by a species of streptomyces bacteria, and named appropriately, streptomycin. This class of antibiotics is termed **aminoglycosides** because of their repeating cyclic sugar rings affixed to an amino substituent. There are over 20 different types of aminoglycosides that have been developed and used in human infections, preferentially against Gram-negative enteric bacteria that may cause abdominal, urinary tract, or bloodstream infections.

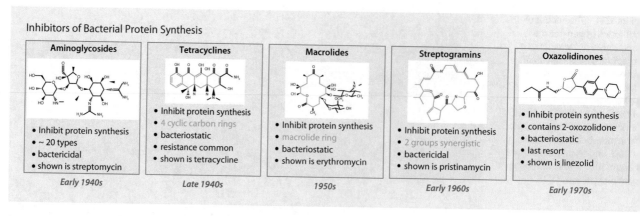

Fig. 16.2   Examples of antibiotics that inhibit bacterial protein synthesis

Another class of antibiotics, discovered (again from streptomyces) and developed a few years after the aminoglycosides, is the **tetracycline subclass**. Characterized by four cyclic hydrocarbon rings, this class of antibiotics has been historically used against a wide range of bacteria, including those that are obligate intracellular pathogens. In the late 1940s and early 1950s, the **macrolide subclass** of antibiotics were discovered. Characterized by a 14–16 carbon macrolide ring, these antibiotics work by binding to the 50S subunit and blocking polypeptide elongation. Its famous member is erythromycin, isolated from soil samples that contained the actinomycete bacterium *Saccharopolyspora erythraea*. There are at least three generations of this class of antibiotics clinically used today, with **extended-spectrum versions** (meaning they have been chemically modified to extend to other strains or species of bacteria) used as therapies for suspected respiratory infections.

The early 1950s and 1960s saw the discovery and introduction of the **streptogramins**, again isolated from soli bacteria. This class of antibiotics function as a two-compound duet that when together are hundreds to thousands of times more potent than each compound individually. The first compound, referred to as the "A" compound, is a large mactolactone with unsaturated bonds. The second compound, the "B" compound, is cyclic hexadepsipeptide. The A version inhibits the binding of the aminoacyl tRNA to the acceptor or A site of the 50S ribosome. The B version inhibits peptide elongation at the P site, often inducing the premature release of the not fully synthesized protein. The two famous members are virginiamycin, isolated from the soil of Virginia, which is commonly used as a feed additive in agriculture, and pristinamycin, which has been used for more than 50 years to treat drug-resistant staphylococcus, enterococcus, and streptococcus infections. A more recently developed class of antibiotics, the **oxazolidinones**, also target bacterial protein synthesis. Characterized by an oxazolidone core structure (5-membered ring with nitrogen and oxygen), this class of antibiotics is completely synthetic, developed in the 1970s and 1980s by pharmaceutical companies. As such, it was the first completely new class of antibiotic in over 30 years. Regarded as a "**last resort**" antibiotic, clinicians primarily use it on Gram-positive bacteria already resistant to other

antibiotics, including vancomycin-resistant enterococci and methicillin-resistant staphylococci. It is believed to inhibit the very first step in protein synthesis, initiation, by binding to the 50S ribosome. Linezolid, the first antibiotic approved for human use in this class (2000), has been used against many Gram-positive bacteria since its approval with overall low rates of resistance reported. Figure 16.3 summarize some of the molecular knowledge of how antibiotics inhibit protein synthesis.

16.4 Inhibition of DNA Synthesis

A second group of antibiotics, made up of three main classes, target nucleic acid, DNA or RNA. The level of inhibition is either at the production of the nucleosides needed to make more DNA, the actual replication or topology of the DNA itself, or the production of the message (RNA). As you might imagine, if DNA cannot be faithfully copied, no daughter cells will be produced. The first class in this group, discovered in the early 1930s, are the **sulfonamides** (Fig. 16.4). Identified by their sulfonamide chemical group (sulfur with two doubly bonded oxygens and an amino substituent), antibiotics in this class target **folate biosynthesis**. Folate is an important nutrient that is used as a building block for the synthesis of thymidine triphosphate, the precursor to thymidine, one of the four essential nucleotides that make up DNA. In bacteria, the enzyme dihydroperoate synthase is necessary for the production of dihydropteroate (DHP) from GTP, a necessary step in the biosynthesis of folate. This enzyme is not made by eukaryotes; this is why humans must acquire folate from their diet and why it is an important nutrient for pregnant mothers. A second enzyme downstream of DHP in the pathway to the synthesis of thymidine is dihydrofolate reductase (DHFR). Both of these enzymes are inhibited by sulfonamide antibiotics and, in some cases, the combinatorial use of these types of antibiotics provides a synergistic and potent inhibition of bacterial growth.

The next class of DNA inhibitors are the **quinolones**, characterized by their heterocyclic aromatic core structure around which numerous substituents are added to induce potency or functionality (Fig. 16.5). They rose to popularity in the

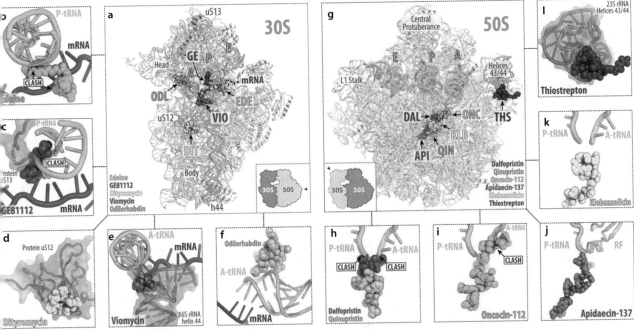

Fig. 16.3 Ribosome-targeting antibiotics. In this panel, the binding sites of several antibiotics that inhibit protein synthesis are shown in relation to the E, P, and A ribosome sites. In several cases, it becomes readily apparent as to how these antibiotics prevent translocation. Overview **a** and close-up views **b–f** of the binding sites of the peptide antibiotics **b** edeine B (EDE, green), **c** GE81112 (GE, red), **d** dityromycin (DIT, yellow), **e** viomycin (VIO, magenta), and **f** odilorhabdin (ODL, orange), which target the small (30S) ribosomal subunit. The mRNA (blue) and anticodon stem loop (ASL) of A-, P-, and E-site tRNAs (cyan) are shown, and 16S rRNA helix h44 as well as ribosomal proteins uS12 and uS13 are highlighted for reference. Overview **g** and close-up views **h–l** of the binding sites of the peptide antibiotics **h** streptogramin type A (dalfoprsitin, DAL, red) and type B (quinupristin, QIN, orange), **i** oncocin-112 (ONC, green), **j** apidaecin-137 (API, magenta), **k** klebsazolicin (KLB, yellow), and **l** thiostrepton (THS, blue), which target the large (50S) ribosomal subunit. The relative position of A, P, and E-site tRNAs (cyan) are shown, and 23S rRNA helices H43/44 is highlighted for reference. (Adapted from Wilson et al. (see *suggested readings*) under a creative commons license. (▶ https://creativecommons.org/licenses/by/4.0/))

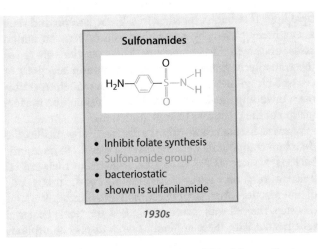

Fig. 16.4 Example of an antibiotic that inhibits folate synthesis

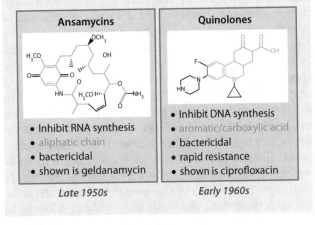

Fig. 16.5 Examples of antibiotics that inhibit bacterial nucleic acid synthesis

1960s after they were discovered as a byproduct in a reaction mechanism aimed at making anti-malarial drugs. Their utility is underscored by their potent action against both Gram-negative and Gram-positive pathogens, particularly in the treatment of urinary tract infections or indwelling devices. Their aromatic frame, a scaffold for the addition of many different combinations of chemical substituents, has meant that thousands of variants have been synthesized and tested for

antibacterial activity. Over the past 70 years, four different generations of this class have been made, each generation either overcoming previous resistance or improving the selectivity towards certain pathogenic bacteria. Their exact mechanism of action is still uncertain, but it is clear that they target DNA replication. Because of its string-like nature of polynucleotides, during replication DNA can become entangled. The cell understands this and has evolved two enzymes, appropriately named DNA gyrase and DNA topoisomerase ("topo"), that help "unwind" the DNA at certain points in its replication. This includes introducing double strand breaks in DNA so that it can be unknotted and then re-ligated back together. Replication can then continue. Quinolones seem to inhibit gyrase and topo's ability to complete this step, and, as such, the cell accumulates double-strand breaks along its DNA that eventually become lethal to the bacterial cell. Quinolones are synthetic, man-made antibiotics. This is interesting because the levels of antimicrobial resistance in this class is high, thereby raising the intriguing question as to whether bacteria have encountered similar chemical warfare from their neighbors in the evolutionary past, or, if the absolutely critical requirement for DNA to be fidel places a strong evolutionary pressure on overcoming its inhibition. The final class of nucleic acid inhibitors are the **ansamycins**. Discovered in the 1960s from what was then called a streptomyces bacterium, this class is characterized by its unusual aliphatic chain forming a loop off a central aromatic core. The recognizable member of this class is rifamycin and its derivatives, which displays activity against pathogenic mycobacteria, including *M. tuberculosis*. This class of antibiotics are unique in that they target RNA polymerase, the enzyme responsible for the synthesis of RNA from a DNA template. By binding strongly to RNA polymerase, it inhibits the ability of the RNA to proceed through the polymerase, which halts production.

16.5   Inhibition of Cell Wall Biosynthesis

The third way antibiotics effect bacteria is through the inhibition of one of the many enzymatic reactions that leads to the synthesis and stability of the cell wall. The cell wall of bacteria, also known as the peptidoglycan, is composed of a repeating series of sugar moieties linked in a long chain with interspersed crossbridges composed of amino acids. These cross bridges impart strength onto the structure and help support the overall shape of the bacterial cell especially in the face of all the osmotic pressures placed on the membrane. As we learned in ▶ Chap. 2, Gram-positive bacteria have a very thick cell wall that is external to their sole membrane. Gram-negative bacteria have a thin cell wall sandwiched between the outer and inner membrane. Antibiotics that target the cell wall of Gram-negatives must first cross the outer membrane, which can be an additional barrier to their effectiveness. Antibiotics disrupt the structure of the cell wall and, in doing so, effect the integrity of the entire bacterial cell. To understand how cell wall modifying antibiotics function, we must first consider the various enzymatic steps that lead to its assembly, using *E. coli* as the model organism. The first step begins in the cytoplasm by a six step enzymatic assembly pathway carried out by the so-called **Mur enzymes** (A through F). The word "mur" comes from murein, another name for the peptidoglycan, which is a derivative of a Greek word that means "wall." The Mur enzymes are responsible for the synthesis of the repeating sugar units and its peptide extension, the basic repeating

component of the cell wall. Mur A and B convert the sugar UDP-N-acetyl-glucosamine (UDP-GlcNAc) to UDP-N-acetyl-muramic acid (UDP-MurNAc), a key modification that primes the glycan to grow a string of amino acids, usually five, often called the **pentapeptide**. This first key step is a target of some cell wall antibiotics, including fosfomycin which inhibits MurA, and is used in the treatment of urinary tract infections. MurC – F next catalyze the formation of UDP-MurNAc-pentapeptide, effectively building, one amino acid at a time, the growing pentapeptide from the precursor UDP-MurNAc.

The second step of cell wall biosynthesis involves the formation of the **lipid I** and **lipid II** components from the UDP-MurNAc-pentapeptide. The objective of these reactions is to turn the glycan-peptide complex into something that is chemically consistent with association with the membrane(s) of the bacterial cell. The first reaction in this sequence is catalyzed by the enzyme MraY, which adds a massive 55-carbon moiety, termed C55-undecaprenyl phosphate, to the activated phosphate of UDP-MurNAc to form lipid I. In the second step, UDP-N-acetyl-glucosamine (UDP-Glc-NAc) is added to lipid I by the glycosyltransferase MurG. This makes lipid II, the fundamental subunit of the peptidoglycan. Several antibiotics inhibit these steps, including tunicamycin, which resembles the substrate of MraY and inhibits its catalysis. The completion of this step in the synthesis of the cell wall occurs after the entire complex of lipid II is transferred from the cytoplasmic side of the membrane to either the periplasm (Gram-negative) or external part of the cell (Gram-positive). After flipping lipid II, the final reaction to complete the cell wall structure includes the linkage of multiple lipid II subunits together in a linear fashion and then strengthening them by covalent crosslinks between amino acids residing in the pentapeptide. These reactions are called the **transglycosylation** and **transpeptidation** reactions of cell wall biosynthesis and are the targets for numerous antibiotics, including the famous penicillins, which inhibit the formation of the crosslinks (transpeptidation).

As was discussed above for the discovery of penicillin, the **β-lactam** compounds were the first to be noted to have antibacterial activity (◘ Fig. 16.6). Characterized by their central β-lactam ring, they are covalent inhibitors of the transpeptidation reaction (final step) in cell wall biosynthesis. Without this step, the cell wall is not crosslinked and weak; bacterial cells treated with these antibiotics often display amorphous cell structures and are unhealthy. They are amongst the most commonly used antibiotics, accounting for most worldwide sales, and have undergone multiple generations of chemical maturation to overcome resistance mechanisms and broaden their activity. Unlike most of the antibiotics discussed thus far, which come from other bacteria or are non-natural and have been chemically synthesized, the β-lactam class originates from fungi. Looking very similar structurally to the dipeptide Ala-Ala, which is a common component of the crossbridge pentapeptide, these antibiotics bind and inactivate the transpeptidation enzymes that recognize the equivalent structure in the pentapeptide.

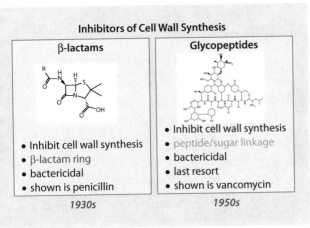

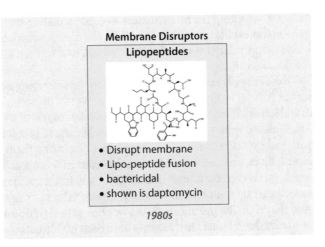

Fig. 16.6 Examples of antibiotics that inhibit bacterial cell wall synthesis

Fig. 16.7 Example of an antibiotic that disrupts bacterial membranes

The second major class of cell wall biosynthesis inhibitors include the **glycopetide** antibiotics, discovered in the early 1950s with the isolation of the best represented antibiotic of this class, vancomycin. Characterized by a peptide linked to a sugar, they resemble in structure the pentapeptide of lipid II, and, as such, bind to the terminal two alanines of free pentapeptide. This inhibits their crosslinking and thus the formation of a strong cell wall. Glycopeptide antibiotics are often considered the second choice antibiotic, used when resistance to β-lactam antibiotics is suspected. They are effective against Gram-positive bacteria, particularly enterococci and staphylococci. The recent emergence of vancomycin resistant forms of these Gram-positive species means that both classes of cell wall modifying antibiotics are ineffective against these pathogens.

16.6 Disruption of Membrane Function

In our final survey of different classes of antibiotics, we finish with the **lipopeptides**, whose star is daptomycin (Fig. 16.7). As the name suggests, daptomycin was also discovered from a streptomyces sample as early as the 1980s, and even tested for safety in human trials. The efforts were put on hold by pharma until the emergence of superbugs of resistant Gram-positive staphylococci emerged, therefore pushing the drive to derive new, and previously under-characterized, antibiotics. Approved in the early 2000s for use against such infections, daptomycin represents a unique class of antibiotics that target the Gram-positive bacterial cell membrane. They are characterized by a lipopeptide structure (essentially a lipid linked to a peptide) that has affinity for bacterial lipids. Thought to form tiny aggregates on the membrane surface, lipopeptide antibiotics disrupt the membrane structure, leading to its depolarization and loss of function, possibly also generating holes that eventually kill the cell. Other membrane-acting antibiotics include **defensins** (produced by eukaryotic organisms) and **lantibiotics** (produced by bacteria). Defensins are antimicrobial peptides produced at mucosal surfaces. In general, they may contain unusual structures and amino acid combinations that make them resistant to proteases but still able to insert into bacterial membranes. Some bacteria also produce peptide antibiotics that also are cationic but hydrophobic enough to insert into membranes; gramicidin and polymyxin are examples. In general, these antibiotics are highly toxic because at high concentrations they can disrupt the membranes of eukaryotic cells. Lantibiotics are peptide antibiotics characterized by a special amino acid peptide combination of cysteine and alanine, termed a lanthionine group. They are made by some Gram-positive bacteria, their mechanism of action also membrane disrupting, and are commonly added to food as a preservative to prevent bacteria spoilage.

16.7 Mechanisms of Antibiotic Resistance

16.7.1 Fairly Alarmed Here

At this point, it may be necessary to provide an emotional backdrop as a lead into the next section. Imagine you are a parent, it is night, and you are at rest in your home. It is a home normally full of peace and silence, only the clocks making their constant tick fill the still air of the evening. It's cold outside but not in.

Then there comes a sound opposite to the tranquility of that moment; a hoarse, irregular, and loud sound. It's the sound of unwell, of unhealthy, of stress and sometimes death. The coughing grows, becoming more frequent. The peace now shattered, you rush into the bedroom hallway and realize its coming from your child's room. Racing towards her, she is hunched over and heaving, each breath a strain. The remainder of the evening is spent in a hospital room. After the evaluation, the physicians know the cause. They even know how to treat it. They try to but more nights pass just like this one. Each new antibiotic fails and test results show most of the antibiotics have no chance of working at all. The underlying cause, a bacterium seated deep in the alveoli, is growing, wrecking the fine structure needed to deliver oxygen to the capillaries which give it to the life-nourishing blood. Supportive therapy of fluids, steroids, and rest are all the doctors can suggest.

This is the new and growing reality. Now, like any story or movie, it's a bit exaggerated. Our bodies, generally, do a wonderful job of killing the invaders that try to take control of us. The immune system has any one of dozens of ways to protect you, and this entire volume has been spent discussing them, especially in what we have already addressed in ▶ Chaps. 4 and 5. But before the advent of antibiotics, any infection that was caused by a bacterium could, in theory, take your life. And they did! The pre-antibiotic era was one with significant mortality due to what until recently have been highly curable infections. Life went on, but it was not uncommon to know of a child, or an adult, that succumbed to a bacterial infection. How many people can you name at the moment that have died from a bacterial infection? And how many times in your life were you or someone you know administered antibiotics and made a full recovery? Children are not an exception. Bacteria cause hundreds of types of infections and in every major tissue or organ of the body. The lungs are one case, but as we saw in ▶ Chap. 14 on sepsis, systemic infections originate from just about everywhere.

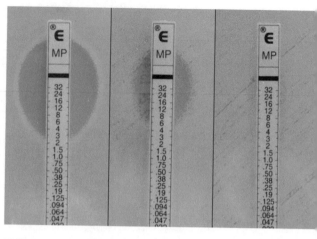

☐ **Fig. 16.8** Antibiotic sensitivity and resistance. A so-called E-test is one way to determine the level of sensitivity or resistance to a particular antibiotic. A strip that contains different levels of antibiotic is embedded into an agar medium seeded with the bacterium in question. The point in which the halo of clearance intersects the strip is a rough estimate of the minimum inhibitory concentration of antibiotic for that strain. Shown here are three strains of *Burkholderia ubonensis* and three different sensitivities (high to low from left to right) to meropenem, a β-lactam antibiotic. Left (an MIC of 3 μg/mL; center an MIC of 6 μg/mL and right a resistant isolate with an MIC of at least 32 μg/mL. (Adapted from Wagner et al. (see *suggested readings*) under a creative commons license. (▶ https://creativecommons.org/licenses/by/4.0/))

16.7.2 Bacterial Advantage

What are the most significant threats to winning or losing the microbial war? We have discussed the need for vaccines for some major bacterial infections of humans, and the emergence or reemergence of bacteria not often encountered by our kind, but at the top of this list must be the failure of some of our most promising drugs to kill them. This concept has been termed **antibiotic resistance** (☐ Fig. 16.8). The phrase is used often in the media and the scientific literature; even the most uninterested in the topic likely know of it. Yet, it is, without a doubt, of the utmost significance in undermining the great advances of containing microbes that have been made over the past 80 years. The evidence that resistance is occurring at significantly high rates is overwhelming. Even before penicillin was synthesized and used to treat infections in people, it was observed certain bacteria could learn to resist it. Within months after its introduction, strains that could overcome its inhibitory properties were isolated. The lifestyle bacteria live means that this very property, adapting to overcome threats against them, is their most successful survival strategy. A good understanding of how we can fix this problem requires knowledge of how bacteria overcome antibiotics.

In general, bacteria have two traits that make them able to overcome resistance. The first is a high replication rate. It takes about 30 minutes for *E. coli* to double. A human generation, in contrast, is about 30 years. This means that bacteria reproduce at a rate that is about 500,000 times faster than humans. With this kind of reproductive productivity, they are much more likely to introduce into a population changes

that might be beneficial simply because they produce many more daughter cells that might have a change. For example, it is known that the mutation rate of *E. coli* is about 1 base change in every 10^7 bases made. Different bacteria have different rates of mutation, some higher, some lower. It is not uncommon to grow *E. coli* in culture to a population of 10^8 total cells or more. This means, in just this culture alone, there will be 10 novel mutants. Now, each of these mutants may not have these changes in each *E. coli* gene; each gene is limited in its contribution to conferring a resistant phenotype. Ten novel mutants implies that about 10 of the roughly 4000 *E. coli* genes have mutations; and, some genes mutate at different rates. But what if you had 10 cultures, or 100? One-hundred cultures implies that now, on a population basis and assuming the mutation rate is equal across the entire genome, that 1000 genes of the approximately 4000 will have novel mutations – one-fourth the entire genome. There are seven billion people on Planet Earth, and another few billion heads of cattle and ten billion or more chickens – all of them harbor *E. coli* in their intestine, not to mention all the many mammals in nature and the *E. coli* in the soil. When considered this way, the number of novel mutations in the genome saturate every possible position of the *E. coli* genome, and many times over.

So, in addition to their prodigious rates of reproduction, bacteria have prodigious rates of making mutations. We discussed in ▶ Chap. 6 the mutagenic tetrasect, that is, the combination of de novo mutation, transduction, transformation, and conjugation, and how all four work together to mutate bacteria. Horizontal gene transfer of genes that confer insensitivity to antibiotics is a major driver of the formation of the resistance pool. Point mutations certainly are drivers; for example, the many that drive the destruction of β-lactam antibiotics. But some antibiotics require entire gene operons or islands to confer resistance; vancomycin is an example. Five genes are necessary for full resistance to this antibiotic. It is possible for this to evolve in a population with enough selective pressure, but it would take time. Many naturally occurring antibiotics, and their semisynthetic derivatives made by the pharmaceutical industry, already have entire operons in existence in the bacterial universe because of the millions, maybe billions of years of chemical warfare that occurred between microbes, before humans arrived on the stage. This implies that it is just a matter of time before these elements drive themselves into clinically significant bacterial pathogens. The reservoir is already there. With enough selective pressure being exerted by our use of antibiotics in nearly every facet of our society, but especially in hospitals and agriculture, if any horizontal gene transfer results in the admittance of this gene or gene cluster into the pressured population, by virtue of natural selection, it will be maintained.

This is thinking about the problem on a population level. It is substantial. But our ability to overcome this challenge will ultimately depend on attaining knowledge as to *how* bacteria overcome our medicines. That is, the molecular mechanisms of resistance. There are three main mechanisms bacteria employ to get around these drugs. They are: i) **export** of the antibiotic from inside the bacterial cell (termed drug **efflux**), ii) **alteration** of the bacterial target

that the antibiotic is supposed to hit, and iii) direct **inactivation** of the antibiotic. Let's talk about each of these more specifically.

16.8 Antibiotic Efflux

Perhaps the easiest way to avoid antibiotics is to pump them out, or even better, don't let them in. Drug influx and efflux are major drivers of antibiotic resistance. Regarding influx, we learned in ▶ Chap. 11 about outer membrane porins. Many antibiotics enter the cell through OMPs. Some OMPs are very selective; that is, most if not all antibiotics will not get through them. Only the ligands they are designed to transport pass through. Others are less selective; that is, like giant holes through which anything smaller than the diameter of the hole seemingly can pass through. The first level of resistance to antibiotics whose mechanism of action is intracellular (e.g. inhibit protein, folate, or DNA synthesis) is to close the gates. Either the OMP does not allow passage of the antibiotic, or, in other cases, the OMP is actually downregulated once the bacterium senses the first few antibiotic molecules.

If the antibiotic does get in, all is not lost, for the bacterium can still pump it out. This is called **antibiotic efflux**. As a survival strategy, efflux is effective at reducing the intracellular concentration of the antibiotic to far below the **minimum inhibitory concentration** for that antibiotic, even though the external concentration might be quite high (🔲 Fig. 16.9). Like OMPs, an efflux pump can be selective or general. It is not surprising that efflux is one of the three main

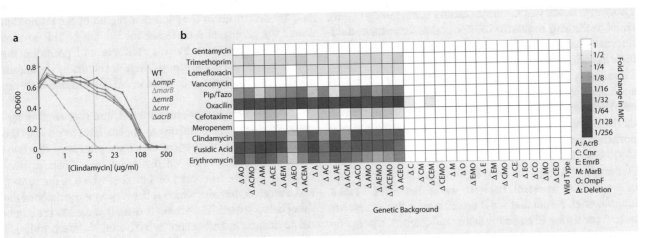

🔲 **Fig. 16.9** The power of the efflux pump. In this study, the authors systematically deleted several membrane proteins or efflux pumps in *E. coli*, and in various combinations, to determine the overall contribution of each to bacterial survival when exposed to the antibiotic clindamycin. In panel **a**, one can see that deletion of genes that encode the AcrAB-TolC (pink line) efflux system is primarily responsible for intrinsic antibiotic resistance. This panel is a representative MIC determination using final optical density at 600 nm (OD600) values at 22 hours of growth with increasing concentration of clindamycin. The left vertical dashed line represents the MIC concentration for the acrB deletion mutant (magenta) while the right vertical dashed line represents the MIC for the remaining strains (WT and the cmr, emrB, marB, ompF

deletion mutants). **b** Heat map showing the normalized mean MIC values for every strain, measured as in **a**. MIC values were normalized using the wild type strain as the reference and depicted colorimetrically with blue representing statistically significant decreases (p < 0.05) in MIC and white representing nonsignificant changes in MIC. Intensity of the blue color indicates the magnitude of MIC change. The loss of AcrA confers some level of resistance to 8 of the 11 antibiotics tested. Almost no resistance is conferred by deletion of any of the other genes (*cmr*, *emrB*, *marB*, and *ompF*). (Adapted from Toprak et al (see suggested readings) under a creative commons license. (▶ https://creativecommons.org/licenses/by/4.0/))

antibiotic pushback strategies. Remember, most antibiotics are either natural compounds or semi-synthetic. They are derived from bacteria and fungi that have been undergoing chemical warfare between each other for eons. It is largely a prerequisite that if you synthesize a chemical warhead, you also have to have the system to export it. If not, your own warhead can detonate in your factory, killing yourself. Thus, efflux pumps have co-evolved with the evolution of natural antibiotics, having been around for as long as antibiotics themselves. Efflux pumps also have functions unrelated to just the export of antibiotics. They also release toxic metabolites, quorum sensing molecules, and sometimes whole proteins themselves. Pathogenic bacteria can acquire these pumps by horizontal gene transfer processes. Many nosocomial pathogens have been evolving in complex biomes with other competitors. They have built up significant efflux capabilities as a result. A good example is *P. aeruginosa*, a nosocomial pathogen of the lungs and wounds that we have visited many times in this text. At last count, sequenced and well-studied strains of *P. aeruginosa* contained more than 60 efflux pumps. It is not surprising then that pseudomonas is one of the leaders in the antibiotic resistance revolution.

16.8.1 Suspects

So what are these efflux pumps? They are the MFS, SMR, RNS, and ABC transporters addressed in ▶ Chap. 11. We approached their description from the point of view of nutrient uptake and metabolism, an important part of a pathogen's lifecycle. Here we view them in the context of explicitly pumping out antibiotics that enter the bacterial periplasm or cytoplasm. Recall that the **major facility superfamily** (MFS), **small multidrug regulator** (SMR), and **resistance/nodulation/cell division** (RND) transporters all couple the efflux of their ligands, in this case antibiotics, to the influx of protons, a chemically favorable process. The **ABC transporters** export antibiotics by hydrolyzing ATP, the high energy phosphate bond providing the energy needed to kick out the antibiotic. Of these, and from studies of the enterobactereciae, the proportion of transporters is about 60–70% MFS, 10–15% RND, 10–15% SMR, and 10–15% ABC. However, the RND members may be the most clinically significant. They are common in multi-drug resistant bacteria associated with human microbiomes. Recall that RND proteins are a three-member system consisting of an outer membrane channel, a periplasmic shuttle protein, and an inner membrane exporter. As such, the antibiotic in question is completely exported out of the cell. The MFS transporters, in contrast, consist of a single component that pumps the compound through the inner membrane and into the cytoplasm. They are mostly involved in the export of the quinolones and the protein synthesis inhibitor chloramphenicol. RNDs, though, can export nearly every major class of antibiotics, including the quinolones, macrolides, sulfonamides, and β-lactam antibiotics. The SMR family can transport quinolones and macrolides whereas the ABC transporters, although perhaps the most infrequent of drug-efflux members, like the RNDs, are also the most versatile, exporting all major classes except for the glycopeptides. The troubling part is not so much that one efflux system can eliminate most of the antibiotic classes as much as it is that many pathogenic bacteria contain representatives of all the efflux families. It is thus possible that a single bacterium could harbor enough efflux mechanisms to confer resistance to all antibiotics.

Although it is clear efflux pumps are ancient and unlikely to have evolved recently to combat the human-driven use of antibiotics, it is possible that mutations that control pump activity or expression have been de novo selected through antibiotic use. Not only can importers garner point mutations that prevent them from binding an antibiotic (which will block entry into the cell), but exporters can acquire mutations that may make them more efficient or more abundant. Most investigation into how mutations cause resistance via efflux pumps has revealed that their expression is often the reason for resistance. Like any gene, transcriptional activators can stimulate the expression of such pumps. Thus, mutations that lead to the increased production of these activators will in turn lead to the increased expression of the pumps. In a similar manner, it is also possible to increase pump production by altering the repressor proteins that shut the pump's production down. It is not uncommon for efflux pumps to be encoded right next to genes that regulate them. Tight control of pumps is an evolved response in bacteria to be able to quickly adjust to the environment and the metabolic flux of their own metabolism. In some cases metabolites are needed; in others, they need to be thrown out quickly due to their toxic effects. Regulation of pump expression is one means to execute this control. In this sense, bacteria can acquire mutations in the promoter region of the pump that lower the affinity of a repressor for the DNA. This in turn relieves the repression by this regulator and promotes the excess expression of the pump. There are clinically significant mutations of these types that confer MDR to human bacterial pathogens.

Another way pumps are regulated, and thus another target for resistance mechanisms to appear, have to do with the other regulatory component of efflux pumps – the two-component systems. As we discussed in ▶ Chap. 6, two-component systems consist of a kinase, which is the sensor, and a receiver domain, which is the response regulator of the thing being sensed. The kinase is usually linked to the external environment and becomes "activated" (phosphorylated) upon sensing this change. The phosphate is then transferred to the regulator which in turn transfers the signal, in the form of a biological action (usually a change in gene expression), to the system that is linked to the environmental change. Two-component systems allow bacteria to sense that antibiotics are near and adjust their efflux capabilities based on this perceived threat. As such, two-component systems should also then be considered important mediators of drug resistance and virulence.

Efflux mediated resistance to tetracycline (tet) is a wonderful example of the many diverse ways bacteria contend with antibiotics. The **tet efflux pump** is tightly repressed by a protein that itself binds tetracycline. When tetracycline enters the cell, the high affinity of this repressor for tet directs it away from the ribosome complex. In fact, the affinity of the repressor for tet is far greater than is the ribosome for tet so that most of the intracellular tet will preferentially be bound not to the ribosome (which would inhibit protein synthesis), but to the repressor. It just so happens that the repressor, when tet is bound, undergoes a dramatic loss of its own affinity for DNA. As a result, it comes off the DNA, and the gene for the efflux pump is made. Should the concentration of tet now build to a point where it is approaching is dissociation constant for its lower affinity target, the ribosome, it will be pumped out and the bacterium protected.

16.9 Chemical Modification of Antibiotics

The second mechanism by which bacteria can become resistant to antibiotics is by chemically modifying the antibiotic. If efflux is throwing the drug in the trash, chemical modification is taking a sledgehammer to it. The outcome of this process is that the antibiotic is destroyed, well, at least in the sense that it cannot perform its intended inhibition of a bacterial enzyme or process. There are hundreds of known chemical reactions of small compounds that either can lead to an altered activity or no activity all together. Not all of these are used to inactivate antibiotics, but many are. These reactions in general can be broken into either addition, alteration or subtraction reactions whereby the antibiotic is either modified by adding another chemical moiety, the compound does not lose atoms but is altered, or the compound has functional substituents removed. In each case, the net result is that the modification renders the compound unable to chemically bind to or modify its target as efficiently (or at all). Here, the inactivating mechanism is directed against the chemical structure of the antibiotic and not the bacterial target or other process.

16.9.1 Ring of Power

The space allocated to this volume will prevent us from discussing all the unique chemical mechanisms bacteria use to destroy antibiotics. To highlight perhaps the most understudied mechanism, let's take a closer look at inactivation of the first discovered class of antibiotics, the β-lactams. Recall that this class of antibiotics is characterized by a central four-atom ring consisting of a nitrogen and carbonyl group (doubly bonded oxygen) termed a β-lactam ring (the nitrogen is in the β position of the ring). The "lact" refers to the fact the structure resembles a lactone heterocycle. As discussed above, the β-lactams are structurally similar to the terminal Ala-Ala peptide of the peptidoglycan subunit NAM-NAG. The critical final step in the assembly of the cell wall peptidoglycan is the crosslinking of the alanine-containing peptide of the NAM-NAG to another alanine-containing peptide NAM-NAG subunit. This imparts a certain structure and form to the cell wall, and it is necessary. The enzyme that carries out this step is termed a transpeptidase. β-lactam antibiotics inhibit their function by fitting into the active site of the transpeptidase and reacting covalently (and irreversibly) with the critical serine residue needed to perform the conjugation of alanine peptides to each other. Thus, the final step in cell wall assembly is prevented. As such, these transpeptidases are also called penicillin-binding proteins.

Even before penicillin was approved for clinical use, researchers were aware of an enzyme that seemingly broke apart the β-lactam before it could disrupt the assembly of the cell wall. These enzymes are termed **β-lactamases**, the "ase" stemming from the finding that their enzymatic activity results in the cleavage, and thus ring-opening, of the four-membered lactam ring. The lactam structure loses its resemblance to Ala-Ala, and its inhibition of the transpeptidase along with it. Lactamases are widespread in the microbial world. Their genes are often mobile, being transferred from bacterium to bacterium via the horizontal processes we revisited above and in-depth in ► Chap. 6. This means bacteria can transfer their resistance to lactam antibiotics like penicillin relatively easily among their peers.

Recognizing that lactamases undermine lactam antibiotics as a class, scientists began searching for ways to inhibit the lactamase. In theory, if the lactamase is neutralized, the lactam antibiotic will remain unmodified and inhibit its target, the transpeptidases. Ingenious solutions were devised. One way was to slow the rate at which the lactamase cleaved the antibiotic. Substituents were added to the lactam ring that did not prevent cleavage but slowed it. If enough functional lactam built up, it may still hit its transpeptidase target. A second way, which has become a chemical hallmark strategy (now used for other antibiotics) was to inactivate the lactamase altogether with another antibiotic – a suicide substrate. The best example may be the use of clavulanate on the β-lactam which covalently reacts with the active site of the lactamase, leading to its inactivation. If combined with a lactam antibiotic, here amoxicillin, the lactam antibiotic is now free to target the bacterial transpeptidase. This has been sometimes termed **augmentation** because the second antibiotic, here clavulanate, augments the first antibiotic (amoxicillin) by inhibiting the lactamase. As such, the amoxicillin-clavulanate combination is trademarked as Augmentin. But the lactamases are comprised of entire families or groups of such enzymes, each group member recognizing a unique chemical structure centered around the lactam ring. As researchers have built more chemical functionality into the lactam antibiotics, the spread of lactamases that inactivate that functionality has increased. As a result, many resistant bacteria have acquired these so-called extended spectrum β-lactamases, organisms that counter a diverse range of lactam structures. And again, a testament to the universe of chemical possibilities that bacteria can invent, they are also able to overcome the inactivation of lactamases by inhibiting the lactamase themselves. Thus, **β-lactamase inhibitory protein** (BLIP) can shield the lactamase by inserting a part of its protein structure into the active site, thereby making it inaccessible to chemical modification by antibiotics. BLIP can then be removed when safe.

16.9.2 Demolition Systems

Resistance is more than just chemical cleavage by a single enzyme. It is an orchestra of distinct parts playing off each other, matching each other's beat and making adjustments where necessary. It's quite easy to believe the only way to stay ahead of these enzymes is to make the next best modification and run with it. As we have appreciated numerous times throughout this chapter, resistance is elegant. Turn to none other than *E. coli* to enjoy the full ensemble. In this pathogen, resistance to β-lactam antibiotics involves not one but four genes. Each gene encodes a protein that carries out a single, yet critical, function to rid the cell of the harmful effects of the antibiotic. When lactams inhibit the cell wall assembly transpeptidases, altered, non-functional peptidoglycan products are produced. One of these is a sugar tripeptide GlcNAc-anhydro-MurNAc-Ala-Glu-DAP. The lactamase gene operon that confers resistance to ampicillin actually encodes four genes, designated ampCDGR. When the modified sugar tripeptide builds, AmpG, a membrane permease, imports the fragment into the *E. coli* cytoplasm. Normally, it will bind immediately to the seclusion protein AmpD. AmpD keeps the intracellular concentration low so the cell does not react for just a small quantity of altered cell wall. But, if many lactams are around causing sweeping damage to the surface, the concentration of the sugar tripeptide grows and overwhelms the seclusion capabilities of AmpD. Excess sugar tripeptide, a sign the bacterium is under attack, now binds to a transcriptional activator, AmpR. This protein activates the expression of the gene ampC, which encodes the functional lactamase which, upon its production, translocates to the periplasm and acts to destroy any lactam antibiotic. Once the concentration of the lactam antibiotic decreases, the altered sugar tripeptide (a sign of stress) also decreases. Less enters the cytoplasm, AmpD binds up what is left, and the lactamase expression is dialed back down, which conserves energy. Here we see that there is a cost-fitness associated with retaining antibiotic resistance; this takes much energy to orchestrate. Thus, the cell would like to know when to turn it on, to save energy, and such a feedback system presumably works well for control. This example also highlights, however, that resistance is more than just enzymes; it's a system, and like any system where parts are dependent on other parts, there are multiple points of therapeutic attack.

The breaking of a chemical link that opens a molecule, essentially the reaction mechanism bacteria use to inactivate lactams, is just one of many diverse chemical ways antibiotics can be modified to render them less effective or inert all together. So the microbe hunter has an appreciation of some other possibilities, we turn now to the aminoglycosides.

Recall that the aminoglycosides are an amino acid-sugar hybrid molecule with many reactive functional substituents capable of receiving and donating electrons in chemical reactions. These properties make this class of molecule ideal for binding to the rRNA in the 30S ribosome, which disrupts its function. The substituents consist of either an amino (NH_2) or hydroxyl (OH) group. They are two of the most reactive chemical moieties in all of biology and participate in essential, everyday cellular processes. It will come as no shock to any chemist to learn that bacteria target these groups to inactivate this class of antibiotics. Aminoglycosides are made inert via the chemical addition to these reactive substituents. The two hydroxyl moieties (OH) can be modified by bacterial phosphotransferases or adenyltransferases. The phosphotransferase will add a phosphate to the hydroxyl. The adenyltransferase will add adenosine monophosphate (AMP) from ATP to the aminoglycoside hydroxyl groups. Finally, an acetyltransferase will ligate an acetyl group (C_2H_3O) to the aminoglycoside amino groups. All of these have the potential to disrupt the interaction of the antibiotic with the ribosome-rRNA complex.

16.10 Target-Mediated Modification

Efflux-mediated resistance aims to cast the antibiotic away. Inactivation-mediated resistance aims to obliterate the antibiotic directly. The final mechanism by which bacteria safeguard themselves from the deadly effects of antibiotics is through modification of not the antibiotic, but its target. This target is a bacterial component, in most cases either the cell wall or ribosome-RNA complex. The objective, from the bacterial standpoint, is to alter the target in such a way that it is impervious to modification by the antibiotic without negatively effecting its job in normal cell physiology. This is not an easy task; imagine the specificity, and subtlety, required to make just the right change to these complex assembly processes without altering efficiency in the process.

To highlight this example, take vancomycin. Prior to the introduction of this antibiotic into clinical practice, bacteria that could survive in its presence were almost never recorded. After about 10 years of its common use through the 1990s, a person was approximately 7–20 times more likely to observe a resistant strain. The main use of vancomycin was to curb the infection with Gram-positive bacteria, particularly *E. faecalis* and *E. faecium*, two opportunistic pathogens whose acquisition of a gene operon to confront vancomycin also led to their meteoric rise as a more frequent cause of human infections. Prominent causes of blood stream infection, and normal inhabitants of the human intestinal microbiome, the enterococci example is one in which the other edge of the antibiotic sword can also sting.

Recall that vancomycin is a glycopeptide antibiotic that binds to the terminal Ala-Ala residue of the free terminal peptide that is involved in crosslinking the NAG-NAM fragments of the cell wall. Resistance arises when vancomycin is no longer able to prevent crosslinking between the peptides.

nvolved is a five-gene bacterial system that encodes an activity that, strikingly, in the nearly dozen reactions that occur to make the cell wall, prevent just a simple, single hydrogen bond from forming. This perceptively insignificant change in a hydrogen bond prevents the antibiotic from binding as strongly to the terminal alanine residue (about a thousand-fold reduction in affinity). It begins with a two-component system, VanS and VanR. VanS is the sensor kinase. It may bind free vancomycin or shed cell wall fragments extracellularly, then transmitting this "message" that antibiotic is around intracellularly by phosphorylating its dimeric binding partner. The phosphate is then transmitted to VanR, the response regulator and transcription factor, which then activates the expression of three additional proteins – VanH, VanA, and VanX. Here is where the real magic happens. VanH is a reductase and adds a single proton to lactate, changing its chirality to D-lactate. VanA is a peptide ligase. It adds a free alanine to the D-lactate to produce Ala-D-lactate. Recall that the normal peptidoglycan produced is Ala-D-Ala. This subtle change in the terminal peptide, when incorporated into the NAG-NAM, becomes recalcitrant to the binding of vancomycin because it disrupts the hydrogen bonding network needed by van to form a tight affinity to the peptide. As a result, the bacterial cell is able to form the crosslinks it needs to build a functional cell wall. Just in case any "normal" dipeptide (Ala-D-Ala) displaces the lactate modified peptide (which would be susceptible to van binding), the third enzyme made, VanX, acts as a peptidase with specificity towards the Ala-D-Ala dipeptide. This ensures that most of the free pool is that of the lactate-modified form, thereby ensuring it gets selectively incorporated into the cell wall.

16.11 Regulation, Industry and Society

The bacterial tetrasect will always find ways to create new mutant strains that show enhanced fitness under certain conditions, especially if the conditions are life or death when faced with small chemical killers. Clinically appreciable resistance to current structural classes is not the exception, it seems to be the rule. Is it no surprise then that the pharmaceutical industry has largely withdrawn from the regular screening, testing and production of new antibiotics? Why invest hundreds of millions of dollars over 10 or more years when the drug you finally introduce becomes obsolete a few years after widespread use? There are 20% fewer companies working on new antibiotics today then there were in the 1960s. The global number of deaths due to resistance per year – estimated at 700,000. If current rates, use, and economic trends hold steady, the United Kingdom's government commission on the topic estimates this number will soar to ten million per year. The cost will be 1 trillion dollars annually, by far higher than the entire GDPs of 90% of the world's countries. These are staggering numbers. Even if the models are wrong by a factor of 10, it means one million lives and 100 billion dollars annually.

So what do we do?

There is the science of a solution, and then there are the politics of it. The latter will require education, regulation, and a global commitment. Our society will need to educate the makers, prescribers, and users of antibiotics about their judicious use. One half of all antibiotics are used in agriculture; the other half in people. Both contribute to resistance but perhaps it is possible to reduce their use and have the same desired clinical benefit. Many respiratory and intestinal infections are causes by viruses whose symptoms mimic that of a bacterial infection. Here we see that better diagnostic standards might be able to inform a physician that the infection is due to a virus, at which point an antibiotic, which does not act on viruses, can be avoided. Antibiotics are often used in agriculture because they protect livestock and foul, even providing a growth advantage which has much economic incentive. Perhaps knowledge of sanitation and regular screening of farms could better inform when antibiotics should and should not be used. Currently, they are often provided without this knowledge and in mass, sweeping quantities. Patients need to be educated about their use as well, including to finish the course and be consistent, to not use antibiotics for other symptoms other than what they were prescribed, and to not share them without clinical evaluation of another person. These topics fall under what is called **antibiotic stewardship**. It is the idea that we have to be careful and specific in our use of these drugs.

Regulation by governments and oversight by ethics groups will also play a part. Nations should look to make incentives for farmers to reduce antibiotic use, perhaps in the form of tax subsidies or assistance programs. Scientific and medical institutions should be funded to track rates of resistance for all major antibiotic classes in agriculture and patients. Regular sampling, testing, and sequencing of strains should be mandated. This will inform whether implemented actions are showing improvement in reducing rates of resistance or are ineffective. Regular investment in new scientific ideas to spawn out-of-the-box solutions should be a priority, as should be continued support for molecular studies to understand the basis of resistance. Guidelines for when and what types of antibiotics should be used for all clinical situations should be made to inform physicians, evaluated regularly by working groups that are experts on the topic. Government action to incentivize the pharmaceutical industry to get back into the antibiotic business is by far a top priority. There simply is too much cost and too low a margin for even the behemoths in this industry to get excited, let alone a small start-up with a great idea. There is data that suggests it takes nearly 20 years for an antibiotic to become profitable to the point that the developing company has found return on the investment. At this point, the patent will have run its life, meaning a competitor can quickly come in a seek reward without the growing pains of development. The government pipeline to approval is also a major barrier. The list of exhaustive studies, from animal efficacy to safety in humans, extends the time to market. No doubt these studies are required; but the process would be made more efficient if redundant rules were merged and there was investment in the number of eyes that could critically evaluate new compounds at the approval stages. Recent buy-in to "fast-track" programs in the U.S. approval process, and discussion to extend patent protections well past the development stage, are good signs legislatures are thinking about these topics. More work is needed.

But what about science? What avenues are there for drug development to counter resistant organisms? Below, we briefly introduce some areas of exploration that the ambitious microbe hunter may one day wish to pursue. The only certainty is that such efforts will be required.

16.12 The Search for New Antibiotics

This is the strategy of choice since antibiotic drug development became enterprise. Second, third, and even fourth generation antibiotics, built by chemical modification of substituents around a central core structure, have yielded most antibiotics that are clinically used today. This process has worked for both natural derivatives as well as synthetic ones. The approach suffers from one major caveat; the core structures have been in circulation for 70 plus years as drugs, and potentially tens to hundreds of millions of years during microbial warfare. Bacteria know them. There is only a finite amount of modifications that can be made around these structures. In the end, the chemical space is rich but perhaps not rich enough to overcome resistance mechanisms.

As we discussed, most of the antibiotics in use are natural product or modified natural product derivatives that originated from soil-dwelling bacteria, particularly the streptomycetes and actinomycetes. It was not uncommon for antibiotic developers to screen large collections of bacteria for compounds that had bactericidal or bacteriostatic properties. Estimates have it that 99% of all possible bacterial species have not been assessed for their ability to inhibit the growth of other bacteria. Considering everything we already have was yielded from just sampling 1% of the bacterial biosphere, this implies there is an untapped world of new chemical discovery in our soils, lakes, and ecosystems. A major obstacle though is that the infrastructure and technologies to capture these organisms has either been retired or is not being maximized to its full potential. Metagenomics of complex microbial communities has taught us that the vast majority of bacterial species do not grow in conventional laboratory media or conditions. Investment is needed in identifying environmental conditions that allow for the large-scale production of diverse bacterial genera and species. Even in our own intestinal tract, the number of cultivatable microorganisms is far fewer than can be cultured. These bacteria may yield chemical diversity in antibiotics never seen before, which would wind new paths to new chemical possibilities and unique structures. Of course, resistance is possible against these structures but it is somewhat comforting to the microbe hunter to know that we can at least keep up with resistance via the continuous discovery of new compounds from this untapped biosource – for the time being.

16.13 Combination of Multiple Antibiotics: Synergy

We learned above that lactam antibiotics are broken by lactamase enzymes. This prevents the antibiotic from stopping the production of the cell wall. Augmentin is an antibiotic that in addition to the cell wall inhibitor amoxicillin, also contains the lactamase inhibitor clavulanic acid. By inhibiting the lactamases, the amoxicillin stays intact and cell wall formation is disrupted. Augmentin is the most prescribed combinatorial antibiotic, a testament to the effectiveness of combining two or more antibiotics to achieve a clinical outcome. There are others. Timentin, unasyn, and prevpac are all composed of two or more antibiotics that are used to treat serious infections, either those related to sepsis or long-term ulcers.

The strategy behind the use of multiple antibiotics in a formulation is based on math. The probability of having or developing resistance against two different antibiotics, each with a distinct mechanism of inhibition of a bacterial process, is less than that against a single antibiotic. The probability against three is even less so, and so on. Now there is a limit as to how many antibiotics can be combined into a single formulation. Some antibiotics **contraindicate**, or may interfere with or make ineffective, other antibiotics. Some are processed differently by the body and have different half-lives. Side effects may be worse when two or more are given, etc. Each combinatorial formulation has to be specifically tested to determine its safety and effectiveness. In the laboratory, this is usually done by adding the two antibiotics together over a concentration range and comparing how well they inhibit or kill bacteria when compared to each antibiotic alone. An **additive effect** is one where the combination of both activities is simply the sum of the two antibiotics alone. A **synergistic effect** is one in which the outcome of both antibiotics together exceeds that observed from the simple addition of both antibiotics individually. Formally, this synergy should show a two-log increase in effectiveness compared to either antibiotic alone. However, even highly synergistic antibiotics must be tested in clinical trials owing to the complexity of what is possible when living, breathing organisms are the test subject. That said, combining antibiotics, especially if they target different bacterial processes, is one exciting avenue to combating drug-resistant bacteria.

16.14 The Cell Process Not Yet Targeted

There are many cellular processes whose inhibition would cripple the cell that have not yet been exploited for antimicrobial development. A few are discussed briefly here. One of them is nutrient uptake. Bacteria must eat. They metabolize what they eat to make energy and more of themselves. This fuels growth in hosts. If small molecule inhibitors prevented their ability to import or process critical nutrients, say metals or sugars or amino acids, they would fail to grow. Some evidence suggests bacteria would enter a state of starvation – not dead, but also not metabolically active. Such a strategy might decrease the production of resistance since the selection is not life or death. By slowing down their growth, it gives the immune system time to catch up. Other avenues are also promising. The inhibition of fatty acid biosynthesis is one. All bacteria require the production of lipids to build their membranes. Without an intact membrane, everything from energy production to cell architecture is altered. The enzymes that synthesize these lipid building blocks would be targets in this case. Some have suggested crippling bacterial stress response. This is a way bacteria deal with environmental hazards, including the production of too much free radicals, or heat, or osmolality. Without the ability to adapt to these stresses, bacteria may die. The adaptation mechanism is a coordinated process with viable targets. Still other avenues include targeting the major metabolic pathways, such as glycolysis or the TCA cycle, thereby crippling energy production, or the electron transport chain. Whatever the process, care must be taken to make sure the developed compounds do not also cripple the host's equivalent of these pathways. This avoids toxicity.

16.15 Inhibitors of Virulence

Elegant studies of the mechanisms of pathogenesis over the past 70 years have taught us that bacterial-induced disease can mostly be distilled to substantial alteration of host physiology as a result of key virulence factors each bacterial species produces during the infection. In some cases for some species, a single virulence factor drives the pathogenesis (think tetanus toxin for *C. tetani*). In other cases, it is the collection of a multitude of virulence factors, each with a different mechanism of action, that drive illness. Many studies show that if these virulence factors are not present or are specifically inhibited, the disease-causing ability of the bacterium is reduced. This implies that medicines that inhibit these factors might prove to be effective antibiotics. The underlying concept behind this approach is that if the medicine prevents the specific disease-causing ability of the pathogen, its ability to continue to grow, divide, and spread throughout the body will be compromised. Similar to our discussion above concerning the inhibition of bacterial growth, such drugs would give the body time to clear the infection, and, as such, may decreases resistance rates since the primary mechanism of bacterial death would be immunological not pharmacological. There are no on-market antibiotics that target virulence factors, but numerous reports in the literature of small molecule inhibitors indicate, at least scientifically and medically, the concept has merit. The lack of development of these approaches by the pharmaceutical industry is based on many factors, perhaps a dominant one being

their preference for small molecules that outright kill bacteria (instead of slowing them down or preventing disease mechanisms via the inhibition of virulence). The inhibition of pathogenic mechanisms without strong life-death selection, albeit a not yet proven concept, may have a longer shelf-life as a strategy. In this regard, the scientific literature suggests that the inhibition of the placement of proteins on the bacteria cell wall, the inhibition of protein secretion systems like the type III needle apparatus, the inhibition of adherence to host tissues, and the inhibition of major disease-causing toxins, all represent promising targets for antibacterial development.

16.16 Human Produced Natural Biologicals

We have not yet addressed what at one point (circa the 1990s) was once an exciting area of antimicrobial development but that now has lost some of its luster; biologicals derived from humans. The forerunner of this group of bacterial antagonists is the human monoclonal antibody, but others include small immunomodulators such as chemokines, antimicrobial peptides, and even enhanced blood complement. The concept here is that the medicine augments the already tried-and-tested ways in which the human immune system combats infection. In theory, since these biological processes have already evolved with your immune system over millions of years, and it's an integral part of your natural defense mechanism, it should be safe and effective. We know that each of these systems already does major damage to a bacterial invader; human antibodies inhibit toxins and induce opsonophagocytosis, complement kills bacteria in the blood and antimicrobial peptides dissolve the bacterial surface at mucosal sites. In the case of monoclonal antibodies, say against a critical protein needed for the assembly or function of the type III secretion system, if the microbe hunter can somehow purify the antigen and develop a hybridoma line that continuously secretes high levels of neutralizing antibody, this antibody can be administered to patients whose infecting bacterium requires the type III secretion system for virulence. There is already some precedence for this clinically so the concept of its medical feasibility is perhaps a bit more accepted than some of the other approaches discussed here. The downside though is that these procedures, especially the quality control in making the inhibitory biologic, can be time-consuming and costly. Resistance is in general possible, although in this case one might argue that any loss or alteration of the virulence factor probably also reduces the bacterium's virulence, which might be considered a welcome outcome. Antibacterial biologicals of human origin may also be substantially influenced by homeostatic processes that naturally dampen the immunological response. Not much is known about how these regulatory systems alter efficacy, but we do know they exist.

16.17 The Evolvable Drug

16.17.1 "Transparent Material"

We end with a final bit of hope in the sea of evolutionary despair. With the mutagenic tetrasect never at end, one wonders if the continuous evolution of resistance against small chemical antibiotics can ever be stopped. Will we simply be resigned to a continuous ebb and flow of small molecule development, one expensive drug arising after another, only then to be discarded once clinically significant resistance forms? Or are their other ways?

In 1917, Fred Twort was trying to find ways to grow vaccinia virus in hopes of making a better smallpox vaccine. Viral research was in its infancy and the methods of investigation into viruses were not as well developed as that of Koch and Pasteur's bacteriologic methods. It would take the 1918 flu epidemic, estimated to have killed between 50 and 100 million people worldwide, for both government and academic interest and support to be put into viral research. Early scientists were using some of the ways bacteria could be grown to propagate viruses. We now know this is generally frivolous. Mammalian viruses need mammalian cells for their growth. Twort noticed that the agar plates he was using seemed to always grow bacteria. Sometimes, however, a "transparent material" would appear in the middle of the bacterial lawn. It could be propagated and transferred to other plates of bacteria. Twort reported this, speculating that it may be an enzyme that killed the bacteria or even a small virus. Twort did not seem to make the extension to the use of this material as a bacterial-killing substance in patients.

The French scientist Felix D' Herelle did just that. Just 2 years later, while investigating an outbreak, he too observed the killing substance, and named it phage, or "eaters of bacteria." The miracle substance was eventually identified; not an enzyme, not a small molecule, not an antibody. A virus, just as Twort had speculated. There are estimates of 10^{25} bacteria on planet Earth. Nothing is more abundant ... except phage. There are 10^{31} of those! They are a plague of bacteria. A bacterial flu that spreads from cell to cell, each infected cell making hundreds of new viruses, each spreading and infecting hundreds of more still. Every infection leaving a corpse of a bacterium behind, its insides ripped apart as new phage progeny seek new victims. It's strange to think that a single-celled organism like a bacterium can actually get sick by an even smaller microorganism, if you can call a phage virus that, but it is true. Bacteria go to great lengths to avoid these infections, just as humans also try to avoid viral infections.

16.17.2 Forgotten Promise

From this period (~1920) to the end of the second World War (1945), phage were being developed as a medicine for bacterial infections. This was still the Wild West of drug development though. As such, the same strict guidelines that allow scientists to determine if a medicine is safe and effec-

tive were not then in place. It was unclear if phage were working well, or even safe. When antibiotics were discovered and they could be made and purified at increased volumes in the 1940s, new regulations about drug control and development were blossoming. Stricter measures were put in place and the biomedical research capacity was ramping up on many levels. The need for a drug to treat a soldier's infections or their wounds was high, and penicillin, fresh off its new production line, thrived. Efforts now turned exclusively to making antibiotics. The golden era of production led to all the classes and derivatives we see today. Except for areas of the world where for political or other reasons antibiotic technologies could not reach, phage was, more or less, forgotten about.

But now we enter a new period. This period is characterized by the failure of our chemical miracles, undermined by the increase in all the different ways bacteria can get around these medicines and propagate this knowledge to their offspring. In desperation, phage has found new backers, and the science around phage development brings renewed hope. In the past few years, there has been numerous reports of the treatment of life-threatening infections, with no other hope, by phage therapy. Specific phages were found, prepared, and given to these patients, some of which showed a clear improvement and recovery after being given the treatment. The number of reports of new phage discoveries and positive results in animal efficacy studies has dramatically risen over the past 10 years. No doubt this renewed interest is driven by the desire to tackle the resistance problem; and unlike the past, the science is in a much better position to answer the key questions on the topic.

16.17.3 The Evobiotic

Why is phage so alluring as a drug candidate? Because they are the only entity on the planet that seems to evolve faster than bacteria. Every time a phage infects a new bacterial cell, it replicates inside the cytoplasm. For phages that are **lytic**, that is, they replicate and then lyse the cell to have the progeny exit and infect a new host, this process may entail the acquisition of new mutations at each successive infection. If there are billions of new particles produced in a large population of cells, one is almost assured some of these phage will have acquired mutations that allow them to even better adapt to their bacterial hosts, *i.e.* become better killers. Since this is natural selection in action, only the best phage survive and continue on. In essence, nature is making the drug in real-time using the greatest biological driver of diversity the universe has ever seen – mutation.

We can call phage that evolve to be even more efficient killers of bacteria, have narrow or more broad host range, and might even be directed or enhanced using methods that promote mutagenesis, evobiotics ("evo" from the word "evolution" to signify that the new killer was essentially evolved and "biotic" referring to it as something that targets life. In this case, it's the life of a pathogenic bacterium). The advantage here is that whereas small molecule inhibitors of a limited number of structural chemical classes have only so much medicinal chemistry that can occur around a core structure, nucleic acid as the template for change is nearly limitless. A typical 100,000 base phage genome can make $4^{100,000}$ possible combinations. There simply is not a conceivable limit as to the number of different ways one can make a new phage. Evobiotics may transcend ways in which we think about the normal drug-making process. It may take 10 years and hundreds of millions of dollars to develop a new chemical antibiotic. Laboratory studies show you can evolve new phage in a culture tube to kill resistant bacteria in hours to days, and at a cost that is orders of magnitude less expensive, and without sophisticated organic chemistry processes. Nature made it this way. One can envision a program whereby every time a pathogenic bacterium evolves to resist a new chemical antibiotic, an evobiotic in turn is evolved in the laboratory to counter this resistant strain. Should resistors to the evobiotic appear, the new bacterial strain can be used to simply evolve a new evobiotic. Phage may be the only rapidly adaptable drug that itself evolves and thus can keep up with, perhaps even exceed, the rate of resistance itself. It is somewhat ironic to think that one day the vary principles bacteria use to cleverly get around our elaborate antibiotics (mutagenesis) may itself be used to turn the tables right back on bacteria. Since phage are so specific for their bacterial hosts and are ubiquitous in our water and food, they are also extremely safe. They can be tailored to each species of bacteria, or even better, each problematic strain of bacteria, thus eliminating the harmful side effects observed with antibiotics, which are not specific and can erase beneficial members of our native microflora. Evobiotics also self-dose; the more bacteria, the more particles that are produced at the site of infection. Their specificity might also allow them to target one single problematic species of the hundreds that live in our intestinal tracts, or other parts of our microbiome. With the adaptable drug on the horizon, from CRISPR-fixing of human mutations to personalized T-cells against one specific tumor, the microbe hunter should also ask why not evolvable medicines for bacterial infections as well.

The microbe hunter will have many challenges ahead as we enter the post-antibiotic era. From new chemical classes to novel human biologicals to evobiotics, the choices will be plentiful. Rigorous scientific and medical testing will lead the way, and should. But the next-generation microbe hunter will also need to be more creative than in the past. After all, bacteria seem to have nearly a limitless amount of creativity themselves.

Summary of Key Concepts

1. Chemical warfare has been waging between microbes and everything else for millions perhaps billions of years. The trials from this period means there are templates to base the development of medicines that kill or stop pathogenic bacteria. It also means, however, that some bacteria have evolved countermeasures to handle such approaches.

2. Natural or synthesized antibiotics fall into four main classes depending on their mode of action and structure. This includes the disruption of protein synthesis, DNA synthesis and topology, cell wall biosynthesis, or membrane function.

3. Bacteria use de novo mutation, conjugation, transformation, and transduction as a means to change their genomic content. As a result, resistance to each antibiotic mechanism of action has emerged.

4. Although there are many ways a bacterium can resist antibiotic pressures, three main ones include efflux of the antibiotic, inactivation of the antibiotic, or alteration of the antibiotic's bacterial target.

5. Great change in the social, political, and regulatory approaches will be needed to thwart the growing increase in antibiotic resistance. Non-molecular strategies include stewardship, education, incentives for smart use or disuse, and streamlining regulatory approval or enhancing incentives for new antibiotic development by pharma.

6. Many novel approaches to treat bacterial infections have arisen. These include the use of novel chemical classes of small molecule inhibitors, human-based biologics such as antibodies or antimicrobial peptides, chemical adjuvation or synergy, and the use of phage, which, by virtue of its ability to evolve itself, can accelerate new drug discovery on an unprecedented scale.

❓ Expand Your Knowledge

1. You are a philanthropist, rich beyond your wildest dreams, made wealthy because the "shame your friend" internet app you created for teenagers went viral. After maturing a bit, you decide to use your fortune to invest in the development of alternatives to antibiotics, especially considering the last clinically useable one just became obsolete with the development of resistance. Devise three distinct areas of new anti-bacterial development that you can invest in and explain why these areas will uniquely address the future development of resistance in ways that are different than conventional antibiotics. Use knowledge of what you have learned throughout this book.

2. As a chemist at a large pharmaceutical company doing Research and Development in the year 2089, you synthesize the fourteenth generation of β-lactam antibiotic series. It goes through rigorous clinical testing but resistance develops quickly. Fearing your program of developing β-lactams is in jeopardy (the

board said 15 generations is all they will allow), you investigate the mechanism of resistance and find that partial inhibition of the cell wall occurs but there are no unique lactamases that destroy the antibiotic. Name three ways resistance could have developed in these strains.

3. The U.S. Food and Drug Administration lobbies congress to pass a law stating that all "health-care providers, the agriculture and livestock industries, and pharmaceutical companies" must reduce by 25% their use and production of a select list of critical antibiotics over the next 5 years. As a policy maker working for the Senate Leadership, what guidelines would you draft for these industries to help implement this law into their respective business practices?

Out of the Box

Tailored Antibiotics in the Era of Precision Medicine

Before medicine evolved in sophistication, cancer was just cancer. It was not classified into colon, or lung, or breast cancer, as it is today. As science illuminated the molecular basis of cancer, we learned cancers can have dozens to hundreds of different varieties, each with a unique cellular biology and etiology. Amazingly, even within the same tumor, cancer cells can have different phenotypes. The same can be said for bacterial infections. In the early days, the type of infection was not readily distinguished; patients were feverous or their wounds putrefied but the underlying tissue and organism did not factor into the diagnosis. Nowadays, clinical microbiology testing can often identify the underlying etiological agent. If there is time to do antibiotic-sensitivity testing, the results can inform which antibiotic to give. Clinicians also understand that some antibiotics seem to work better than others for certain types of infections – say urinary tract versus bacterial bronchitis. As we learn more about how bacteria cause disease, we find that each pathogen is different, even among those of the same species.

For many bacteria that cause routine infections of humans, pathogenesis is the summation of their virulence arsenal, their ability to resist treatment, and the host's genetics. The first two change often because of horizontal gene transfer. The future of medicine may be one in which antibiotics are not empirically applied in hopes of having treatment success. The ability to rapidly culture and sequence genomes may allow for an assessment of the exact drug to be used for *that* type of infection and agent, and this may be different for another similar infection of the same species of bacterium in another person. For those chronically infected, often with in-dwelling devices or other debilitating conditions, drug resistance over the course of the infection may limit treatment options unless the drug itself can adapt to the bacterium (like our evobiotic example above) or there is an extensive repertoire of a combination of antibiotics one can turn to (synergy). In 150 years, science has moved from a complete lack of understanding that bacteria underlie disease to understanding the various molecules they produce to *cause* the disease. As technology improves, the speed in which a diagnosis is made and genomes are sequenced will also improve, and so too will technology generate advanced anti-bacterial options that work and change in real-time, with specific targeting of the *strain* of pathogen ever the more likely. As we close this important chapter, and ultimately this entire volume, the microbe hunter will need to be a little bit of a visionary. He or she will need to imagine what medicines will (and should) be a part of our future. It has been 150 years since Koch and Pasteur and we have come far. What medicines will be made in the next 150 years? You will be part of that decision.

Suggested Reading

Aminov RI (2010) A brief history of the antibiotic era: lessons learned and challenges for the future. Front Microbiol 1:134. https://doi.org/10.3389/fmicb.2010.00134

Ayhan DH et al (2016) Sequence-specific targeting of bacterial resistance genes increases antibiotic efficacy. PLoS Biol 14:e1002552. https://doi.org/10.1371/journal.pbio.1002552

Blair JM, Richmond GE, Piddock LJ (2014) Multidrug efflux pumps in Gram-negative bacteria and their role in antibiotic resistance. Future Microbiol 9:1165–1177. https://doi.org/10.2217/fmb.14.66

Clardy J, Fischbach MA, Walsh CT (2006) New antibiotics from bacterial natural products. Nat Biotechnol 24:1541–1550. https://doi.org/10.1038/nbt1266

Lewis K (2013) Platforms for antibiotic discovery. Nat Rev Drug Discov 12:371–387. https://doi.org/10.1038/nrd3975

Piddock LJ (2006) Clinically relevant chromosomally encoded multidrug resistance efflux pumps in bacteria. Clin Microbiol Rev 19:382–402. https://doi.org/10.1128/CMR.19.2.382-402.2006

Polikanov YS, Aleksashin NA, Beckert B, Wilson DN (2018) The mechanisms of action of ribosome-targeting peptide antibiotics. Front Mol Biosci 5:48. https://doi.org/10.3389/fmolb.2018.00048

Price EP et al (2017) Phylogeographic, genomic, and meropenem susceptibility analysis of Burkholderia ubonensis. PLoS Negl Trop Dis 11:e0005928. https://doi.org/10.1371/journal.pntd.0005928

Rybak MJ (2006) The efficacy and safety of daptomycin: first in a new class of antibiotics for Gram-positive bacteria. Clin Microbiol Infect 12(Suppl 1):24–32. https://doi.org/10.1111/j.1469-0691.2006.01342.x

Walsh C (2003) Antibiotics: actions, origins, and resistance. ASM Press